# Hemoglobinopathies in Children

Progress in Pediatric Hematology/Oncology, Volume III

# HEMOGLOBINOPATHIES IN CHILDREN

**Elias Schwartz, M.D., Editor**
Professor of Pediatrics
University of Pennsylvania School of Medicine
Director, Division of Hematology
The Children's Hospital of Philadelphia
Philadelphia, Pennsylvania

**Carl Pochedly, M.D.**
**Denis R. Miller, M.D.**
Series Editors

PSG Publishing Company, Inc.
Littleton, Massachusetts

Library of Congress Cataloging in Publication Data
Main entry under title:

Hemoglobinopathies in children.

   (Progress in pediatric hematology/oncology ; v. 3)
   Includes index.
   1.   Hemoglobinopathy in children.   I.   Schwartz,
Elias, 1935–        II.   Series.   [DNLM:  1.   Hemo-
globinopathies — In infancy and childhood.
W1  PR677E  v. 3 / WS300 H489]
RJ416.H43H45                 618.9'21'5                 78-55277
ISBN  0-88416-204-4

Printed in the United States of America.

International Standard Book Number: 0-88416-204-4

Library of Congress Catalog Card Number: 78-55277

57855

In memory of
Irving J. Wolman, M.D.,
a pioneer in the treatment
of children with hemoglobinopathies

# EDITORS AND CONTRIBUTORS

Progress in Pediatric Hematology/Oncology
Volume III
HEMOGLOBINOPATHIES IN CHILDREN

**Series Editors**

Carl Pochedly, M.D.
Denis R. Miller, M.D.

**Guest Editor**

Elias Schwartz, M.D.

**Contributors**

Kazuhiko Adachi, Ph.D.
Assistant Professor of Pediatrics
University of Pennsylvania
  School of Medicine
Division of Hematology
The Children's Hospital
  of Philadelphia
Philadelphia, Pennsylvania

Blanche P. Alter, M.D.
Associate Professor of Pediatrics
Harvard Medical School
Associate in Medicine
  (Hematology/Oncology)
Children's Hospital
  Medical Center
Senior Clinical Associate
Sidney Farber Cancer Institute
Boston, Massachusetts

Toshio Asakura, M.D., Ph.D.
Professor of Pediatrics,
  Biochemistry, and Biophysics
University of Pennsylvania
  School of Medicine
Division of Hematology
The Children's Hospital
  of Philadelphia
Philadelphia, Pennsylvania

Jean Atwater, B.S., M.T. (ASCP)
Assistant Professor of Medicine
Jefferson Medical College
Cardeza Foundation
  for Hematologic Research
Philadelphia, Pennsylvania

Robert L. Baehner, M.D.
Hugh McK. Landon Professor
  of Pediatrics and Clinical
  Pathology
Director, Division of Pediatric
  Hematology/Oncology
James Whitcomb Riley Hospital
  for Children
Indiana University
  School of Medicine
Indianapolis, Indiana

Alan Cohen, M.D.
Assistant Professor of Pediatrics
University of Pennsylvania
  School of Medicine
Assistant Hematologist
The Children's Hospital
  of Philadelphia
Philadelphia, Pennsylvania

Julian R. Davis, Jr., M.D.
Associate Hematologist
Director, Sickle Cell
  Counselor Training Program
Children's Hospital Medical Center
Oakland, California

Robert S. Festa, M.D.
Assistant Professor of Pediatrics
University of New York
  at Stony Brook Medical School
Pediatric Hematologist-Oncologist
Long Island-Jewish Medical Center
New Hyde Park, New York

Shlomo Friedman, M.D.
Associate Professor of Pediatrics
State University of New York
  at Buffalo
Pediatric Hematologist
Children's Hospital of Buffalo
Buffalo, New York

Frances M. Gill, M.D.
Assistant Professor of Pediatrics
University of Pennsylvania
  School of Medicine
Associate Hematologist
The Children's Hospital
  of Philadelphia
Philadelphia, Pennsylvania

George R. Honig, M.D., Ph.D.
Professor of Pediatrics
Northwestern University
  School of Medicine
Director, Division of Hematology
The Children's Memorial Hospital
Chicago, Illinois

Klaus Hummeler, M.D.
Professor of Pediatrics
University of Pennsylvania
  School of Medicine
Director, Joseph Stokes, Jr.
  Research Institute
The Children's Hospital
  of Philadelphia
Philadelphia, Pennsylvania

Yuet Wai Kan, M.D.
Professor of Medicine
University of California
  at San Francisco
Director, Howard Hughes
  Medical Institute Laboratory
San Francisco General Hospital
San Francisco, California

John F. Kelleher, Jr., M.D.
Research Fellow in Pediatric
  Hematology
The Children's Hospital
  of Philadelphia
Philadelphia, Pennsylvania

Haewon C. Kim, M.D.
Assistant Professor of Pediatrics
University of Pennsylvania
  School of Medicine
Assistant Hematologist
The Children's Hospital
  of Philadelphia
Philadelphia, Pennsylvania

Thomas R. Kinney, M.D.
Assistant Professor of Pediatrics
Duke University School of Medicine
Durham, North Carolina

Bertram H. Lubin, M.D.
Chief, Division of Hematology
Director, Sickle Cell Screening,
  Counseling and Education Center
Children's Hospital Medical Center
Oakland, California
Associate Clinical Professor
  of Pediatrics
University of California
  at San Francisco

William C. Mentzer, Jr., M.D.
Associate Professor of Pediatrics
University of California
  at San Francisco
Chief, Pediatric Hematology
San Francisco General Hospital
Director, Northern California
  Comprehensive Sickle Cell Center
San Francisco, California

Denis R. Miller, M.D.
Professor of Pediatrics
Cornell University Medical College
Chairman, Department of Pediatrics
Memorial Sloan-Kettering
  Cancer Center
New York, New York

Kwaku Ohene-Frempong, M.D.
Research Fellow in Pediatric
  Hematology
The Children's Hospital
  of Philadelphia
Philadelphia, Pennsylvania

Arthur J. Provisor, M.D.
Assistant Professor of Pediatrics
Indiana University
   School of Medicine
Division of Pediatric
   Hematology/Oncology
James Whitcomb Riley Hospital
   for Children
Indianapolis, Indiana


Clarice D. Reid, M.D.
Coordinator, National Sickle Cell
   Disease Program
Chief, Sickle Cell Disease Branch
Division of Blood Diseases
   and Resources
National Heart, Lung and Blood
   Institute
National Institutes of Health
Bethesda, Maryland


Marie O. Russell, M.D.
Assistant Professor of Pediatrics
University of Pennsylvania
   School of Medicine
Director, Sickle Cell Project
The Children's Hospital
   of Philadelphia
Philadelphia, Pennsylvania

Fredric T. Serota, M.D.
Research Fellow in Pediatric
   Hematology
The Children's Hospital
   of Philadelphia
Philadelphia, Pennsylvania

Gary F. Temple, M.D.
Assistant Research Physician
University of California
   at San Francisco
San Francisco General Hospital
San Francisco, California

Natale Tomassini
Research Associate
   in Experimental Pathology
The Children's Hospital
   of Philadelphia
Philadelphia, Pennsylvania

Winfred Wang, M.D.
Assistant Clinical Professor
   of Pediatrics
University of California
   at San Francisco
Pediatric Hematologist
San Francisco General Hospital
Assistant Director
Northern California Comprehensive
   Sickle Cell Center
San Francisco, California

# CONTENTS

# INTRODUCTION

In the past several years there have been major advances in the biochemistry, molecular biology, and genetics of human hemoglobins and in the care of patients with hemoglobinopathies. The purpose of this volume in the Progress in Pediatric Hematology/Oncology Series is to summarize this knowledge as it relates to affected children. The information presented here is meant to provide hematologists, pediatricians, geneticists, and all others interested in the care of children with hemoglobin disorders with information on many of the exciting advances in basic research in this area as well as on the many facets of diagnosis and care.

The first two chapters summarize current knowledge of the relationship of hemoglobin structure and function and the role that the identification of the profusion of abnormal hemoglobins has played in our knowledge of hemoglobin function. The following four chapters are concerned with diagnosis, including the use of the clinical laboratory and red cell morphology, the current status of prenatal diagnosis, and the sensitive and important area of community education and screening. Following a discussion of structurally abnormal hemoglobins which cause clinical disease in heterozygotes, two major sections are devoted to sickle cell disease and to thalassemia, including clinical features, complications, genetic variants, and treatment. A chapter deals with the role of federal programs in stimulating increased attention to many aspects of sickle cell disease, while another discusses the current status of the increasingly important area of investigations of abnormalities in RNA and DNA in the many forms of thalassemia.

I am indebted to the many colleagues whose contributions to this volume reflect their own dedication to treatment of children with hemoglobinopathies and to the advancement of knowledge in this field. I am grateful to Janet Fithian for invaluable assistance in editing and to Carol Way for expert secretarial help.

Elias Schwartz, M.D.

# PART I

# Human Hemoglobins
## and
# Hemoglobinopathies

# 1 Hemoglobin Structure and Function*

Toshio Asakura, M.D., Ph.D.
Robert S. Festa, M.D.

An adult requires 15 liters of pure oxygen per hour, or 250 ml per minute, which must be transported by about 5 liters of blood. If this much oxygen were to be transported only by plasma, 100 liters of plasma per minute would have to be circulated, assuming that all oxygen physically dissolved in plasma is totally extracted at the tissue and that the heart could pump this much fluid without additional energy and oxygen consumption. In reality, however, blood carries 80 times more oxygen than does plasma. This amazing difference between the oxygen carrying capacities of plasma and of blood is due to the presence of hemoglobin in red cells; 1 gram of hemoglobin carries 1.36 ml of oxygen while 1 gram of plasma carries only 0.0026 ml of oxygen.[1]

Tissues cannot obtain a sufficient supply of oxygen by diffusion from air surrounding the organism. Oxygen diffuses roughly 1 million

*The authors wish to acknowledge the editorial assistance of Janet Fithian and the preparation of the chapter by Margaret E. Nagle. This work was supported by NIH grants HL18226 and HL20750.

3

times more slowly through animal tissues than through air[2]; only if the body were paper-thin could an organism obtain sufficient oxygen without the assistance of an oxygen carrier.

It is generally believed that the primitive forms of life had only one oxygen binding heme-protein, probably one that resembled myoglobin, and that only after many mutations genes for the production of $\alpha$ and $\beta$ chains of hemoglobin evolved. Human hemoglobin not only is one of the most efficient oxygen carriers, but is also involved in the transport of hydrogen ion and carbon dioxide.

## STRUCTURE OF HUMAN HEMOGLOBIN

Hemoglobin is a complex protein composed of four polypeptide chains and four prosthetic groups (heme). Although the specific amino acid sequences of the polypeptide chains differ between animals, there is a fundamental structure common to almost all hemoglobins in various organisms.

Human red blood cells normally contain at least three different types of hemoglobins, all having two $\alpha$ and two non-$\alpha$ chains:

$$Hb\ A = \alpha_2\beta_2$$

$$Hb\ F = \alpha_2\gamma_2$$

$$Hb\ A_2 = \alpha_2\delta_2$$

Hb A is the major adult hemoglobin and comprises more than 95% of the total hemoglobin in red cells. Hb $A_2$ makes up about 2.5% of the total hemoglobin. Hb F is the major hemoglobin in the fetus; it is gradually replaced by Hb A during the last two months of fetal life and the first six months after birth. About 20% of Hb F molecules have an acetylated N terminus of the $\alpha$ chain (Hb $F_1$).[3] Hb $A_{1c}$ is a modified form of Hb A in which the N terminus of the $\beta$ chain is combined with glucose.[4,5] About 5% of the total hemoglobin in normal subjects is Hb $A_{1c}$, but the amount is doubled in patients with diabetes mellitus.[6,7] Other modified hemoglobins, called Hb $A_{1a}$, Hb $A_{1b}$, and Hb $A_{1e}$, are present in lesser amounts and are of unknown significance.

### Structure of Heme

Aside from containing either an $\alpha$ or $\beta$ chain, each subunit of hemoglobin contains iron-protoporphyrin IX, or protoheme, as the prosthetic group. As shown in Figure 1-1A, protoheme contains four pyrrole rings connected by four methene bridges. Oxygen combines with the iron in the center of the porphyrin ring.

The vinyl groups at positions 2 and 4 of the porphyrin ring are deeply embedded in the heme pocket of globin. The interaction of these two vinyl groups with the amino acid residues of the pocket seem to be important for the proper binding of oxygen; when these two groups or the amino acid residues interacting with these groups are modified, the oxygen binding property is significantly altered.[8,9] In contrast, the two propionic acid groups at positions 6 and 7 are oriented toward the outside of the heme pocket. Modification of these two groups does not affect the oxygen binding properties of hemoglobin.[10,11]

For reversible oxygen binding by hemoglobin, it is essential for the heme-iron to be kept in the ferrous state. When heme-iron is oxidized to the ferric form, hemoglobin becomes methemoglobin and can no longer carry oxygen. The oxidation of ferrous heme-iron occurs rapidly when heme is isolated from protein or when certain amino acids near the heme are genetically replaced, suggesting that the special amino acid arrangement in the globin pocket prevents the oxidation of heme-iron.

Methemoglobin is formed constantly even under physiologic conditions in circulating blood, but it is reduced again to the active ferrous form constantly by methemoglobin reducing enzymes. Whenever hemoglobin leaves the red blood cell, it is fairly rapidly oxidized to the ferric forms, as evidenced by the color change from red (oxy-form) to brown (ferric-form) seen routinely in regions of trauma.

Certain sea worms circulate a cell-free hemoglobin solution as an oxygen carrier and have no problems with oxidation.[12] Structural studies of the prosthetic groups of hemoglobin from these worms have shown that the side chain at position 2 of this heme differs from protoheme; instead of a vinyl group, the worm heme has a formyl group (Figure 1-1B),[13,14] which changes the color of hemoglobin to green and provides increased resistance to oxidation.

## Primary and Secondary Structure of Hemoglobin

Both $\alpha$ and $\beta$ chains of hemoglobin are long linear chains of amino acids linked by peptide bonds. Twenty different amino acids may make up thousands of different proteins simply by changes in the sequence and length of polypeptide chains. All of these amino acids have the same basic structure: an amino group, a hydrogen atom, a carboxyl group, and a side chain (R-group) bound to a carbon atom:

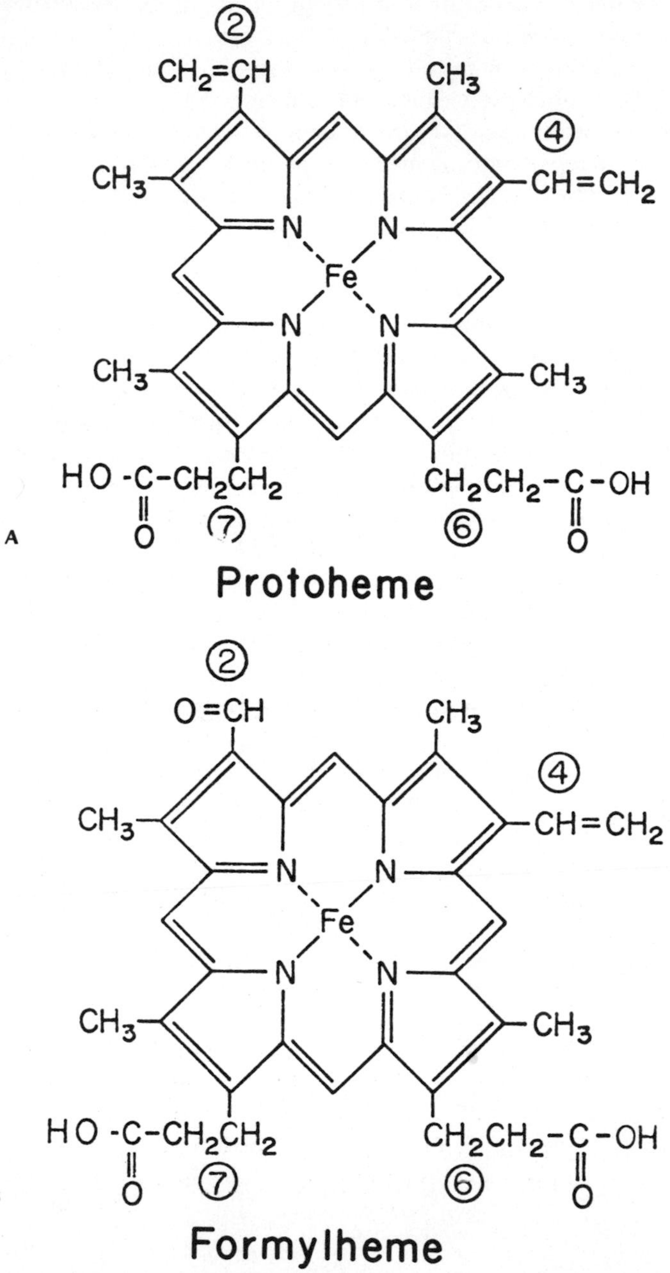

**Figure 1-1.** Structures of protoheme and formylheme. **(A)** Protoheme is the prosthetic group of hemoglobin, myoglobin, peroxidase, and catalase. **(B)** 2-Formyl-4-vinylheme (cruoroheme) exists in nature as the prosthetic group of green hemoglobin found in polychaete worms. The conversion of the vinyl group to the formyl group not only prevents the heme from oxidation but decreases the oxygen affinity of this worm hemoglobin significantly.

The -COOH group of one amino acid can be connected with the -NH₂ group of the next amino acid by a linkage -CO-NH-, called a peptide bond. As a result of each linkage, two potentially charged groups (-NH₃⁺, -COO⁻) of amino acids are removed; the charged groups remaining in the polypeptide are the amino group of the N terminus, the carboxyl group of the C terminus, and any ionizable groups in the R side chains (Figure 1-2). The net charge of a protein is determined by the relative numbers of acidic and basic amino acids. Two acidic amino acids and three basic amino acids are listed in Figure 1-2. Generally, most of these hydrophilic amino acids are exposed at the outside of the molecule, and the number of these amino acids determines the solubility and electrophoretic mobility of a protein.

Amino acid chains are more stable in a coil, or helical, configuration. This configuration was first proposed by Pauling and Corey in 1951.[15] One type of coil is called the α-helix, in which 3.6 amino acids are found per turn of the helix with a 5.4 Å pitch. The helix is stabilized by hydrogen bonding between the carboxyl group of each residue and the amino group four residues away. This helical structure is the "secondary structure," while the amino acid sequential structure is the "primary structure" (Figure 1-3).

The two α chains of hemoglobin each contain 141 amino acids while the β chains contain 146 amino acids. The complete sequences of human α and β chains are shown in Figure 1-4. The helical regions are

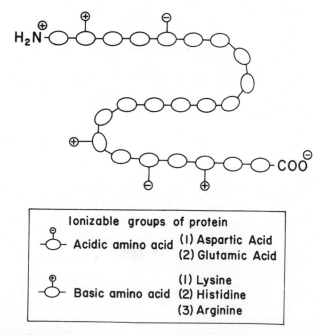

**Figure 1-2.** Charged groups of polypeptide chain.

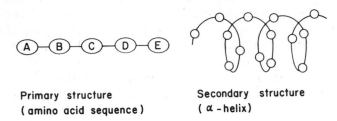

Primary structure
(amino acid sequence)

Secondary structure
(α-helix)

**Figure 1-3.** Primary and secondary structures of polypeptide chain.

designated by single capital letters (A to H) and the nonhelical regions are designated by two letters, from the preceding and succeeding helices. The nonhelical regions at the N terminal and C terminal are called NA and HC, respectively. The helical region corresponds to about 75% of the total molecule in the native state. Upon removal of heme, the helical content of apohemoglobin decreases to about 50%.[16]

The heme group is bound covalently with the imidazole groups of the 87th histidine in the α chain and the 92nd histidine in the β chain and helps maintain the helical structure of the protein.[17] These amino acids are called the proximal histidines and are essential to all animal hemoglobins. Other histidine residues, the so-called distal histidines at α-58 and β-63, also play important roles in the proper binding of oxygen by hemoglobin.

## Tertiary and Quaternary Structures of Hemoglobin

The helical and nonhelical segments of globin chains contribute to a three-dimensional configuration that provides a hydrophobic pocket to accommodate heme and allows the four globin subunits to have smooth interlocking contact. The tertiary structure of hemoglobin refers to the configuration of each subunit in three-dimensional space, while the quaternary structure refers to the overall structure created by four subunits.

The packing of four subunits into the hemoglobin molecule is such that there is a close, interlocking contact of side chains between unlike chains but virtually no contact between like chains. The molecule is roughly spherical with a dimension of $64 \times 55 \times 50$ Å. The nature of the intersubunit bonding is mainly hydrophobic, except for a few hydrogen bonds and ionic interaction.

As shown in Figure 1-4, 34 side chains are involved with the $\alpha_1\beta_1$ contact in contrast to only 19 with the $\alpha_1\beta_2$ contact. It is interesting that the amino acid contact at the $\alpha_1\beta_2$ interface moves considerably during oxygenation while that at the $\alpha_1\beta_1$ interface remains relatively fixed.

The abnormal oxygen binding properties of many hemoglobins that have a substitution at the $\alpha_1\beta_2$ interface, in contrast to those having substitutions at the $\alpha_1\beta_1$ interface, may be related to the need for retaining mobility at the $\alpha_1\beta_2$ interface.[17]

## Conformational Change and Heme-Heme Interaction

The most characteristic functional property of hemoglobin is its cooperative binding with oxygen. This unique property of hemoglobin has important physiologic significance for both the binding of oxygen at the lung and for efficient release of oxygen at the tissue level. Since the binding of oxygen to one heme increases the affinity of the second, third, and fourth hemes progressively, this cooperative binding of oxygen by hemoglobin is called heme-heme interaction.

This interaction results in the efficient unloading of oxygen to tissues. When one molecule of oxygen is released from a hemoglobin, then the second, third, and fourth oxygens in the same hemoglobin molecule are released progressively more easily. The efficiency of heme-heme interaction may be seen clearly by comparing the oxygen equilibrium curves of two hemoglobins with or without cooperativity.

In Figure 1-5, the oxygen equilibrium curve of native cooperative hemoglobin is compared with two synthetic noncooperative curves having high and low affinities. All of these hemoglobins bind the same amount of oxygen at high oxygen pressure and release all oxygen at zero oxygen pressure. The important fact is that the arterial oxygen tension at the lung is not extremely high (about 100 mm Hg) and that the average oxygen tension at the tissue is only 40 mm Hg. The most ideal oxygen carrier may be the one which is fully saturated with oxygen at the lung and which releases all oxygen at the tissue. Human blood with hemoglobin having cooperativity does not totally fulfil this criteria, but performs very well compared with a noncooperative oxygen carrier. First, under normal lung conditions more than 95% of the total heme becomes saturated with oxygen. Secondly, our blood releases 25% to 30% of the total oxygen at the tissues, with the remaining oxygen (70% to 75%) being reserved for circumstances when tissue oxygen requirements increase. Another advantage of human blood is that the oxygen equilibrium curve changes sharply near tissue oxygen tensions, indicating that the amount of oxygen released can be easily adjusted by a small change of tissue oxygen tension or by a slight shift of the oxygen equilibrium curve. For instance, a slight change in the red cell 2,3-diphosphoglyceric acid level shifts the curve to the right, resulting in increased oxygen release at the tissues. This compensatory mechanism has practical physiologic significance for patients with anemia or for persons who live in areas of high altitude where the oxygen tension is low.

What would happen if hemoglobin had no heme-heme interaction? If such a hemoglobin had a high oxygen affinity, as does muscle myoglobin (curve I in Figure 1-5), it would bind well with oxygen at the lung but it would not release enough oxygen at the tissue. Hb H, Hb Köln, and many noncooperative abnormal hemoglobins show this kind of oxygen equilibrium curve. Even if myoglobin had the same $P_{50}$ value as normal hemoglobin, it could not deliver sufficient oxygen because

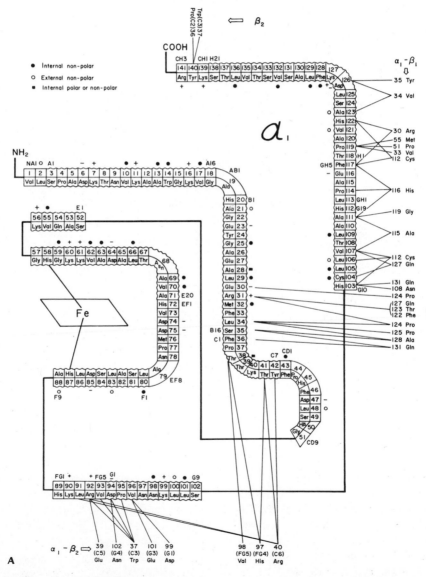

**Figure 1-4.** Primary amino acid sequence of α chain (**A**) and β chain (**B**) of human Hb A. The names of helical (A-H) and nonhelical (such as AB) segments, and the contacts

such an oxygen carrier cannot bind enough oxygen at the lung (curve III in Figure 1-5). Hb M Boston, Hb M Iwate, and Hb Kansas are hemoglobins with a low oxygen affinity and therefore the ferrous heme of these hemoglobins cannot be saturated with oxygen at the lung.

The mechanism of heme-heme interaction has been the focus of research interest for the last ten years. Although the precise mechanism is not yet known, it is certain that the transmittance of information about oxygen binding from site to site is not by a direct means such as electromagnetism, but rather that oxygen affinities are changed by the conformational changes of the protein. Two representative models for the mechanism of heme-heme interaction of hemoglobin are the allosteric two-state model described by Monod,

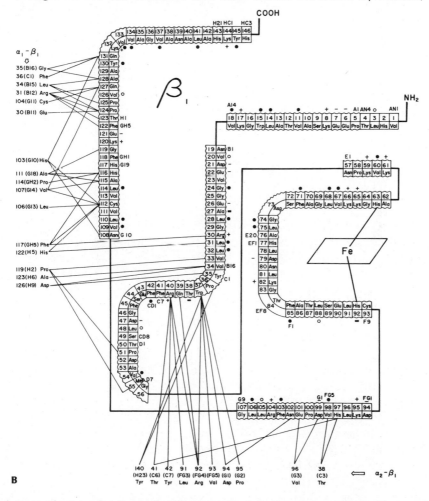

between the two subunits are also illustrated. The helical portions are denoted by wave and nonhelical portions by straight lines.

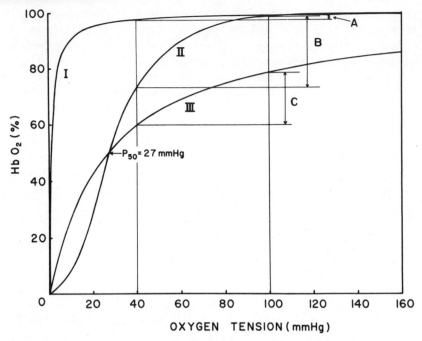

**Figure 1-5.** Comparison of oxygen equilibrium curves of high affinity noncooperative hemoglobin (I), sigmoidal normal hemoglobin (II), and low affinity noncooperative hemoglobin (III). The $P_{50}$ of I is 1 mm Hg, and $P_{50}$ of II and III are 27 mm Hg. The n-value of I and III is 1 while that of II is 2.7. Note the difference in the amount of oxygen delivered to tissue (A,B,C).

Wyman, and Changeux,[18] and the sequential model such as that reported by Koshland, Némethy, and Filmer.[19] In the two-state model hemoglobin exists in two equilibrium states, the R (relaxed) and T (tense) states. The hemoglobin with R structure has a high affinity for oxygen while that with T structure has a low affinity. The sequential model is based on the fact that protein exists in more than two conformational states; i.e., that the binding of a ligand to a subunit changes the tertiary structure of that subunit, which then affects the conformation of the unliganded subunits. In the sequential model, therefore, hemoglobin produces several intermediate conformational species. The x-ray crystallography results by Perutz[17] showed that the conformations of oxy (R) and deoxy (T) hemoglobins are clearly different, supporting the two-state model. This technique, however, cannot provide information about the intermediates during the R to T transformation. Evidence by kinetic, equilibrium, and other physical techniques is accumulating to support the presence of intermediate structures.

## OXYGEN BINDING PROPERTIES OF HEMOGLOBIN AND BLOOD

The standard method of determining the $P_{50}$ value is tonometry, as described by Astrup et al.[20] A sample of blood (usually several cc) is equilibrated with several gases of various oxygen tensions at 37°C and the hemoglobin saturation is measured. The values are corrected to pH 7.4 and plotted on graph paper. When several points have been obtained on the straight portion of the curve (saturations between 25% and 60%), a line is drawn to connect them and the oxygen tension corresponding to 50% hemoglobin saturation ($P_{50}$) is determined. Recent progress in electronics and other technology has made it possible to construct machines which draw a full oxygen equilibrium curve automatically and continuously.[11,21,22] The advantage of these machines is that they provide information on the shape of the curve which may be altered by the presence of an abnormal hemoglobin. For example, the presence of an abnormal hemoglobin component, such as Hb H, produces a biphasic curve that would not be detected by the mixing technique.

Examples of oxygen equilibrium curves determined with an automatic apparatus are shown in Figure 1-6. The position of the curve

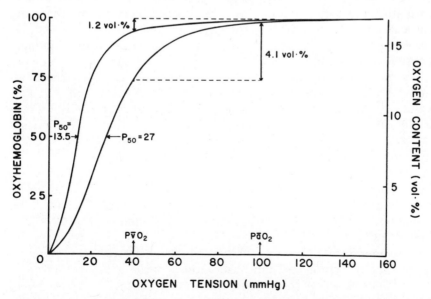

**Figure 1-6.** Oxygen equilibrium curves of free hemoglobin and whole blood. The oxygen affinity of hemoglobin within the erythrocyte ($P_{50}$ = 27.0 mm Hg) allows a more than three-fold increase in oxygen release compared to hemoglobin in solution ($P_{50}$ = 13.5 mm Hg).

for free hemoglobin in solution differs from that for red cell suspensions. Since 1 gram of hemoglobin binds 1.36 ml of oxygen, the oxygen-carrying capacity of the blood from a 10-year-old child with a hemoglobin level of 12.5 g/dl is 17 ml of oxygen per 100 ml of blood, i.e., 17 vol%. Assuming an oxygen tension of 100 mm Hg after blood is oxygenated in the lung and 40 mm Hg after blood has circulated through the tissues (normal mixed venous $PO_2$), hemoglobin within the red cell releases about 25% of its oxygen, or 4.1 vol%. A hemoglobin solution of 12.5 g/dl would release only about 30% of this amount. The difference in the oxygen releasing capacity of hemoglobin solutions and hemoglobin within the red cell demonstrates that certain substances within the erythrocyte modify hemoglobin oxygen binding to allow suitable amounts of oxygen to be released to tissues.

## Determinants of Oxygen Affinity

In order to express the affinity of hemoglobin for oxygen in some quantitative manner, the term $P_{50}$ is used to describe the position of the oxygen equilibrium curve. The $P_{50}$ value of the oxygen equilibrium curve is defined as the oxygen tension at which hemoglobin is half saturated. This value does not provide information about the shape of the curve. As oxygen affinity increases, the $P_{50}$ value decreases; as oxygen affinity decreases, the $P_{50}$ value increases. Under normal physiologic conditions (37°C, pH 7.4, $pCO_2$ 40 mm Hg), the $P_{50}$ value of blood from adults is about 27 mm Hg, while children between 6 months and 12 years of age have somewhat higher (1 to 3 mm Hg) $P_{50}$ values.[23,24] Since a shift of 1.0 mm Hg in the $P_{50}$ value compensates for a 1.0 g/dl change in the hemoglobin concentration,[25] the modest decrease in oxygen affinity reported in children would appear appropriate for the lower hemoglobin levels in childhood.

There are a number of factors which alter the oxygen affinity of human blood and thus significantly affect the $P_{50}$ value of the oxygen equilibrium curve. The major determinants of oxygen affinity are temperature, pH, and 2,3–DPG; less important factors are ATP, $CO_2$, and MCHC.

**Temperature**    Oxygen affinity varies inversely with temperature. Severinghaus[26] combined the observations of six groups of investigators and obtained the relationship ($\Delta \log P_{50}/\Delta T = 0.024$) at a constant pH. The relationship between temperature and oxygen affinity would appear to be physiologically appropriate. During pyrexia the decrease in oxygen affinity results in enhanced oxygen unloading to help meet the increased oxygen requirement of tissues. For example, a 3°C increase in temperature would increase the $P_{50}$ value of a normal individual from 27 mm Hg (pH 7.4, 37°C) to approximately

32 mm Hg (pH 7.4, 40°C). This would increase oxygen unloading in the normal individual by 35% to 40%.

**pH (Bohr Effect) and CO$_2$**    In 1974, Bohr published two papers, one describing the sigmoid shape of the oxygen equilibrium curve[27] and the other demonstrating that the position of the curve changed with alterations in partial pressure of carbon dioxide.[28] Subsequent investigations showed that CO$_2$ exerts its effects on oxygen affinity by two mechanisms. The first, and most important, is due to the effect of P$_{CO_2}$ on pH. The second is the binding of CO$_2$ to free amino groups of hemoglobin to form carbamino compounds. Over a pH range of 6.5 to 7.5, P$_{50}$ varies inversely with pH, and this is a measure of the alkaline Bohr effect (Figure 1-7). This phenomenon can be expressed as a chemical equation. Under physiologic conditions, hemoglobin releases approximately 2.4 protons upon oxygenation, i.e., oxyhemoglobin is a stronger acid than deoxyhemoglobin. Thus, the effect of pH on hemoglobin can be expressed as follows:

$$Hb\,(H^+)_{2.4} + 4O_2 \rightleftharpoons Hb\,(O_2)_4 + 2.4\,H^+$$

It can be seen from this equation that any increase in hydrogen ion favors the formation of deoxyhemoglobin via reaction 2 and thus lowers oxygen affinity; any decrease in hydrogen ion favors formation of oxyhemoglobin via reaction 1 and increases oxygen affinity.

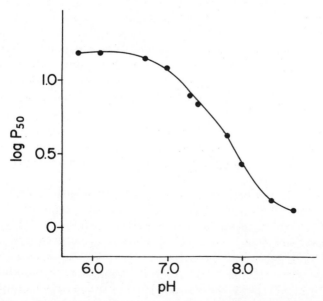

**Figure 1-7.**    Effect of pH on the oxygen affinity of human hemoglobin. The slope of the line between pH 6.5 and 7.5 is a measure of the alkaline Bohr effect.

A quantitative expression of the change in oxygen affinity with pH is the Bohr effect ($\Delta\log P_{50}/\Delta pH$). The value of the Bohr effect is $\Delta\log P_{50}/\Delta pH = -.40$ when the pH change is induced by metabolic acids.[29] The Bohr effect produced by varying carbon dioxide tension is somewhat larger ($\Delta\log P_{50}/\Delta pH = -.48$) because $CO_2$ affects oxygen affinity by altering pH and combining with the N terminal amino acids of hemoglobin as carbamino compounds.[29]

The Bohr effect is physiologically advantageous for oxygen transport. As blood circulates through the capillaries, $CO_2$ from the tissues enters the plasma and red cells, resulting in a lowering of red cell pH, which through the Bohr effect lowers oxygen affinity. This decrease in oxygen affinity enhances oxygen unloading to tissues. Conversely, as $CO_2$ is expelled during circulation through the lungs, there is an increase in pH which increases oxygen affinity and favors the binding of oxygen to hemoglobin. Therefore, the interaction of hemoglobin with hydrogen ions results in a physiologically appropriate mechanism for the transport of oxygen and carbon dioxide.

**2,3-Diphosphoglycerate (2,3-DPG)** If one compares the $P_{50}$ value of hemoglobin solutions with that of intact red cells, the oxygen equilibrium curve of red cells is considerably more right-shifted (Figure 1-6). Benesch and Benesch[30] and Chanutin and Curnish[31] demonstrated that 2,3-DPG and to a lesser extent other organic phosphates are potent modifiers of oxygen affinity and account for this difference. The addition of increasing amounts of 2,3-DPG to a solution of Hb A results in a progressive lowering of oxygen affinity. This organic phosphate is present within red cells at a concentration of about 4.5 mM/liter red cells, roughly equivalent to the concentration of the hemoglobin tetramer. Benesch and Benesch[32] further showed that under physiologic conditions of pH and ionic strength, 2,3-DPG lowers oxygen affinity by binding avidly to deoxyhemoglobin A in 1:1 molar ratio. By x-ray analysis technique,[33] 2,3-DPG has been shown to bind to the N terminal amino groups of the $\beta$ chains, the imidazoles of $\beta$143-histidine, and the amino groups of the $\beta$82-lysine. DPG stabilizes the deoxy conformation and lowers oxygen affinity, as shown schematically in Figure 1-8. The binding of 2,3-DPG to hemoglobin can be expressed as follows:

$$Hb \cdot DPG + 4O_2 \rightleftharpoons Hb(O_2)_4 + DPG$$

In addition to this direct effect on oxygen affinity, 2,3-DPG also lowers the oxygen affinity indirectly by decreasing intracellular pH. As pointed out by several investigators,[34,35] 2,3-DPG is a negatively charged impermeable anion, and any increase in this compound within the red cell lowers intracellular pH relative to plasma pH as a manifestation of the Gibbs-Donnan equilibrium. This decrease in red cell pH lowers oxygen affinity by the Bohr effect. Duhm[36] has demonstrated that with a 2,3-DPG level up to 5.0 μmoles/ml red blood cells, oxygen affinity is lowered both by preferential binding to deoxyhemoglobin and indirectly by the Bohr effect. At levels greater than 5.0 μmoles/ml red blood cells, 2,3-DPG has a small effect on oxygen affinity which is attributed almost solely to a progressive lowering of intracellular pH.

Red cell 2,3-DPG is produced through the Rapoport-Luebering pathway, which is a detour from the main road of red cell glycolysis (Figure 1-9). Normally, the main metabolism of 1,3-diphosphoglycerate (1,3-DPG) is to 3-phosphoglyceric acid (3-PGA) with the formation of high energy ATP. Some 1,3-DPG is converted to 2,3-DPG by the action of DPG mutase. Removal of a phosphate from 2,3-DPG by a DPG phosphatase brings the substrate back to the main glycolytic pathway in the form of 3-PGA. The major difference in these two pathways is that the one route produces high energy ATP while the other does not.

The level of 2,3-DPG is regulated by three factors: 1) the rate of synthesis of 1,3-DPG; 2) the relative amount of 1,3-DPG going into the Rapoport-Luebering shunt versus that going through the main glycolytic pathway; and 3) the rate at which 2,3-DPG is hydrolyzed. Although the mechanism of the elevation of blood 2,3-DPG in patients with various types of hypoxia is not completely understood, factors that affect the level of 2,3-DPG are summarized in Table 1-1. For instance, 2,3-DPG levels sharply decrease upon incubating cells in an acid medium.[37] The ligand state of hemoglobin also affects the levels of red cell 2,3-DPG.[38]

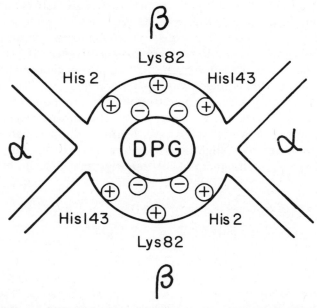

**Figure 1-8.** Schematic drawing of 2,3-DPG binding with hemoglobin. 2,3-DPG is kept in the central cavity created by four subunits.

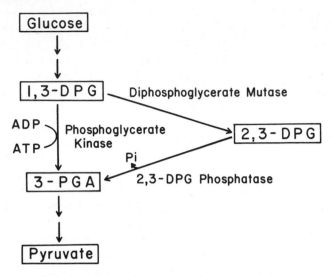

**Figure 1-9.** Metabolism of 2,3-DPG via the Rapoport-Luebering pathway. 1,3-Diphospho-glycerate (DPG) can be isomerized to 2,3-DPG or converted directly to 3-phosphoglyceric acid (3-PGA).

**ATP and Other Organic Phosphates**    While red cell 2,3-DPG is by far the most important organic phosphate as far as oxygen affinity is concerned, other organic phosphates can also lower the oxygen affinity of hemoglobin. On a molar basis, their degree of interaction with hemoglobin is 2,3-DPG > ATP > ADP > AMP. Although there is almost one-third as much ATP as 2,3-DPG in human red cells, the majority of ATP is bound to magnesium. The Mg-ATP complex does not interact with hemoglobin and thus has no effect on oxygen affinity.[39] The other organic phosphates are present in such small quantities that they have no significant effect on hemoglobin-oxygen binding.

**MCHC**    The intracellular concentration of hemoglobin does not seem to play a significant role in the oxygen binding properties of red cells. Benesch et al[40] showed that the oxygen affinity of phosphate-free hemoglobin increases only slightly with increasing hemoglobin concentration. However, Bellingham et al[41] reported a significant effect

**Table 1-1**
**Factors Which Affect the Level of Red Cell 2,3-DPG**

| Increase 2,3-DPG level | Decrease 2,3-DPG level |
| --- | --- |
| 1,3-DPG | Orthophosphate |
| Alkalosis | Acidosis |
| 3-PGA | Sulfite |
| Sulfate | Dithionite |
| Deoxyhemoglobin | Glycolate-2-P |

and positive correlation between $P_{50}$ and MCHC. Subsequent work by May and Huehns[42] and Murphy et al[43] could find no significant change in $P_{50}$ when the MCHC of red cells was varied with hyper- and hypotonic solutions. More recently the effect of MCHC on $P_{50}$ was studied by altering plasma osmolarity. The effect of MCHC on $P_{50}$ was very small at normal 2,3-DPG levels, and at high 2,3-DPG levels no correlation was found between $P_{50}$ and MCHC.[44]

These investigations would seem to indicate that MCHC plays no significant role in the oxygen binding properties of red cells containing Hb A, and it is unlikely that the range of MCHC encountered clinically can significantly affect hemoglobin function. The normal levels of 2,3-DPG with increased $P_{50}$ values in splenectomized patients with hereditary spherocytosis[45] would appear not to be due to the increase in MCHC but to some other as yet unidentified mechanism.

**In Vitro $P_{50}$ vs In Vivo $P_{50}$**  The position of the oxygen equilibrium curve (in vitro $P_{50}$) obtained under standard physiologic conditions of pH, temperature, and $P_{CO_2}$ will reflect red cell 2,3-DPG levels. In clinical disorders in which significant abnormalities in pH and temperature are not present, the $P_{50}$ value in vitro will closely approximate the $P_{50}$ value in vivo. In these instances the oxygen equilibrium curve in vitro will give a good estimate of the oxygen releasing capacity of the blood in vivo. However, if significant acidosis or alkalosis is present, or if the patient has high fever, the $P_{50}$ in vitro will be significantly different from the $P_{50}$ in vivo. In these situations the position of the curve obtained under standard conditions should be recalculated with the correct ion factors for temperature and pH as follows:

$$Log\ P_{50}\ in\ vivo = Log\ P_{50}\ in\ vitro + 0.48\ (7.4 - pH) + 0.024\ (T\text{-}37)$$

if the change in pH is due to alterations in $P_{CO_2}$, or:

$$Log\ P_{50}\ in\ vivo = Log\ P_{50}\ in\ vitro + 0.40\ (7.4 - pH) + 0.024\ (T\text{-}37)$$

if the change in pH is due to a metabolic acidosis with a near normal $P_{CO_2}$.

These corrections will give a more accurate assessment of oxygen unloading in vivo.

## Tissue Oxygen Delivery

The unloading of oxygen to tissues ($\bar{v}O_2$ in ml/min) is expressed by the Fick equation:

$$\bar{v}O_2 = 1.36 \cdot Q \cdot Hb \cdot (S_{\bar{a}}O_2 - S_{\bar{v}}O_2)$$

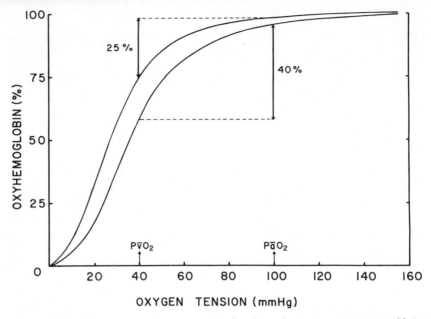

**Figure 1-10.** Enhancement of oxygen unloading by a decrease in oxygen equilibrium curve allows a greater fraction of oxygen to be released to tissues at any given oxygen tension.

where 1.36 is the number of ml of $O_2$ that can bind to 1 gram of hemoglobin, Q is the blood flow (liters/min), Hb is the hemoglobin concentration (g/dl) and $S_{\bar{a}} O_2$ and $S_{\bar{v}} O_2$ are the arterial and mixed venous oxygen saturations (%). Thus, the three major variables in oxygen delivery are cardiac output, red cell mass, and the arterio-venous oxygen difference, which is determined by the position of the oxygen equilibrium curve. During hypoxia of any type, a compensatory increase in oxygen unloading can occur by:

1. Increase in cardiac output (↑ Q).
2. Increase in red cell mass (↑ Hb).
3. Decrease in oxygen affinity (↑ [$S_{\bar{a}} O_2 - S_{\bar{v}} O_2$]).

The decrease in oxygen affinity mediated by elevated red cell 2,3-DPG is recognized as a rapid and efficient means of increasing tissue oxygen delivery in a variety of hypoxic states. The decrease in oxygen affinity allows a greater fraction of oxygen to be released from hemoglobin at any given $PO_2$ (Figure 1-10) and lessens the requirement for an increase in blood flow, decrease in tissue oxygen tension, and increase in red cell mass.

## Alterations in Whole Blood Oxygen Affinity in Clinical Disorders

A large number of clinical disorders have been identified in which a displacement of the oxygen equilibrium curve occurs. Those disease states associated with an increase in 2,3-DPG and $P_{50}$, and thus a decrease in oxygen affinity, include anemia, chronic pulmonary disease, cyanotic heart disease with right to left shunt, congestive heart failure, cirrhosis, thyrotoxicosis, uremia, hyperphosphatemia, and pyruvate kinase deficiency. An increase in oxygen affinity with low 2,3-DPG levels has been reported in acidosis, transfusion of stored blood, hypophosphatemia, panhypopituitarism, hypothyroidism, and hexokinase deficiency. Oxygen affinity is also altered by the presence of increased amounts of normal hemoglobin components with structural changes at the 2,3-DPG binding site, such as Hb F in the neonate and Hb $A_{1C}$ in juvenile diabetics. For an extensive discussion of these entities, the reader is referred to several review articles which have appeared in recent years.[46-48]

## REFERENCES

1. Altman, P.L., and Dittmer, D.S., Editors. *Respiration and Circulation.* Bethesda: Federation of American Societies for Experimental Biology, 1970.
2. Lehman, H., and Huntsman, R.G. *Man's Haemoglobins.* Philadelphia: J.B. Lippincott Co., 1974, p. 18.
3. Schroeder, W.A., Chua, J., Metsuda, G., et al. Hemoglobin $F_I$, an acetyl-containing hemoglobin. *Biochim. Biophys. Acta* 63:532–534, 1962.
4. Bookchin, R.M., and Gallop, P.M. Structure of hemoglobin $A_{1C}$. Nature of the N-terminal $\beta$-chain blocking group. *Biochem. Biophys. Res. Commun.* 33:86–95, 1968.
5. Holmquist, W.R., and Schroeder, W.A. A new N terminal blocking group involving a Schiff base in hemoglobin $A_{1C}$. *Biochemistry* 5:2489–2503, 1966.
6. Rahbar, S. An abnormal hemoglobin in red cells of diabetics. *Clin. Chim. Acta* 22:296–298, 1968.
7. Trivelli, L.A., Ranney, H.M., and Lai, H. Hemoglobin components in patients with diabetes mellitus. *N. Engl. J. Med.* 284:353–357, 1971.
8. Antonini, E., Brunori, M., Caputo, A., et al. Studies on the structure of hemoglobin. III. Physiochemical properties of reconstituted hemoglobins. *Biochim. Biophys. Acta* 79:284–292, 1964.
9. Asakura, T., and Sono, M. Optical and oxygen binding properties of spirographis, isospirographis and 2,4-diformyl hemoglobins. *J. Biol. Chem.* 249:7087–7093, 1974.
10. Sugita, Y., and Yoneyama, Y. Oxygen equilibrium of hemoglobins containing unnatural hemes: Effect of modification of heme carboxyl groups and side chains at positions 2 and 4. *J. Biol. Chem.* 246:389–394, 1971.
11. Asakura, T., and Tamura, M. Heme–spin-label studies of hemoglobin. II. Spin-labeled oxy- and deoxyhemoglobins. *J. Biol. Chem.* 249:4504–4506, 1974.

22

12. Fox, H.M. The oxygen affinity of chlorocruorin. *Proc. R. Soc. Lond.* B111:358–363, 1932.

13. Fischer, H., and Von Seemann, C. Die konstitution des spirographishamins. *Z. Physiol. Chem.* 242:133–157, 1936.

14. Antonini, E., Rossi-Fanelli, A., and Caputo, A. Studies on chlorocruorin. I. The oxygen equilibrium of spirographis chlorocruorin. *Arch. Biochem. Biophys.* 97:336–342, 1962.

15. Pauling, L., and Corey, R.B. Atomic coordinates and structure factors for two helical configurations of polypeptide chains. *Proc. Natl. Acad. Sci. USA* 37:235–240, 1951.

16. Asakura, T., Minakami, S., Yoneyama, Y., et al. Combination of globin and its derivatives with hemins and porphyrins. *J. Biochem. (Tokyo)* 56:594–600, 1964.

17. Perutz, M.F., Stereochemistry of cooperative effects in haemoglobin. *Nature* 228:726–739, 1970.

18. Monod, J., Wyman, J., and Changeux, J.P. On the nature of allosteric transitions: A plausible model. *J. Mol. Biol.* 12:88–118, 1965.

19. Koshland, D.E., Némethy, G., and Filmer, D. Comparison of experimental binding data and theoretical models in proteins containing subunits. *Biochemistry* 5:365–385, 1966.

20. Astrup, P., Engel, K., Severinghaus, J.W., and Munson, E. The influence of temperature and pH on the dissociation curve of oxyhemoglobin of human blood. *Scand. J. Clin. Lab. Invest.* 17:515, 1965.

21. Duvelleroy, M.A., Buckles, R.G., Rosenkaimer, S., et al. An oxyhemoglobin dissociation analyzer. *J. Appl. Physiol.* 28:227–233, 1970.

22. Imai, K., Morimoto, H., Kotani, M., et al. Studies on the function of abnormal hemoglobins. *Biochim. Biophys. Acta* 200:189–196, 1970.

23. Card, R.T., and Brain, M.C. The anemia of childhood. *N. Engl. J. Med.* 288:388–392, 1973.

24. Oski, F.A. Designation of anemia on a functional basis. *J. Pediatr.* 83:353–354, 1973.

25. Edwards, M.J., and Canon, B. Oxygen transport during erythropoietic response to moderate blood loss. *N. Engl. J. Med.* 287:115–119, 1972.

26. Severinghaus, J.W. Blood gas calculator. *J. Appl. Physiol.* 21:1108–1116, 1966.

27. Bohr, C. Theoretische Behandlung der quantitativen Verhältnisse bei der Sauerstoffaufnahme der Hamoglobins. *Zentralbl. Physiol.* 17:682–691, 1904.

28. Bohr, C., Hasselbach, K., and Krogh, A. Veber einen in biologischer Beziehung wichtigen Einfluss den die Kohlensaurespannung des Blutes auf dessen sauerstoffbinding übt. *Skand. Arch. Physiol.* 16:402–412, 1904.

29. Naerraa, N., Strange Peterson, E., Boye, E., et al. pH and molecular $CO_2$ components of the Bohr effect in human blood. *Scand. J. Clin. Lab. Invest.* 18:96–102, 1966.

30. Benesch, R., and Benesch, R.E. The effect of organic phosphates from human erythrocytes on the allosteric properties of hemoglobin. *Biochem. Biophys. Res. Commun.* 26:162–167, 1967.

31. Chanutin, A., and Curnish, R.R. Effect of organic and inorganic phosphates on the oxygen equilibrium of human erythrocytes. *Arch. Biochem. Biophys.* 121:96–102, 1967.

32. Benesch, R., and Benesch, R.E. Intracellular organic phosphates as regulators of oxygen release by hemoglobin. *Nature* 221:618–622, 1969.

33. Arnone, A. X-ray diffraction study of binding of 2,3-diphosphoglycerate to human deoxyhemoglobin. *Nature* 237:146–149, 1972.

34. Guest, G.M., and Rapoport, S. Role of acid soluble phosphorous compounds in red blood cells in experimental rickets, renal insufficiency, pyloric obstruction, gastroenteritis, ammonium chloride acidosis, and diabetes acidosis. *Am. J. Dis. Child.* 58:1072–1089, 1939.

35. Battaglia, F.C., McGaughey, H., Makowski, E.L., et al. Postnatal changes in oxygen affinity of sheep red cells: A dual role of 2,3-diphosphoglyceric acid. *Am. J. Physiol.* 219:217–221, 1970.

36. Duhm, J. Effects of 2,3-diphosphoglycerate and other organic phosphate compounds on oxygen affinity and intracellular pH of human erythrocytes. *Pfluegers. Arch.* 326:341–356, 1971.

37. Asakura, T., Sato, Y., Minakami, S., et al. pH Dependency of 2,3-diphosphoglycerate content in red blood cells. *Clin. Chim. Acta* 14:840–841, 1966.

38. Asakura, T., Sato, Y., Minakami, S., et al. Effect of deoxygenation of intracellular hemoglobin on red cell glycolysis. *J. Biochem. (Tokyo)* 5:524–526, 1966.

39. Bunn, H.F., Ransil, M.J., and Chao, A.O. The interaction between erythrocyte organic phosphates, magnesium ion, and hemoglobin. *J. Biol. Chem.* 246:5273–5279, 1971.

40. Benesch, R., Benesch, R.E., and Yu, C.I.O. The oxygenation of hemoglobin in the presence of diphosphoglycerate: Effect of temperature, pH, ionic strength, and hemoglobin concentration. *Biochemistry* 8:2567–2571, 1969.

41. Bellingham, A.I., Detter, J.C., and Lenfant, C. Regulatory mechanism of hemoglobin oxygen affinity in acidosis and alkalosis. *J. Clin. Invest.* 50:700–706, 1971.

42. May, A., and Huehns, E.R. The mechanism of the low oxygen affinity of red cells in sickle cell disease. *Haematol. Bluttransfus.* 10:279–283, 1972.

43. Murphy, J.R., Wengerd, M., and Kellermeyer, R.W. Erythrocyte $O_2$ affinity: Influence of cell density and *in vitro* changes in hemoglobin concentration. *J. Lab. Clin. Med.* 84:218–224, 1974.

44. Woodson, R.D., Wranne, B., and Detter, J.C. Effect of osmotic shrinking and swelling of red cells on whole blood oxygen affinity. *Scand. J. Clin. Lab. Invest.* 33:261–267, 1974.

45. Fernandez, L.A., and Erslev, A.J. Oxygen affinity and compensated hemolysis in hereditary spherocytosis. *J. Lab. Clin. Med.* 80:780–785, 1972.

46. Oski, F.A., and Gottlieb, A.J. The interrelationships between red blood cell metabolites, hemoglobin and the oxygen-equilibrium curve. *Prog. Hematol.* 7:33–67, 1971.

47. Thomas, H.M., Lefrak, S.S., Irwin, R.S., et al. The oxyhemoglobin dissociation curve in health and disease. *Am. J. Med.* 57:331–348, 1974.

48. Harken, A.D. The surgical significance of the oxyhemoglobin dissociation curve. *Surg. Gynecol. Obstet.* 144:935–955, 1977.

# 2 Human Hemoglobin Variants*

Kazuhiko Adachi, Ph.D.
John F. Kelleher, Jr., M.D.

Human hemoglobin variants have become increasingly interesting and important to physicians, as evidence has accumulated that a number of distinct clinical syndromes can be attributed to the presence of an abnormal hemoglobin. At present, more than 300 varieties of abnormal hemoglobins have been reported (Table 2-1). Although the majority of these are not associated with clinical abnormalities, many do cause disease.

All hemoglobin variants, except for approximately the first ten, which were given letter names, are named for the hospital, city, province, or country where they were discovered; family names are also used. Not surprisingly, the same variant has been discovered in different laboratories and therefore has acquired several names. For instance, Hb $\alpha_2$ 47 Asp→Gly$\beta_2$ has nine different names, but is generally called Hb L Ferrara after the place where it was first described.

*The authors wish to acknowledge the editorial assistance of Janet Fithian and the typing of this chapter by Margaret E. Nagle. This work was supported by NIH grants HL18226 and HL20750.

**Table 2-1**
**Human Hemoglobin Variants**

|  | Total | Unstable | Abnormal $O_2$ affinity |
|---|---|---|---|
| $\alpha$ Chain | 96 | 10 | 13 |
| $\beta$ Chain | 183 | 58 | 63 |
| $\delta$ Chain | 9 | – | – |
| $\gamma$ Chain | 16 | 1 | – |
| Fusion | 8 | – | 2 |
| Total | 312 | 69 | 78 |

Table compiled March, 1978.

After the finding of Hb S, sickle hemoglobin, which has a single amino acid substitution in the $\beta$ chain ($\beta$6 Glu→Val), electrophoresis became widely employed in the search for human hemoglobin variants. Methods of hemoglobin identification by electrophoresis are mainly based on the electrical charge of hemoglobin. The molecular location of the substituted residue, as well as the substitution itself, can determine the mobility of a mutant hemoglobin. For instance, Hb C and Hb E each migrate differently on citrate agar gel electrophoresis despite the identical Glu→Lys mutation at $\beta$6 and $\beta$26, respectively. Hemoglobin variants that migrate exactly the same distance as normal hemoglobin are called electrophoretically silent hemoglobins. Detection of these abnormal molecules involves other techniques, including isoelectric focusing, determination of oxygen binding curves, reactivity of sulfhydryl groups, and measurement of the rate of denaturation by heat, alkali, or mechanical agitation. The mutation site must be determined by amino acid analysis. The structural analysis of the mutation site in many hemoglobin variants has aided in the evaluation of the structure-function relationship of hemoglobin.

## CLASSIFICATION OF HEMOGLOBIN VARIANTS

Hemoglobins can be classified according to several criteria. Hemoglobin variants that are clinically significant are shown in Table 2-2. Abnormal hemoglobins can also be categorized on the basis of the mutation site on the hemoglobin molecule (Table 2-3; see pp. 28–41). Hemoglobins with a mutation at the heme contact region or the $\alpha_1\beta_2$ contact region tend to have abnormal oxygen binding properties, with some of these hemoglobins being unstable. Many abnormal hemoglobins that produce symptoms have an internally directed replacement in the hemoglobin molecule, while those with a substitution at external positions usually do not produce symptoms. All variants in

**Table 2-2**
**Clinically Important Hemoglobin Variants**

A. The Sickle Syndromes

B. The Unstable Hemoglobins
 (approximately 70 variants)

C. Hemoglobins with Abnormal Oxygen Affinity
 1. High affinity (familial erythrocytosis)
  (approximately 30 variants)
 2. Low affinity
  (approximately 15 variants)

D. The M Hemoglobins (familial cyanosis)
 (5 variants)

E. Structural Variants Which Result in a Thalassemic Phenotype
 1. Lepore hemoglobins ($\beta$-thalassemia phenotype)
 2. Chain termination mutants (i.e., Hb Constant Spring: $\alpha$-thalassemia phenotype)

F. Other Hemoglobins (Hb C, D, E, G, O)

G. Abnormal Hemoglobins Interacting with Thalassemia

which the amino acid sequence has been listed by the International Hemoglobin Information Center[1] as well as additional variants reported in recent publications are shown in Table 2-3.

We have grouped the chemical replacements of amino acid residues according to their position in tridimensional structures: (1) replacement of residues in contact with heme, including replacements of nonpolar residues interacting with the porphyrin and replacements of the proximal and distal histidine; (2) replacement of residues at the interfaces between the subunits, including those in the $\alpha_1\beta_1$, $\alpha_2\beta_2$, $\alpha_1\alpha_2$, and $\beta_1\beta_2$ regions of contact; (3) replacement of residues at other positions, which are still associated with large changes in structure and function (internal residues); and (4) replacement of residues in the outer parts of the molecule, which generally have no direct effect on the structure and function, although their presence may be accompanied by pathologic symptoms in homozygotes (external residues, like Hb S).

Human hemoglobin variants can also be classified according to their genetic abnormality (Table 2-4). These are (1) variants in which the structural alteration can be explained by a single base substitution in the corresponding triplet codon of the globin gene DNA (and its corresponding mRNA); (2) variants in which the already existing chain has been extended at the carboxy terminus, probably resulting from a single point mutation in the codon for termination of the chain allowing amino acids to be coded until the next termination codon is read; (3) variants in which one or more amino acids are missing due to deletion

**Table 2-3**
**Classification of Abnormal Hemoglobins**

| Designation | Residue number | Position | Replacement | Abnormal properties |
|---|---|---|---|---|
| | | A. Residues in Contact with Heme Groups | | |
| *α Chain* | | | | |
| Torino | 43 | CD1 | Phe→Val | Unstable ↓ O₂ affinity |
| Hirosaki | 43 | CD1 | Phe→Leu | |
| Fort de France³ | 45 | CD3 | His→Arg | |
| M Boston | 58 | E7 | His→Tyr | ↓ O₂ affinity |
| M Iwate | 87 | F8 | His→Tyr | Ferri Hb |
| Bibba | 136 | H19 | Leu→Pro | Unstable ↑ dissociation |
| *β Chain* | | | | |
| Mequon | 41 | C7 | Phe→Tyr | |
| Hammersmith | 42 | CD1 | Phe→Ser | Unstable ↓ O₂ affinity |
| Louisville | 42 | CD1 | Phe→Leu | Unstable ↓ O₂ affinity |
| M. Saskatoon | 63 | E7 | His→Tyr | Ferri Hb |
| | | | | Unstable ↑ O₂ affinity |
| Zürich | 63 | E7 | His→Arg | Unstable ↑ O₂ affinity |
| Bicetre | 63 | E7 | His→Pro | Unstable |
| I Toulouse | 66 | E10 | Lys→Glu | Unstable Ferri Hb |
| M Milwaukee-T | 67 | E11 | Val→Glu | |
| Bristol | 67 | E11 | Val→Asp | Ferri Hb, ↓ O₂ affinity |
| Sydney | 67 | E11 | Val→Ala | Unstable |
| Seattle | 70 | E14 | Ala→Asp | ↓ O₂ affinity |
| Christchurch | 71 | E15 | Phe→Ser | Unstable |

| Designation | Residue number | Position | Replacement | Structural site | Abnormal properties |
|---|---|---|---|---|---|
| Santa Ana | 88 | F4 | Leu→Pro | | Unstable |
| Borås | 88 | F4 | Leu→Arg | | Unstable |
| Sabine | 91 | F7 | Leu→Pro | | Unstable |
| Caribbean | 91 | F7 | Leu→Arg | | Unstable ↓ $O_2$ affinity |
| M Hyde Park | 92 | F8 | His→Tyr | | Ferri Hb Normal $O_2$ |
| St. Etienne | 92 | F8 | His→Gln | | Unstable ↑ $O_2$ affinity ↑ dissociation |
| J. Altgeld Gardens | 92 | F8 | His→Asp | | Normal $O_2$ affinity |
| Newcastle | 92 | F8 | His→Pro | | |
| Köln | 98 | FG5 | Val→Met | | Unstable ↑ $O_2$ affinity |
| Nottingham | 98 | FG5 | Val→Gly | | Unstable ↑ $O_2$ affinity |
| Djelta | 98 | FG5 | Val→Ala | | Unstable ↑ $O_2$ affinity |
| Richmond | 102 | G4 | Asn→Lys | | Asymmetric hybrids |
| Kansas | 102 | G4 | Asn→Thr | | ↓ $O_2$ affinity ↑ dissociation |
| Beth Israel | 102 | G4 | Asn→Ser | | ↓ $O_2$ affinity |
| Heathrow | 103 | G5 | Phe→Leu | | ↑ $O_2$ affinity |
| Southampton | 106 | G8 | Leu→Pro | | ↑ $O_2$ affinity |
| Tübingen | 106 | G8 | Leu→Gln | | Unstable ↑ $O_2$ affinity |
| Olmstead | 141 | H19 | Leu→Arg | | |
| Coventry | 141 | H19 | Leu Deleted | | Unstable |
| B. Residues at Contacts Between Subunits | | | | | |
| α Chain | | | | | |
| Memphis | 23 | B4 | Glu→Gln | $α_1α_2$ | |

**Table 2-3** (continued)

| Designation | Residue number | Position | Replacement | Structural site | Abnormal properties |
|---|---|---|---|---|---|
| G Audhali | 23 | B4 | Glu→Val | $\alpha_1\alpha_2$ | |
| Chad | 23 | B4 | Glu→Lys | $\alpha_1\alpha_2$ | |
| O Padova | 30 | B11 | Glu→Lys | $\alpha_1\beta_1$ | |
| G Chinese | 30 | B11 | Glu→Gln | $\alpha_1\beta_1$ | |
| J. Sardegna | 50 | CD8 | His→Asp | $\alpha_1\alpha_2$ | |
| Port Phillip | 91 | FG3 | Leu→Pro | $\alpha_1\beta_2$ (Oxy) | Unstable |
| J Capetown | 92 | FG4 | Arg→Gln | $\alpha_1\beta_2$ | ↑ O₂ affinity |
| Chesapeake | 92 | FG4 | Arg→Leu | $\alpha_1\beta_2$ | ↑ O₂ affinity |
| Setif | 94 | G1 | Asp→Tyr | $\alpha_1\beta_2$ | Unstable |
| Titusville | 94 | G1 | Asp→Asn | $\alpha_1\beta_2$ | ↓ O₂ affinity ↑ dissociation |
| G Georgia | 95 | G2 | Pro→Leu | $\alpha_1\beta_2$ | ↑ dissociation |
| Rampa | 95 | G2 | Pro→Ser | $\alpha_1\beta_2$ | ↑ dissociation |
| Denmark Hill | 95 | G2 | Pro→Ala | $\alpha_1\beta_2$ | ↑ O₂ affinity |
| St. Luke's | 95 | G2 | Pro→Arg | $\alpha_1\beta_2$ | ↑ dissociation |
| Chiapas | 114 | GH2 | Pro→Arg | $\alpha_1\beta_1$ | |
| Hopkins-2-II | 112 | G19 | His→Asp | | |
| | 114 | GH2 | Pro→Ser | $\alpha_1\beta_1$ | |
| | 118 | GH6 | Thr→Gly | | |
| Tarrant | 126 | H9 | Asp→Asn | $\alpha_1\beta_1$ | |
| St. Claude | 127 | H10 | Lys→Thr | $\alpha_1\alpha_2$ | |
| Jackson | 127 | H10 | Lys→Asp | $\alpha_1\alpha_2$ | |
| Singapore | 141 | HC3 | Arg→Pro | $\alpha_1\alpha_2$ | |

| Name | Position | Chain | Substitution | Contact | Effect |
|---|---|---|---|---|---|
| Surenes | 141 | HC3 | Arg→His | $\alpha_1\alpha_2$ | |
| J Camagüey | 141 | HC3 | Arg→Gly | $\alpha_1\alpha_2$ | |
| J Cabujuqui[4] | 141 | HC3 | Arg→Ser | $\alpha_1\alpha_2$ | |
| Legnano | 141 | HC3 | Arg→Leu | $\alpha_1\alpha_2$ | ↑ $O_2$ affinity |
| *β Chain* | | | | | |
| Nagasaki | 17 | A14 | Lys→Glu | $\beta_1\beta_2$ | |
| E | 26 | B8 | Glu→Lys | $\beta_1\beta_2$ | |
| Henri Mandor | 26 | B8 | Glu→Val | $\beta_1\beta_2$ | Unstable (slight) |
| Tacoma | 30 | B12 | Arg→Ser | $\alpha_1\beta_1$ | Unstable ↓ Bohr |
| Philly | 35 | B12 | Tyr→Phe | $\alpha_1\beta_1$ | Unstable ↑ $O_2$ affinity |
| Hirose | 37 | C3 | Trp→Ser | $\alpha_1\beta_2$ | ↑ $O_2$ affinity |
| Rothchild | 37 | C3 | Trp→Arg | $\alpha_1\beta_2$ | |
| Alabama | 39 | C5 | Gln→Lys | $\alpha_1\beta_2$ Oxy | |
| Vaasa | 39 | C5 | Gln→Glu | $\alpha_1\beta_2$ Oxy | |
| Athens-Georgia | 40 | C6 | Arg→Lys | $\alpha_1\beta_2$ | ↑ $O_2$ affinity |
| Austin | 40 | C6 | Arg→Ser | $\alpha_1\beta_2$ | |
| Williamette | 51 | D2 | Pro→Arg | $\alpha_1\beta_1$ | |
| Seattle | 61 | E5 | Lys→Glu | $\beta_1\beta_2$ | |
| Hikari | 61 | E5 | Lys→Asn | $\beta_1\beta_2$ | |
| G Hsi-Tsou | 79 | EF3 | Asp→Gly | $\beta_1\beta_2$ Deoxy | |
| Yakima | 99 | G1 | Asp→His | $\alpha_1\beta_2$ | ↑ $O_2$ affinity |
| Kempsey | 99 | G1 | Asp→Asn | $\alpha_1\beta_2$ | ↑ $O_2$ affinity |
| Radcliffe[3] | 99 | G1 | Asp→Ala | $\alpha_1\beta_2$ | ↑ $O_2$ affinity |
| Ypsilanti | 99 | G1 | Asp→Tyr | $\alpha_1\beta_2$ | ↑ $O_2$ affinity |
| Rush | 101 | G3 | Glu→Gln | $\alpha_1\beta_2$ | Unstable |
| British Columbia | 101 | G3 | Glu→Lys | $\alpha_1\beta_2$ | ↑ $O_2$ affinity |

**Table 2-3** (continued)

| Designation | Residue number | Position | Replacement | Structural site | Abnormal properties |
|---|---|---|---|---|---|
| Alberta | 101 | G3 | Glu→Gly | $\alpha_1\beta_2$ | ↑ $O_2$ affinity |
| Potomac[5] | 101 | G3 | Glu→Asp | $\alpha_1\beta_2$ | ↑ $O_2$ affinity |
| Yoshizuka | 108 | G10 | Asn→Asp | $\alpha_1\beta_1$ | ↓ $O_2$ affinity |
| Madrid | 115 | G17 | Ala→Pro | $\alpha_1\beta_1$ | Unstable |
| Fannin-Lubbock | 119 | GH2 | Gly→Asp | $\alpha_1\beta_1$ | Unstable (slight) |
| D | 121 | GH4 | Glu→Gln | $\beta_1\beta_2$ | ↑ $O_2$ affinity |
| O Arab | 121 | GH4 | Glu→Lys | $\beta_1\beta_2$ | |
| Beograd | 121 | GH4 | Glu→Val | $\beta_1\beta_2$ | |
| Khartoum | 124 | H2 | Pro→Arg | $\alpha_1\beta_1$ | Unstable |
| Hacettepe | 127 | H5 | Gln→Glu | $\alpha_1\beta_1$ | |
| J Taichung | 129 | H7 | Ala→Asp | $\alpha_1\beta_1$ | |
| K Cameroon | 129 | H7 | Ala→Glu or Asp | $\alpha_1\beta_1$ | |
| Tokuchi | 131 | H9 | Gln→Glu | $\alpha_1\beta_1$ | |
| Deaconess | 131 | H9 | Glu→Deleted | $\alpha_1\beta_1$ | Unstable |
| Woolwich | 132 | H10 | Lys→Gln | $\beta_1\beta_2$ | |
| Bethesda | 145 | HC2 | Tyr→His | $\beta_1\beta_2$ | ↑ $O_2$ affinity |
| Rainier | 145 | HC2 | Tyr→Cys | $\beta_1\beta_2$ | ↑ $O_2$ affinity |
| Osler | 145 | HC2 | Tyr→Asp | $\beta_1\beta_2$ | ↑ $O_2$ affinity |
| Hiroshima | 146 | HC3 | His→Asp | $\alpha_1\beta_2$ Deoxy | ↑ $O_2$ affinity |
| York | 146 | HC3 | His→Pro | $\alpha_1\beta_2$ Deoxy | ↑ $O_2$ affinity |
| Cochin-Port Royal | 146 | HC3 | His→Arg | $\alpha_1\beta_2$ Deoxy | ↑ $O_2$ affinity |

| Designation | Residue number | Position | Replacement | Abnormal Properties |
|---|---|---|---|---|
| γ Chain | | | | |
| F Auckland | 7 | A4 | Asp→Asn | $\gamma_1\gamma_2$ Deoxy (136,Gly) |
| F Jamaica | 61 | E5 | Lys→Glu | $\gamma_1\gamma_2$ (136, Ala) |
| F Dickinson | 97 | FG4 | His→Arg | $\gamma_1\gamma_2$ (136, Ala) |
| F Hull | 121 | GH4 | Gly→Lys | $\gamma_1\gamma_2$ (136,Ala) |
| F Carlton | 121 | GH4 | Gly→Lys | $\gamma_1\gamma_2$ (136,Gly) |
| F Port Royal | 125 | H3 | Glu→Ala | $\gamma_1\gamma_1$ (136,Gly) |
| δ Chain | | | | |
| A₂ Coburg | 116 | G18 | Arg→His | $\delta_1\delta_1$ |

C. Residues at Internal Replacement and Internal (*) and Central Cavity (**)

| Designation | Residue number | Position | Replacement | Abnormal Properties |
|---|---|---|---|---|
| α Chain | | | | |
| Lapin[3] | 29 | B10 | Leu→Val | |
| G Waimanalo | 64 | E13 | Asp→Asn | |
| Q India | 64 | E13 | Asp→His | |
| Perspolis | 64 | E13 | Asp→Tyr | |
| Etobicoke | 84 | F5 | Ser→Arg | ↑ $O_2$ affinity |
| β Chain | | | | |
| Raleigh | 1 | NA1* | Val→Ala | |
| Deer Lodge | 2 | NA2* | His→Arg | |
| Belfast | 15 | A12 | Trp→Arg | Unstable ↑ $O_2$ affinity |
| Freiburg | 23 | B5 | Val→Deleted | Ferri Hb ↑ $O_2$ affinity |
| Riverdale-Bronx | 24 | B6 | Gly→Arg | Unstable |
| Savannah | 24 | B6 | Gly→Val | Unstable |

**Table 2-3** (continued)

| Designation | Residue number | Position | Replacement | Abnormal properties |
|---|---|---|---|---|
| Moscva | 24 | B6 | Gly→Asp | Unstable ↓ $O_2$ affinity |
| Volga | 27 | B9 | Ala→Asp | Unstable |
| St. Louis | 28 | B10 | Leu→Gln | Ferri Hb Unstable ↑ $O_2$ affinity |
| Genova | 28 | B10 | Leu→Pro | Unstable ↑ $O_2$ affinity |
| Perth | 32 | B14 | Leu→Pro | Unstable |
| Castilla | 32 | B14 | Leu→Arg | Unstable |
| J Calobria | 64 | E8 | Gly→Asp | Unstable |
| Mizuho | 68 | E12 | Leu→Pro | Unstable |
| Atlanta | 75 | E19 | Leu→Pro | Unstable |
| Baylor | 81 | EF5 | Leu→Arg | Unstable (slight) |
| Providence | 82 | EF6** | Lys→Asn→Asp | ↓ $O_2$ affinity |
| Rahere | 82 | EF6** | Lys→Thr | ↑ $O_2$ affinity |
| Helsinki | 82 | EF6** | Lys→Met | ↑ $O_2$ affinity |
| Bryn Mawr | 85 | F1 | Phe→Ser | Unstable ↑ $O_2$ affinity |
| Vanderbilt | 89 | F5 | Ser→Arg | |
| Creteil | 89 | F5 | Ser→Asn | ↑ $O_2$ affinity |
| Brigham | 100 | G2* | Pro→Leu | ↑ $O_2$ affinity |
| Camperdown | 104 | G6** | Arg→Ser | Unstable (slight) |
| Sherwood Forest | 104 | G6 | Arg→Thr | |
| Burke | 107 | G9 | Gly→Arg | |
| San Diego | 109 | G11 | Val→Met | ↑ $O_2$ affinity |

| | | | | |
|---|---|---|---|---|
| Peterborough | 111 | G13 | Val→Phe | Unstable ↓ $O_2$ affinity |
| New York | 113 | G15 | Val→Glu | Unstable |
| Wien | 130 | H8 | Tyr→Asp | Unstable |
| North Shore | 134 | H12 | Val→Glu | Unstable |
| Altdorf | 135 | H13** | Ala→Pro | Unstable ↑$O_2$ affinity |
| Hope | 136 | H14 | Gly→Asp | Unstable |
| Abruzzo | 143 | H21** | His→Arg | ↑ $O_2$ affinity |
| Little Rock | 143 | H21** | His→Gln | ↑ $O_2$ affinity |
| Syracuse | 143 | H21** | His→Pro | ↑ $O_2$ affinity |
| *γ Chain* | | | | |
| F Malaysia | 1 | NA1 | Gly→Cys | |
| F Texas I | 5 | A2 | Glu→Lys | |
| F Sardinia | 75 | E19 | Ile→Thr | |
| F Poole | 130 | H8 | Trp→Gly | Unstable |
| *δ Chain* | | | | |
| $A_2$ Sphakia | 2 | NA2** | His→Arg | |
| $A_2$ Babinga | 136 | H14 | Gly→Asp | |

D. Residues at External Replacement and Surface Crevice (*)

| | | | |
|---|---|---|---|
| *α Chain* | | | |
| J Toronto | 5 | A3 | Ala→Asp |
| Sawara | 6 | A4 | Asp→Ala |
| J Paris I | 12 | A10 | Ala→Asp |
| Anantharaj | 13 | A11* | Lys→Glu |
| J Oxford | 15 | A13 | Gly→Asp |
| Ottawa | 15 | A13 | Gly→Arg |

**Table 2-3** *(continued)*

| Designation | Residue number | Position | Replacement | Abnormal properties |
|---|---|---|---|---|
| I | 16 | A14 | Lys→Glu | |
| Handsworth | 18 | A16 | Gly→Arg | |
| J Kurosh | 19 | A17 | Ala→Asp | |
| J Nyanza | 21 | B2 | Ala→Asp | |
| J Medellin | 22 | B3 | Gly→Asp | |
| Spanish Town | 27 | B8 | Glu→Val | |
| G Fort Worth | 27 | B8 | Glu→Gly | |
| Umi | 47 | CE5 | Asp→Gly | |
| L Ferrara | 47 | CE5 | Asp→His | Unstable |
| Arya | 47 | CE5 | Asp→Asn | Unstable (slight) |
| Montgomery | 48 | CE6 | Leu→Arg | |
| Russ | 51 | CE9 | Gly→Arg | |
| J Abidjan | 51 | CE9 | Gly→Asp | |
| J Rovigo | 53 | E2 | Ala→Asp | Unstable |
| Shimonoseki | 54 | E3 | Gln→Arg | |
| Mexico | 54 | E3 | Gln→Glu | |
| Thailand | 56 | E5 | Lys→Thr | |
| Norfolk | 57 | E6 | Gly→Asp | |
| L Persian Gulf | 57 | E6 | Gly→Arg | |
| Zambia | 60 | E9 | Lys→Asn | |
| J Buda | 61 | E10 | Lys→Asn | |
| G Philadelphia | 68 | E17 | Asn→Lys | |

| Name | Position | Helix | Substitution | Comments |
|---|---|---|---|---|
| Ube II | 68 | E17 | Asn→Asp | |
| J Habana | 71 | E20 | Ala→Glu | |
| Daneskgah-Tehran | 72 | EF1 | His→Arg | |
| G Taichung | 74 | EF3 | Asp→His | |
| G Pest | 74 | EF3 | Asp→Asn | |
| Chapel Hill | 74 | EF3 | Asp→Gly | |
| Q Iran | 75 | EF4 | Asp→His | |
| Winnipeg | 75 | EF4 | Asp→Tyr | |
| Matsue-Oki | 75 | EF4 | Asp→Asn | |
| Stanleyville-II | 78 | EF7 | Asn→Lys | |
| Singapore | 78, 79 | EF7 | Asn→Asp, Ala→Gly | |
| Ann Arbor | 80 | F1* | Leu→Arg | Unstable |
| Garden State | 82 | F3 | Ala→Asp | |
| Atago | 85 | F6 | Asp→Tyr | |
| G Norfolk | 85 | F6 | Asp→Asn | |
| Inkster | 85 | F6 | Asp→Val | |
| Broussais | 90 | FG2 | Lys→Asn | |
| J Rajappen | 90 | FG2 | Lys→Thr | |
| Manitoba | 102 | G9 | Ser→Arg | |
| Hopkins-II | 112 | G19 | His→Asp | Unstable ↑ O₂ affinity |
| Serbia | 112 | G19 | His→Arp | |
| Dakar | 112 | G19 | His→Gln | Unstable |
| J Tongariki | 115 | GH3 | Ala→Asp | |
| O Indonesia | 116 | GH4 | Glu→Lys | |
| Ube-4 | 116 | GH4 | Glu→Ala | |
| J Birmingham | 120 | H3 | Ala→Glu | |

**Table 2-3** (continued)

| Designation | Residue number | Position | Replacement | Abnormal properties |
|---|---|---|---|---|
| β Chain | | | | |
| S | 6 | A3 | Glu→Val | Sickling, mechanically unstable |
| C | 6 | A3 | Glu→Lys | |
| G Makassar | 6 | A3 | Glu→Ala | Mechanically unstable |
| Leiden | 6 or 7 | A3 or 4 | Glu→Deleted | |
| Travis | 6 | A3 | Glu→Val | |
| | 142 | H20 | Ala→Val | |
| G San Jose | 7 | A4 | Glu→Gly | |
| Siriraj | 7 | A4 | Glu→Lys | |
| Porto Alegre | 9 | A6 | Ser→Cys | |
| Ankara | 10 | A7 | Ala→Asp | |
| Sögn | 14 | A11 | Leu→Arg | |
| Saki | 14 | A11 | Leu→Pro | Unstable |
| J Baltimore | 16 | A13 | Gly→Asp | |
| D Bushman | 16 | A13 | Gly→Arg | |
| D Ouled Rabah | 19 | B1 | Asn→Lys | |
| Alamo | 19 | B1 | Asn→Asp | |
| Olympia | 20 | B2 | Val→Met | ↑ $O_2$ affinity |
| Strasbourg | 20 | B2 | Val→Asp | Unstable (slight) |
| E Saskatoon | 22 | B4 | Glu→Lys | |
| G Coushatta | 22 | B4 | Glu→Ala | |
| G Taipei | 22 | B4 | Glu→Gly | |

| Name | Position | Helix | Substitution | Comment |
|---|---|---|---|---|
| D Iran | 22 | B4 | Glu→Gln | |
| G Taiwan Ami | 25 | B7 | Gly→Arg | |
| Lufkin | 29 | B11 | Gly→Asp | |
| G Galveston | 43 | CD2 | Glu→Ala | |
| K Ibadan | 46 | CD5 | Gly→Glu | |
| G Copenhagen | 47 | CD6 | Asp→Asn | |
| Gavello | 47 | CD6 | Asp→Gly | |
| Edmonton | 50 | D1 | Thr→Lys | |
| Osu Christiansborg | 52 | D3 | Asp→Asn | |
| Ocho Rios | 52 | D3 | Asp→Ala | |
| J Bangkok | 56 | D7 | Gly→Asp | |
| Hamadan | 56 | D7 | Gly→Arg | |
| G Ferrara | 57 | E1 | Asn→Lys | |
| C Ziguinchor | 6 | A3 | Glu→Val | Sickle normal $O_2$ |
| Dhofar | 58 | E2 | Pro→Arg | |
| I High Wycombe | 59 | E3 | Lys→Glu | |
| J Kaohsiung | 59 | E3 | Lys→Thr | |
| J Lome | 59 | E3 | Lys→Asn | |
| Duarte | 62 | E6 | Ala→Pro | Unstable ↑ $O_2$ affinity |
| J Sicilia | 65 | E9 | Lys→Asn | |
| J Cairo | 65 | E9 | Lys→Gln | |
| J Cambridge | 69 | E13 | Gly→Asp | |
| Vancouver | 73 | E17 | Asp→Tyr | ↓ $O_2$ affinity |
| Korle Bu | 73 | E17 | Asp→Asn | |
| Mobile | 73 | E17 | Asp→Val | ↓ $O_2$ affinity |
| C Harlem | 6 | A3 | Glu→Val | Sickling, mechanically unstable |

40

**Table 2-3** *(continued)*

| Designation | Residue number | Position | Replacement | Abnormal properties |
|---|---|---|---|---|
| Shepherds Bush | 73 | E17 | Asp→Asn | Unstable, $O_2$ affinity |
| Bushwich | 74 | E18 | Gly→Asp | |
| J Chicago | 74 | E18 | Gly→Val | |
| J Iran | 76 | E20 | Ala→Asp | |
|  | 77 | EF1 | His→Asp | |
| G Szuhu | 80 | EF4 | Asn→Lys | ↑ $O_2$ affinity |
| Ta-Li | 83 | EF7 | Gly→Cys | |
| Pyrgos | 83 | EF7 | Gly→Asp | |
| Tours | 87 | F3 | Thr→Deleted | ↑ $O_2$ affinity |
| D Ibadan | 87 | F3 | Thr→Lys | |
| Agenogi | 90 | F6 | Glu→Lys | ↓ $O_2$ affinity |
| N Baltimore | 95 | FG2 | Lys→Glu | |
| Arlington Park | 6 | A3 | Glu→Lys | |
|  | 95 | FG2 | Lys→Glu | |
| P Galveston | 117 | G19 | His→Arg | |
| Hijiyama | 120 | GH3 | Lys→Glu | |
| Riyadh | 120 | GH3 | Lys→Asn | |
| Andrew Minneapolis | 144 | HC1 | Lys→Asn | ↑ $O_2$ affinity |
| *γ Chain* | | | | |
| F Texas II | 6 | A3 | Glu→Lys | |
| F Alexander | 12 | A9 | Thr→Lys | |

| | | | |
|---|---|---|---|
| F Melbourne | 16 | A13 | Gly→Arg |
| F Kuala Lumpur | 22 | B4 | Asp→Gly |
| F Victoria Jubilee | 80 | EF4 | Asp→Tyr |
| F Malta | 117 | G19 | His→Arg |
| $\delta$ Chain | | | |
| A$_2$ NYU | 12 | A9* | Asn→Lys |
| A$_2$ (B$_2$) | 16 | A13 | Gly→Arg |
| A$_2$ Roosevelt | 20 | B2 | Val→Glu |
| A$_2$ Flatbush | 22 | B4 | Ala→Glu |
| A$_2$ Melbourne | 43 | CD2 | Glu→Lys |
| A$_2$ Indonesia | 69 | E13 | Gly→Arg |

**Table 2-4**
**Hemoglobins Classified by Genetic Abnormality**

A. Single Base Substitution (approximately 275 variants)

B. Stop Codon Mutations
1. Hb Constant Spring:  31 additional residues (172 amino acids)
2. Hb Icaria:  31 additional residues (172 amino acids)
3. Hb Koya Dora:  31 additional residues (172 amino acids)
4. Hb Seal Rock:  30 additional residues (171 amino acids)

C. Deletion
1. Hb Leiden   ($\beta$6 or 7, Glu→O)
2. Hb Lyon   ($\beta$17-18, Lys-Val→O)
3. Hb Freiburg   ($\beta$23, Val→O)
4. Hb Niteroi   ($\beta$42-44, Phe-Glu-Ser→O)
   ($\beta$43 or 45, Glu-Ser-Pher→O)
5. Hb Tochigi   ($\beta$56-59, Gly-Asp-Pro-Lys→O)
6. Hb St. Antoine   ($\beta$74-75, Gly-Lys→O)
7. Hb Tours   ($\beta$87, Thr→O)
8. Hb Gun Hill   ($\beta$91-95, Leu-His-Cys-Asp-Lys→O)
9. Hb Leslie Deaconess   ($\beta$131, Gln→O)
10. Hb Coventry   ($\beta$141, Leu→O)
11. Hb Mickees Hock   ($\beta$145-146, Tyr-His→O)

D. Frameshift
1. Hb Wayne $\alpha$ 139-141
   140
   Thr-Ser-Asn-Thr-Val-Lys-Leu-Glu-Pro
2. Hb Cranston $\beta$145
   144                                                                157
   Lys-Ser-Ile-Thr-Lys-Leu-Ala-Phe-Leu-Leu-Ser-Asn-Phe-Tyr-COOH
3. Hb Tak $\beta$147
   144                                                                157
   Lys-Tyr-His-Thr-Lys-Leu-Ala-Phe-Leu-Leu-Ser-Asn-Phe-Tyr-COOH

E. Insertion

Hb Grady α 115-118

|  | 115 | 116 | 117 | 118 | 119 |
|---|---|---|---|---|---|
|  | Ala | Glu | Phe | Thr | Clu-Phe-Thr-Pro |

F. Fusion

| | A6 9 | A9 12 | B4 22 | D1 50 | F2 86 | F3 87 | G18 116 | G19 117 | H2 124 | H4 126 |
|---|---|---|---|---|---|---|---|---|---|---|
| 1. α Chain → | Thr | Asn | Ala | Ser | Ser | Gln | Arg | Asn | Glu | Met |
| 2. β Chain → | Ser | Thr | Glu | Thr | Ala | Thr | His | His | Pro | Val |
| 3. Lepore-Hollandia | | | δ | β | | | | | | |
| 4. Lepore-Baltimore | | | | δ | β | | | | | |
| 5. Lepore-Washington–Boston | | | | | | δ | β | | | |
| 6. Miyada | | β | δ | | | | | | | |
| 7. Lincoln Park[6] | | | β | δ | | | | | | |
| 8. P-Congo | | | β | | | | | | | |
| 9. P-Nilotie | | | β | δ | | | | | | |

| | NA1 1 | EF4 80 | EF5 81 | F2 86 | F3 87 |
|---|---|---|---|---|---|
| 10. γ Chain → | Gly | Asp | Leu | Ala | Gln |
| 11. β Chain → | Val | Asn | Leu | Ala | Thr |
| 12. Kenya | γ | | | β | |

Except those otherwise designated, from IHC.[1]

of three base pairs (or a multiple thereof) in the structural gene; (4) variants which are the result of a "frameshift" of the codon triplets caused by the deletion or insertion of one or two nucleotides; (5) variants with an elongated chain due to an insertion of amino acid residues because of a tandem duplication of base pairs; and (6) variants with fused or hybrid globin chains.

## ABNORMAL HEMOGLOBINS OF CLINICAL SIGNIFICANCE

The clinical manifestations and laboratory findings of the abnormal hemoglobins listed in Table 2-2, sections F and G, are discussed in this chapter. Other clinical disorders due to hemoglobin abnormalities—including those involving sickle hemoglobin, $\beta$ and $\alpha$ thalassemia and related disorders, unstable hemoglobins, and hemoglobin abnormalities causing erythrocytosis or cyanosis—are discussed in other chapters.

### Hemoglobin C

In Hb C, lysine is substituted for glutamic acid in position 6 of the $\beta$ chain. On cellulose acetate at pH 8.6, Hb C migrates with Hb $A_2$. The maximal frequency of Hb C is in northern Ghana, where the carrier rate exceeds 20%.[7,8] It has also been reported in other black populations, Lumbee Indians, Algerians, Saudi and Kuwait Arabs, Dutch, and Italians.[9] The incidence in American blacks is 2% to 3%.[10,11]

**Heterozygotes** Persons with Hb C trait have no significant abnormalities. Hemoglobin values are normal. Reticulocyte counts are usually normal, but may be slightly increased. Red cell survival is slightly decreased in some patients.[12] Hematuria has been reported in three patients and priapism in two patients with Hb C trait,[10,13] but it is not known whether this represents an increased incidence. The peripheral smear may show increased targeting, but no other abnormalities are noted.

Hemoglobin C Harlem (Hb C Georgetown) migrates to the same position as Hb C on cellulose acetate electrophoresis at alkaline pH, and the heterozygous condition for these may be confused. These abnormal hemoglobins may be clearly differentiated by citrate agar gel electrophoresis. In Hb C Harlem, there is a substitution of valine for glutamic acid at position 6 (the same abnormality as in Hb S) and asparagine for aspartic acid at position 73 of the $\beta$ chain. Occasional target cells may be seen on the peripheral smear and sickling occurs in 2% Na metabisulfite. Persons heterozygous for Hb C Harlem develop a renal concentrating defect and hematuria may occur.[14,15]

**Homozygotes** Hemoglobin CC disease (Hb CC) is a mild disorder that is usually recognized during the investigation of an unrelated medical problem. Complaints of arthralgia and frequent headaches are common, but their relationship to the hemoglobinopathy is unclear. Vaso-occlusive crises are extremely unusual.[16] Growth and development are appropriate for age, and a normal life span is expected. Pregnancy is not associated with increased morbidity, although folate deficiency may develop and supplementation with daily oral folic acid during this period is advised.[16] The incidence of cholelithiasis is increased.[16,17] Surgery, in general, seems to be well tolerated.[18]

Splenomegaly, which develops during childhood, occurs in 90% of patients. Hypersplenism develops in 25%.[10,16] Functional asplenia and increased susceptibility to infection do not occur. Splenectomy will correct leukopenia or thrombocytopenia due to hypersplenism but has little effect on baseline hemoglobin values.[10] Hepatomegaly, presumably due to reticuloendothelial hyperplasia, is common.[16] Retinal abnormalities, which are common in Hb SC disease, do not occur.[16] Renal concentrating ability is not impaired.[19]

Anemia is generally not severe, with hemoglobin values of 8 to 14 g/dl reported.[16,20] Patients with hemoglobin values below 10 g/dl should be investigated for concomitant iron or folate deficiency and for infection. Treatment of these conditions in one series of 15 patients increased the mean hemoglobin value from 9.3 to 11.3 g/dl.[16] The most striking feature of the peripheral smear is the presence of 30% to 100% target cells. Numerous microspherocytes are found. Intra-erythrocytic crystals are common and can be found in all patients after incubation of blood overnight with 3% NaCl solution. Reticulocyte counts average 3% to 6%. Erythrocyte survival is moderately shortened[12] and osmotic fragility is decreased. Hemoglobin F is usually normal, but may be mildly increased.

**Variants of Hb C Disease** Hemoglobin C in combination with other hemoglobin abnormalities results in a generally milder disorder than Hb CC. These conditions include Hb C-O Arab, Hb C-N Baltimore, Hb C-E, and Hb C-$\alpha$ thalassemia.[21-24] Hemoglobin C-$\beta$ thalassemia in blacks produces no clinical symptoms, and hemoglobin levels are similar to those found with $\beta$-thalassemia trait. Microcytosis and targeting are noted on smear, and Hb F is increased.[10,25,26] No satisfactory method is available for separating Hb $A_2$ and Hb C, so that Hb $A_2$ levels have not been determined. In Italian, Algerian, and Turkish persons, Hb C-$\beta$ thalassemia may be more severe, resembling thalassemia of intermediate severity.[26]

**Pathophysiology** Hemoglobin C is less soluble than Hb A in hemolysates and intact red cells. This decreased solubility may be due to electrostatic interaction between the positively charged $\beta$6 amino groups and the negatively charged groups on adjacent molecules. Red cells from homozygotes are more rigid than normal, and differences are exaggerated if mean corpuscular hemoglobin concentration is increased by suspension in hypertonic solution.[27] Crystalloid inclusions become evident in virtually every red cell after incubation in 3% saline solution.[28] The increased rigidity leads to fragmentation, formation of microspherocytes, splenic sequestration, and shortened red cell survival.[27]

As noted previously, most homozygotes are anemic. The rate of marrow hemoglobin production is 2.5 to 3 times that of normal, yet marrow is usually capable of 6 to 8 times normal production before anemia becomes evident.[20] This suboptimal erythropoietic response appears to be a consequence of a right-shifted oxygen dissociation curve. Levels of 2,3-DPG are, surprisingly, not elevated and the lessened oxygen affinity is due to intracellular acidosis. It is thought that this acidosis may be a result of the biochemical properties of Hb C.[29]

## Hemoglobin D

Hemoglobin D migrates to the same position as Hb S on cellulose acetate at pH 8.6, but Hb D red cells do not sickle. In agar gel, at acid pH, Hb D migrates with Hb A. There are variants of Hb D, the most common being Hb D Punjab (D Los Angeles), in which glycine replaces glutamic acid at position 126 of the $\beta$ chain. Hemoglobin D Punjab occurs in 1% to 3% of western Indian populations and in small numbers in European groups with colonial ties to India.[30,31] Hemoglobin D Punjab is rare in American blacks; Hb G Philadelphia, an $\alpha$ chain abnormality, is the most common variant with the electrophoretic mobility of Hb D found in this population.[30]

**Heterozygotes** Hemoglobin D trait is benign and no associated clinical or hematologic abnormalities have been reported.

**Homozygotes** Homozygous Hb D patients have not been clearly identified, since careful family studies to rule out heterozygosity for Hb D-$\beta^O$ thalassemia have not been obtained. It is of interest that one of the first patients reported to have homozygous Hb D was later found to have had HbD-$\beta^O$ thalassemia.[32,33] Several patients with only Hb D on electrophoresis and without elevation of A$_2$ or F levels are described.[34-36] Their clinical features are identical to those of the Hb D-$\beta$ thalassemia heterozygotes described below.

**Variants of Hb D Disease** Double heterozygosity for Hb D and $\beta$ thalassemia is clearly documented.[37-40] Hemoglobin F and A$_2$ levels are elevated and Hb D is the predominant hemoglobin. Hemoglobin values range from 9.5 to 13.9 g/dl, and reticulocyte counts from 1.3% to 2.7%. Microcytosis and large numbers of target cells are seen on peripheral smear. Osmotic fragility is decreased. Several patients had moderate splenomegaly. None had clinical symptoms which could be attributed to their hemoglobinopathy. Other D hemoglobins include Hb D Bushman (16 Glycine → Arginine), Hb D Iran (22 Glutamic acid → Glutamine), and Hb D Ibadan (87 Threonine → Lysine). These variants are generally milder than Hb D Punjab when interacting with other abnormal hemoglobins.

**Pathophysiology**  The pathophysiologic aspects of this hemoglobinopathy have not been well studied. $\beta D$ and $\beta A$ chains are synthesized at similar rates in heterozygotes and no increased destruction of $\beta D$ chains is noted. In Hb D-$\beta^o$ thalassemia, $\beta D/\alpha$ globin synthesis ratios greater than or equal to 0.5 are usual. It is thought that the maintenance of a relatively high $\beta/\alpha$ synthesis ratio in the presence of a stable structural mutation accounts for the mildness of the Hb D-$\beta$ thalassemia syndrome.[41,42]

## Hemoglobin E

Hemoglobin E is due to the substitution of lysine for glutamic acid at position 26 of the $\beta$ chain. Hemoglobin E migrates with Hb C on cellulose acetate at pH 8.6, but may be separated from Hb C on agar gel at pH 6.2. The maximal gene frequency of 30% to 40% occurs in the Khmer region of Thailand and Cambodia. It is relatively common in the regions from Bengal to Vietnam and from Laos to Malaysia, and it occasionally occurs in China, India, Turkey, Egypt, and Greece. Hemoglobin E has not been reported in tropical Africa, Japan, or in American Indians.[43] More than 20 million people are carriers. A selective advantage for the heterozygote may result from protection against malaria,[43] although clinical studies offer conflicting results.[44,45]

**Heterozygotes**  No clinical symptoms are noted in Hb E trait. Hemoglobin values are normal and red cell morphology has been considered unremarkable. However, a recent report described hypochromia in nine iron-replete heterozygotes.[46] Osmotic fragility may be decreased. The percentage of Hb E ranges from 20% to 40%.[47,48]

**Homozygotes**  Most patients are in excellent health, although some complain of fatigue.[43,49-51] There is no increased morbidity in pregnancy.[52] Physical condition is entirely normal except for mild splenomegaly in a few patients. Hemoglobin values range from 10 to 16 g/dl in those patients not obviously iron deficient. Red cells are typically microcytic and hypochromic with many target cells present. Osmotic fragility is decreased. Reticulocyte counts are normal. Red cell survival is slightly reduced.[43]

**Variants of Hb E Disease**  In surprising contrast to the homozygote, the Hb E-$\beta$ thalassemia heterozygote is severely affected, with symptoms being evident in early childhood. Growth and development are severely retarded and sexual maturation rarely occurs. Affected children are described as "chronically ill with wasted extremities and protuberant abdomens."[48] Massive splenomegaly is universal and marked hepatomegaly is frequent. Hypersplenism may develop. Thalassemic facies are sometimes found. Spinal cord compression with paraparesis due to extramedullary hematopoiesis has been reported.[53] The natural history is not well studied, but life expectancy appears to be significantly decreased.[49] Autopsy findings are similar to those for homozygous $\beta$ thalassemia.[54]

Hemoglobin levels are between 3.0 and 7.0 g/dl in untransfused patients, and reticulocyte counts average 5% to 10%.[43,49,55,56] The peripheral smear shows extreme anisopoikilocytosis, hypochromia, and basophilic stippling, with large numbers of target cells and nucleated red blood cells. All cases from Southeast Asia appear to be of the $\beta^O$ thalassemia type with 15% to 40% Hb F and the remainder Hb E. One case of Hb E-$\beta^+$ thalassemia is described from Turkey with findings identical to those of Hb E-$\beta^O$ thalassemia patients.[55]

Transfusion therapy is frequently necessary, although the transfusion requirement may not be as great as in homozygous $\beta$ thalassemia.[49] Splenectomy may eliminate or decrease the transfusion requirements in some patients.[49]

Hemoglobin H disease is described in Chapter 16; it results from an $\alpha_{thal\ 1}/\alpha_{thal\ 2}$ genotype. Hemoglobin H disease has been described in association with Hb E in approximately 25 patients[57,58] and appears to be intermediate in severity between Hb E-$\beta$ thalassemia and Hb H disease. Average hemoglobin values are 6.9 g/dl, and mean reticulocyte counts are 5% to 10%. Hemoglobin electrophoresis reveals predominantly Hb A, with 13% to 15% Hb E, 8% to 10% Hb Bart's, 4% to 7% Hb F, and small amounts of Hb H ($\beta_4$). Beta$^E{}_4$ tetramers do not occur.[57] Hypochromia, microcytosis, anisopoikilocytosis, and targeting are noted on peripheral smear. A few cells will show typical Hb H inclusions. Hepatosplenomegaly is universal, and hypersplenism may develop. Most patients are not transfusion dependent, although the typical thalassemic facies may develop.[58] Life expectancy for this disease has not been determined.

**Pathophysiology** Initial reports suggested that the oxygen affinity of Hb E was low,[59] perhaps explaining the mild anemia in homozygotes. More recent studies,[60-61] however, do not confirm this finding. Pure Hb E behaves identically to Hb A in respect to oxygen dissociation, Bohr shifts, and interaction with 2,3-DPG.

Hemoglobin E production does not match that of Hb A in heterozygotes. Hemoglobin E values of 20% to 40% are usual, which is less than the percentage of abnormal hemoglobin noted in heterozygotes for Hbs S, C, and D. This difference is accentuated when $\alpha$-thalassemia trait[57] or iron deficiency[31,48] is superimposed.

Hemoglobin E levels may be as low as 15% in these conditions. Hemoglobin E also appears to be relatively unstable.[62] Globin synthesis studies on peripheral blood of Hb E heterozygotes suggest that Hb E is synthesized in relatively greater amounts than is found in peripheral blood and is preferentially destroyed during maturation of the erythrocyte.[56] Two patients with Hb E-$\beta^0$ thalassemia have had $\beta^E/\alpha$ synthesis ratios of 0.26 and 0.27,[63] although another study reports a 0.74 ratio.[56] Large excesses of $\alpha$ chain production as compared to the combined amounts of $\gamma$ and $\beta^E$ chains in Hb E-$\beta$ thalassemia results in a large intracellular pool of free $\alpha$ chains.[26] This unbalanced globin synthesis combined with the relative instability of Hb E could be responsible for the severe clinical manifestations of Hb E-$\beta$ thalassemia, although the number of patients studied is too small to draw firm conclusions.

## Other Abnormal Hemoglobins

Only a small number of abnormal hemoglobins are described in the homozygous state. Homozygosity for Hbs C, D, and E have been discussed previously in this chapter; homozygous Hb S is discussed in Chapter 8. A homozygote for Hb O Arab has recently been described who has mild anemia and reticulocytosis with frequent episodes of acute hemolysis and hyperbilirubinemia. Splenectomy was performed because of splenomegaly and the episodic hemolysis. The peripheral blood smear showed anisopoikilocytosis and polychromasia with many target cells and nucleated red cells.[64] Other $\beta$-chain variants, Hbs Porto Alegre, Korle Bu, and G Szuhu, have been described in the homozygous state, but are not associated with clinical disease.[64-66] Homozygotes for three $\alpha$-chain variants, J Mexico, J Tongariki, and G Philadelphia, have been reported and have not been associated with clinical abnormalities.[67-69]

Abnormal hemoglobins of clinical significance in the heterozygous state are those with abnormal oxygen affinity, the unstable hemoglobins, and those causing methemoglobinemia or cyanosis (Chapter 7). Abnormal hemoglobins that may sickle under appropriate conditions are C Harlem, I, Bart's, Porto Alegre, and F Alexandra, although only C Harlem is of clinical significance.

Several abnormal hemoglobins have been described in association with $\beta$-thalassemia trait. Hemoglobin Beograd-$\beta$ thalassemia and Hb O Arab-$\beta$ thalassemia result in a clinical picture of $\beta$ thalassemia of intermediate severity. Hepatosplenomegaly is noted on physical examination. Moderate anemia with reticulocytosis is present, and red cell survival is markedly decreased.[70,71]

The unstable hemoglobins Leslie and Saki, which cause minimal abnormality in the heterozygote, interact with $\beta$-thalassemia trait to produce a moderate hemolytic anemia with reticulocyte counts of 8% to 10%.[72,73] Severe anemia (Hb 5.8 g/dl) and massive splenomegaly developed in one of these patients who contracted infectious mononucleosis.[72] Hemoglobin Duarte, an unstable hemoglobin with increased oxygen affinity, when associated with β thalassemia resulted in a marked reticulocytosis (10.4%)[74] and a normal hemoglobin level (15.1 g/dl).[74]

Clinical and hematologic findings similar to those in β-thalassemia trait result from the association of other β-chain variants, including Hbs G San Jose, [75] J Georgia,[76] and J Baltimore,[77] with β thalassemia. β-thalassemia trait interacts with four α-chain variants, Hbs O Indonesia, Hasharon, Q India, and J Paris, to decrease the relative amount of abnormal hemoglobin,[78] although there is no such interaction with other α-chain variants.[26] Alpha-thalassemia trait also interacts with β-chain variants to lower the percentage of abnormal hemoglobin. This relationship has been demonstrated with hemoglobins S, C, D, and E.

## REFERENCES

1. Wrightstone, R.N. *Bulletin of the International Hemoglobin Information Center.* Augusta, Georgia, October 1977 and March 1978 (suppl).

2. Perutz, M.F., and Lehmann, H. Molecular pathology of human hemoglobin. *Nature* 219:902–909, 1968.

3. Lehmann, H., and Kynock, P.A.M. *Human Haemoglobin Variants and Their Characteristics.* Amsterdam: North Holland Publishing Co., 1976. pp. 50–53, 149.

4. Martinez, G., Lima, F., Residenti, C., and Colombo, B. A new abnormal hemoglobin, Hb Cahaguey. $\alpha_2$141 (HC) Arg→Gly$\beta_2$. *Hemoglobin* 2:47-52, 1978.

5. Charache, S., Jacobson, R., Brimhall, B., et al. Hb Potomac (101 Glu→Asp): Speculation on placental oxygen transport in carriers of high affinity hemoglobins. *Blood* 51:331–338, 1978.

6. Honig, G.R., Shamsuddin, M., Mason, R.G., et al. Hemoglobin Lincoln Park: A βδ fusion (anti-Lepore) variant with an amino acid deletion in the δ chain-derived segment. *Proc. Natl. Acad. Sci. USA* 75:1475–1479, 1978.

7. Eddington, G.M., and Laing, W.N. Relationship between haemoglobin C and S and malaria in Ghana. *Br. Med. J.* 2:143–145, 1957.

8. Neel, J.V. Human hemoglobin types, their epidemiologic implications. *N. Engl. J. Med.* 256:161–170, 1957.

9. Mulla, N., and Chrobak, L. Haemoglobin C in Arabs in Kuwait. *Acta Haematol.* 50:112–115, 1973.

10. Smith, E.W., and Krevans, J.R. Clinical manifestations of hemoglobin C disorders. *Bull. J. Hopkins Hosp.* 104:17–43, 1958.

11. Schneider, R.G. Incidence of C trait in 505 normal Negroes: A family with homozygous hemoglobin C and sickle cell trait union. *J. Lab. Clin. Med.* 44:133–144, 1954.

12. Prindle, K.H., and McCurdy, P.R. Red cell life span in hemoglobin C disorders. *Blood* 36:14–19, 1970.

13. Robertson, M.G. Priapism and painless hematuria in hemoglobin C trait. *JAMA* 216:677, 1971.

14. Bookchin, R., Davis, R., and Ranney, H.M. Clinical features of hemoglobin C Harlem, a new sickling hemoglobin variant. *Ann. Intern. Med.* 68:8–19, 1968.

15. Wong, Y., Tanaka, K., Greenberg, L., et al. Hematuria associated with hemoglobin C Harlem: A sickling hemoglobin variant. *J. Urol.* 102:762–763, 1969.

16. Redetzki, J.E., Bickers, J.N., and Samuels, M.S. Homozygous hemoglobin C disease: Clinical review of 15 patients. *South. Med. J.* 61:238–242, 1968.

17. Anderson, M., Bluestone, R., and Milner, P.F. Pregnancy in homozygous haemoglobin C disease. *J. Obstet. Gynecol. Br. Common.* 74:694–696, 1967.

18. Fuller, A.M., Hunt, R., and Barelli, P. Tonsillectomy and hemoglobin CC disease. *Arch. Otolaryngol.* 85:121–123, 1967.

19. VanEps, L.W., Schouten, H., Romeny-Wachter, T.H., et al. The relationship between age and renal concentrating capacity in sickle cell disease and hemoglobin C disease. *Clin. Chim. Acta* 27:501–511, 1970.

20. Williams, W., Editor. *Hematology.* New York: McGraw-Hill Book Company, 1972.

21. Milner, P.F., Miller, M., Greg, R., et al. Hemoglobin O Arab in four Negro families and its interaction with hemoglobin S and hemoglobin C. *N. Engl. J. Med.* 283:1417–1425, 1970.

22. Johnson, C., Powars, D., and Schroeder, W. A case with both haemoglobin C and N Baltimore. *Acta Haematol.* 56:183–188, 1976.

23. Steinberg, M. Haemoglobin C/β thalassaemia: Haematological and biosynthetic studies. *Br. J. Haematol.* 30:337–341, 1975.

24. Schroeder, W.A., Powars, D., Reynolds, R.D., et al. Hemoglobin E in combination with Hb S and Hb C in a black family. *Hemoglobin* 1:287–289, 1977.

25. Konoty-Ahulu, P., and Ringelhann, B. Sickle cell anaemia, sickle cell thalassaemia, sickle cell haemoglobin C disease, and asymptomatic haemoglobin C thalassaemia in one Ghanian family. *Br. Med. J.* 1:607–612, 1969.

26. Weatherall, D.J., and Clegg, J.B. *The Thalassaemia Syndromes.* London: Blackwell Scientific Publications, 1972.

27. Charache, S., Conley, C.L., Waugh, D.F., et al. Pathogenesis of hemolytic anemia in homozygous hemoglobin C disease. *J. Clin. Invest.* 46:1795–1811, 1967.

28. Kraus, A.P., and Diggs, L.W. In vitro crystalization of hemoglobin occurring in citrated blood from patients with hemoglobin C. *J. Lab. Clin. Med.* 47:700–705, 1956.

29. Murphy, J.R. Hemoglobin CC erythrocytes: Decreased intracellular pH and decreased $O_2$ affinity-anemia. *Semin. Hematol.* 13:177–180, 1976.

30. Vella, F., and Lehmann, H. Haemoglobin D Punjab. *J. Med. Genet.* 11:341–345, 1974.

31. Chatterjea, J.B. Haemoglobinopathies, glucose-6-phosphate dehydrogenase deficiency, and allied problems in the Indian subcontinent. *Bull. WHO* 35:837–856, 1966.

32. Bird, G., and Lehmann, H. Haemoglobin D in India. *Br. Med. J.* 1:514, 1956.

33. Lehmann, H. *Man's Haemoglobins.* Philadelphia: J.B. Lippincott Co., 1969.

34. Chernoff, A. The hemoglobin D syndromes. *Blood* 12:116–127, 1958.

35. Stout, C., and Holland, C. Hemoglobin D in an Oklahoma family.

*Arch. Intern. Med.* 114:296–300, 1961.
36. Ozsoylu, S. Homozygous haemoglobin D Punjab. *Acta Haematol.* 43:353–359, 1976.
37. Schneider, R.G., Ueda, S., Alperin, J., et al. Hemoglobin D Los Angeles in two Caucasian families: Hemoglobin SD disease and hemoglobin D-thalassemia. *Blood* 32:250–259, 1968.
38. Rohe, R.A., Sharma, V., and Ranney, H.M. Hemoglobin D Iran in association with thalassemia. *Blood* 42:455–462, 1973.
39. Deliyannis, G., Ballis, A., and Christakis, I. Haemoglobin D in a Greek family. *Acta Haematol.* 41:121–125, 1967.
40. Tsistrakis, G.A., Scampardonis, G.J., Clonizakis, J.P., et al. Haemoglobin D and D-thalassaemia. *Acta Haematol.* 54:172–179, 1975.
41. Rieder, R. Globin chain synthesis in Hb D Punjab-$\beta$ thalassemia. *Blood* 47:113–120, 1976.
42. Ballis, S.K., Atwater, J., and Norris, D.G. The interaction of $\beta^0$ thalassemia with hemoglobin D Punjab: A study of globin chain synthesis in an Indian family. *Hemoglobin* 1:697–701, 1977.
43. Flatz, G. Hemoglobin E: Distribution and population genetics. *Humangenetik* 3:189–234, 1967.
44. Ray, R.N., Chatterjea, J.B., and Chaudhuri, R. Observations on resistance of hemoglobin E-thalassemia disease to induced infection with P. vivax. *Bull. WHO* 30:51–55, 1964.
45. Kruatrachue, M., Na-Nakorn, S., Charoenlarp, P., et al. Hemoglobin E and malaria in southeast Thailand. *Ann. Trop. Med. Parasitol.* 55:468–473, 1961.
46. Keller, P., and Kohne, E. Hypochromie due Erythrozyten bei Heterozygotem, Hamoglobin E. *Acta Haematol.* 56:276–284, 1976.
47. Anderson, J.E., Jr. Anemia and hemoglobin E trait in the Republic of Vietnam. *Mil. Med.* 13:148–149, 1968.
48. Wasi, P., Disthasongchan, P., and Na-Nakorn, S. The effect of iron deficiency on the levels of hemoglobins A$_2$ and E. *J. Lab. Clin. Med.* 71:85–91, 1968.
49. Chernoff, A., Minnich, V., Na-Nakorn, S., et al. Studies on hemoglobin E. I. The clinical, hematologic, and genetic characteristics of the hemoglobin E syndromes. *J. Lab. Clin. Med.* 47:455–489, 1956.
50. Lehmann, H., and Story, P. Haemoglobin E in Burmese, two cases of haemoglobin E disease. *Br. Med. J.* 1:544–547, 1956.
51. Eng., L.L., and Gok, O.H. Homozygous haemoglobin E disease in Indonesia. *Lancet* 1:20–23, 1957.
52. Ong, H.C. Maternal and fetal outcome associated with hemoglobin E trait and hemoglobin E disease. *Obstet. Gynecol.* 45:672–674, 1975.
53. Mihindukulasuriya, J., Chanmugam, D., Machado, V., et al. A case of paraparesis due to extramedullary hemopoesis in hemoglobin E-thalassemia. *Postgrad. Med. J.* 53:393–397, 1977.
54. Bhamarapravati, N., Na-Nakorn, S., Wasi, P., et al. Pathology of abnormal hemoglobin diseases seen in Thailand. I. Pathology of $\beta$ thalassemia-hemoglobin E disease. *Am. J. Clin. Pathol.* 47:745–758, 1967.
55. Okcuoglu, A., Minnich, V., and Arcasoy, A. A further example of thalassaemia-haemoglobin E disease in Turkey. *Acta Haematol.* 34:354–359, 1965.
56. Feldman, R., and Rieder, R. The interaction of hemoglobin E with $\beta$-thalassemia: A study of hemoglobin synthesis in a family of mixed Burmese and Iranian origin. *Blood* 42:783–791, 1973.
57. Tuchinda, S., Beale, D., and Lehmann, H. The suppression of haemoglobin E synthesis when haemoglobin H disease and haemoglobin E trait

occur together. *Humangenetik* 3:312–318, 1967.

58. Wasi, P., Sookanek, M., Pootrakul, S., et al. Haemoglobin E and α-thalassaemia. *Br. Med. J.* 4:29–32, 1967.

59. Stamatoyannopoulos, G.A., Bellingham, A., Lenfant, C., et al. Abnormal hemoglobins with high and low oxygen affinity. *Ann. Rev. Med.* 22:221–234, 1971.

60. Bunn, H.F., Meriweather, W.D., Balcerzak, S.T., et al. Oxygen equilibrium of hemoglobin E. *J. Clin. Invest.* 51:2984–2997, 1972.

61. May, A., and Huehns, E.R. The oxygen affinity of haemoglobin E. *Br. J. Haematol.* 30:177–184, 1975.

62. Frischer, H., and Bowman, J. Hemoglobin E, an oxidatively unstable mutation. *J. Lab. Clin. Med.* 85:531–539, 1975.

63. Weatherall, D.J., and Clegg, J.D. The pattern of disordered haemoglobin synthesis in homozygous and heterozygous β-thalassaemia. *Br. J. Haematol.* 16:251–262, 1967.

64. Efremov, G.D., Sadikario, W., Stayancov, A., et al. Homozygous O Arab in a gypsy family in Yugoslavia. *Hemoglobin* 1:389–394, 1977.

65. Lehmann, H., Beale, D., Bai-Daku, F.S. Haemoglobin G Accra. *Nature* 203:363–365, 1964.

66. Kaufman, S., Leiba, H., Clejan, L., et al. Homozygous Hb G Szuhu. *Hum. Hered.* 25:60–68, 1975.

67. Trabuchet, G., Pagnier, J., Benabadji, M., et al. Homozygous cases for hemoglobin J Mexico, evidence for a duplicated α gene with unequal expression. *Hemoglobin* 1:13–25, 1976.

68. Abramson, R.K., Rucknagel, D.L., and Sheffler, D.C. Homozygous J Tongariki: Evidence for only one alpha chain structural locus in Melanesians. *Science* 169:194–196, 1976.

69. Huisman, T.H.J., and Jonxis, J.H. *The Hemoglobinopathies: Techniques of Identification.* New York: Marcel Dekker, Inc., 1977, pp. 325–331.

70. Ruvidic, R., Efremov, G.D., Juricic, Z., et al. Haemoglobin Beograd interacting with β thalassaemia. *Acta Haematol.* 56:183–188, 1976.

71. Kantchev, K., Tcholakov, B., Casey, R., et al. Twelve families with Hb O Arab in the Burgas district of Bulgaria. Observations on 16 examples of hemoglobin O Arab β⁰ thalassemia. *Humangenetik* 26:93–97, 1975.

72. Lutcher, C.L., Wilson, J.B., Gravely, M.E., et al. Hb Leslie, an unstable hemoglobin due to deletion of glutamyl residue β131 occurring in association with β⁰ thalassemia, Hb C, and Hb S. *Blood* 47:99–112, 1976.

73. Milner, P.F., Corley, C.C., Pomoroy, W.L., et al. Thalassemia intermedia caused by heterozygosity for both β-thalassemia and hemoglobin Saki. *Am. J. Hematol.* 1:283–292, 1976.

74. Beutler, E., Lang, A., and Lehmann, H. Hemoglobin Duarte: A new unstable hemoglobin with increased oxygen affinity. *Blood* 43:527–535, 1974.

75. Schwartz, H.C., Spaet, T.H., Zuelzer, W.U., et al. Combination of hemoglobin G, hemoglobin S, and thalassemia occurring in one family. *Blood* 12:238–250, 1969.

76. Syndenstricker, V.P., Horton, B., Payne, R.A., et al. Studies on a fast hemoglobin variant found in a Negro family in association with thalassemia. *Clin. Chim. Acta* 6:677–685, 1961.

77. Wilkinson, T., Kronenberg, H., Isaacs, W.A., et al. Haemoglobin J Baltimore interacting with β-thalassaemia in an Australian family. *Med. J. Aust.* 54:907–910, 1967.

78. Marinucci, M., Mavilio, F., Tentori, L., et al. Hb O Indonesia in association with β thalassaemia. *Hemoglobin* 2:59–63, 1978.

# 3 Laboratory Evaluation of Hemoglobin Disorders

Shlomo Friedman, M.D.
Thomas R. Kinney, M.D.
Jean Atwater, B.S., M.T. (ASCP)

A large variety of laboratory methods are available to detect and diagnose both abnormal hemoglobins and the thalassemic syndromes. In this chapter emphasis will be placed on the more commonly used techniques, which can be performed in most hospital laboratories. These include hemoglobin electrophoresis, quantitation of minor hemoglobin fractions, and tests for the stability of hemoglobin and for intraerythrocytic inclusion bodies. More sophisticated techniques that are used for the definitive diagnosis of the hemoglobinopathies, such as structural analysis of abnormal hemoglobins and globin synthesis studies, both of which are best performed in a research laboratory, will also be discussed.

No single simple test can accurately diagnose either an abnormal hemoglobin or a thalassemic disorder; therefore, several techniques are required to characterize a specific disorder. For instance, when an abnormal hemoglobin is suspected, the initial evaluation should include a cellulose acetate hemoglobin electrophoresis at pH 8.4. If there is an abnormal band, the hemoglobin electrophoresis should be repeated employing a different medium and pH, such as citrate agar gel, pH 6.0. If the abnormal hemoglobin still cannot be identified, further analysis by globin chain electrophoresis is required.

Unstable hemoglobins that cause hemolysis or polycythemia and that may exhibit an abnormal fraction on electrophoresis may be detected by heat or isopropanol precipitation, the presence of intra-erythrocytic inclusions, forceful shaking, analysis of spectra, and by oxygen dissociation. When the combination of some or all of these techniques fails to identify a mutant, identification must be done by some specialized procedures. The mutant can be isolated, aminoethylated, digested with trypsin, and chromatographed or finger-printed. Amino acid analysis of the abnormal peptide may be necessary to identify the substitution.

If thalassemia is suspected from the medical history, physical examination, and results of the complete blood count, evaluation should include cellulose acetate and starch gel electrophoresis, quantitation of Hb $A_2$ and Hb F, serum iron and total iron binding capacity, and family studies. Further studies to diagnose a thalassemic disorder definitively should include a methyl violet stain of a bone marrow aspirate for intranormoblast inclusions, globin synthesis studies, and quantitation of the free radioactive $\alpha$ chain pool.

Methods for the various tests will not be outlined fully in this chapter; only important features of each method will be stressed. All methods will be evaluated for simplicity and accuracy. For more detailed information, the reader is referred to several other texts.[1-6]

## LABORATORY DIAGNOSIS OF ABNORMAL HEMOGLOBINS

### Preparation of Hemolysate

A clear, stroma-free hemolysate should be prepared. The red cells are washed with isotonic saline (0.85 gm NaCl in 100 cc distilled water) and hemolyzed by the addition of 5 volumes of 5 mM phosphate buffer, pH 7.4, containing 0.5 mM EDTA.[7] The stromata are partially precipitated after the addition of 1 volume of 9% NaCl and centrifugation for 10 minutes at 6000 rpm or at a higher speed. The hemolysate is removed with a Pasteur pipette and filtered through two layers of Whatman No. 1 filter paper. Hemolysates may be stored at 4°C after adding 50 microliters of a 0.1 M KCN (6.53 gm/liter) to each ml of a 10% hemoglobin solution.[3] Hemoglobin H is precipitated irreversibly when chloroform or freezing and thawing are used instead of phosphate buffer to induce hemolysis. The use of toluene should be avoided because it accelerates denaturation of most hemoglobins.

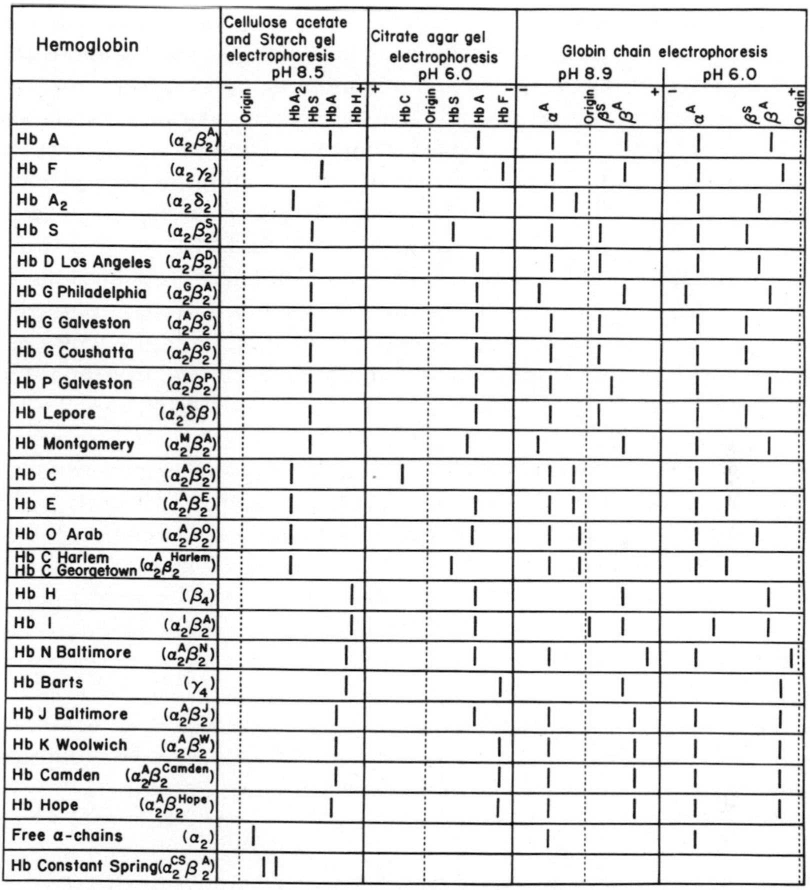

| Hemoglobin | Cellulose acetate and Starch gel electrophoresis pH 8.5 | | | | | Citrate agar gel electrophoresis pH 6.0 | | | | | Globin chain electrophoresis | | | | | |
|---|---|---|---|---|---|---|---|---|---|---|---|---|---|---|---|---|
| | − Origin | HbA₂ | HbS | HbA | HbH + | HbC + | Origin | HbS | HbA | HbF − | pH 8.9 αᴬ − | Origin βˢ βᴬ + | | pH 6.0 αᴬ − | βˢ βᴬ | Origin + |

Hb A $(\alpha_2\beta_2^A)$
Hb F $(\alpha_2\gamma_2)$
Hb A₂ $(\alpha_2\delta_2)$
Hb S $(\alpha_2\beta_2^S)$
Hb D Los Angeles $(\alpha_2^A\beta_2^D)$
Hb G Philadelphia $(\alpha_2^G\beta_2^A)$
Hb G Galveston $(\alpha_2^A\beta_2^G)$
Hb G Coushatta $(\alpha_2^A\beta_2^G)$
Hb P Galveston $(\alpha_2^A\beta_2^P)$
Hb Lepore $(\alpha_2^A\delta\beta)$
Hb Montgomery $(\alpha_2^M\beta_2^A)$
Hb C $(\alpha_2^A\beta_2^C)$
Hb E $(\alpha_2^A\beta_2^E)$
Hb O Arab $(\alpha_2^A\beta_2^O)$
Hb C Harlem / Hb C Georgetown $(\alpha_2^A\beta_2^{Harlem})$
Hb H $(\beta_4)$
Hb I $(\alpha_2^I\beta_2^A)$
Hb N Baltimore $(\alpha_2^A\beta_2^N)$
Hb Barts $(\gamma_4)$
Hb J Baltimore $(\alpha_2^A\beta_2^J)$
Hb K Woolwich $(\alpha_2^A\beta_2^W)$
Hb Camden $(\alpha_2^A\beta_2^{Camden})$
Hb Hope $(\alpha_2^A\beta_2^{Hope})$
Free α-chains $(\alpha_2)$
Hb Constant Spring $(\alpha_2^{CS}\beta_2^A)$

**Figure 3-1.** Mobilities of normal and abnormal hemoglobins and globin chains on cellulose acetate, citrate agar gel, and urea globin chain electrophoresis. [Modified from Schneider.[8,9,14,16]]

## Electrophoretic Studies

Electrophoresis is the most useful method of detecting mutant hemoglobins. The mobilities of normal and mutant hemoglobins on cellulose acetate, agar gel, and globin chain electrophoresis can be found in Figure 3-1.

## Cellulose Acetate Electrophoresis

Cellulose acetate hemoglobin electrophoresis with TRIS-EDTA borate (TEB) buffer, pH 8.4, is, at present, the most widely used method for the preliminary screening of abnormal hemoglobins, because it is simple, fast, and sensitive. However, starch gel electrophoresis is the method of choice for the detection of minor hemoglobin fractions. The Zip Zone electrophoresis apparatus, Titan III cellulose acetate plates, and Super-Heme buffer (Helena Laboratories, Beaumont, Texas) are used. Electrophoresis is performed at room temperature using 350 volts for 15 to 20 minutes. The plates are stained with ponceau S, which stains all proteins, and cleared with 5% acetic acid. When ponceau S is used without benzidene, minor hemoglobins are not always visible or may be hidden under the carbonic anhydrase band. Hemoglobin H is not visualized when electrophoresis is carried out in a Microzone Electrophoresis Cell (Beckman Instruments, Inc., Fullerton, California); it denatures and precipitates as a result of the intense heat generated during electrophoresis.[8]

It is essential that each electrophoretic run include proper controls, such as an artificial mixture of Hbs J, A, F, S, and C, to indicate the exact migration position of the variant hemoglobin in relation to the known hemoglobins.

**Citrate Agar Gel Electrophoresis**

Citrate agar gel hemoglobin electrophoresis in a 0.05 M citrate buffer, pH 6.0, should be used in conjunction with cellulose acetate electrophoresis for the presumptive identification of a majority of mutant hemoglobins.[9] Agar gel electrophoresis differentiates Hb S from mutants that migrate with Hb S on cellulose acetate electrophoresis, serves as a confirmatory test for sickle hemoglobin, and differentiates Hb C from mutants that migrate with Hb C on cellulose acetate electrophoresis. Citrate agar gel electrophoresis is also useful in the presumptive identification of abnormal hemoglobins that migrate anodally to Hb A on cellulose acetate electrophoresis (Fig. 3-1). In addition, it differentiates Hbs H, I, N Baltimore, and J Baltimore from Hbs Bart's, K Woolwich, Camden, and Hope.

Since Hbs F, A, S, and C separate distinctly on citrate agar gel and small amounts of these hemoglobins can be easily visualized, this method is useful for the screening of homozygous sickle cell disease in the neonate.[10] CM-cellulose microchromatography is also useful for the detection of Hb S at birth.[11]

Titan IV citrate agar plates may be purchased (Helena Laboratories) or prepared by impregnating cellulose acetate plates with agar.[12] Electrophoresis is run at room temperature applying 60 to 90 volts for 15 to 45 minutes. The plates are stained with o-dianisidine stain.

## Starch Gel Electrophoresis

Starch gel is useful for the detection of small amounts of Hb A in the presence of large amounts of Hb F. This increased sensitivity of starch gel allows the identification of patients with Hb S-$\beta^+$ thalassemia or Hb C-$\beta^+$ thalassemia whose red cells contain small amounts of Hb A (approximately 1% to 2%), but who exhibit a pattern of Hb SF or Hb CF on cellulose acetate and are thus erroneously considered to have homozygous Hb S or Hb C disease.

Vertical starch gel hemoglobin electrophoresis is performed in a TRIS-EDTA borate buffer, pH 8.6, at 4°C for 15 to 20 hours, at 25 mamp, 200 volts, using Electro Starch (Electro Starch Company, Madison, Wisconsin). This method gives excellent resolution of minor hemoglobin components, such as Hb Bart's, Hb H, Hb $A_2$ variants, free $\alpha$ chains, unstable hemoglobins, and Hb Constant Spring, and is recommended for the screening of neonates for $\alpha$ thalassemia and hemoglobinopathies other than Hb S.[13,14] Free $\alpha$ chains and Hb Constant Spring migrate cathodally to Hb $A_2$ (Fig. 3-1). For the detection of Hb Constant Spring and free $\alpha$ chains, fresh and very concentrated hemolysate should be loaded onto the gel. Starch gel or cellulose acetate electrophoresis in a phosphate buffer system, pH 7.0, is useful for confirming small amounts of Hb H, but the system is too sensitive for Hb Bart's, which may show up in every cord blood sample.

A horizontal apparatus that holds 30 to 40 specimens in three rows and uses a voltage of 500 to 600 volts which reduces electrophoresis time to 4 to 5 hours has been described.[5] When high voltage is used, the gel should be covered with ice or cold water.[5]

## Globin Chain Electrophoresis

Hemoglobins E and O cannot be differentiated by the combination of cellulose acetate and citrate agar gel electrophoresis, but can be differentiated by acid globin chain electrophoresis (Fig. 3-1). On acid globin chain electrophoresis, $\beta^O$ migrates toward the anode and $\beta^E$ toward the cathode. Hemoglobins I and N, which cannot be differentiated by the combination of cellulose acetate and citrate agar gel electrophoresis, can be differentiated by alkaline globin chain electrophoresis.

Globin chain separation by electrophoresis may be performed on cellulose acetate strips using TEB buffers at pH 8.9 and 6.0[15] or on starch gel using TEB buffers at pH 8.0[16] in the presence of 6 molar urea and 0.05 M $\beta$-mercaptoethanol. This method separates normal $\alpha$ and $\beta$ chains as well as abnormal globin chains. Comparison with known variants run on the same strip or gel enables a presumptive identification of the mutant chain to be made.

When presumptive identification by four methods of electrophoresis was compared to structural analysis of a large number of mutant hemoglobins, no discrepancies were found.[17]

## Structural Analysis of Abnormal Hemoglobins

When a mutant hemoglobin cannot be identified by the combination of cellulose acetate, agar gel, and urea gel electrophoresis, identification must be done in a laboratory equipped to do structural analysis of hemoglobins. Column chromatography on carboxymethyl-cellulose (CM52) can be used to separate large amounts of globin which can be collected with a fraction collector[35]; $\beta$-mercaptoethanol, rather than dithiothreitol, should be used in this separation. Tubes containing each chain can be pooled, aminoethylated with ethyleneimine,[37] digested with trypsin, and "fingerprinted." "Fingerprint" is the term used to describe the two-dimensional peptide map produced by paper electrophoresis in one direction and chromatography in a second direction at right angles to the first.[37,38]

Ingram found that for Hb A, Hb S, and Hb C, there were specific arrangements of the peptide spots.[37] An amino acid substitution that results in a net charge difference will cause the involved peptide to move to a different position on the peptide map compared to the position of the corresponding peptide in normal adult Hb A. Papers are dried without heat, stained with ninhydrin, and exposed to heat in a drying oven to develop the peptide spots. There are five amino acids that can be recognized by specific staining reactions: arginine, histidine, methionine, tryptophan, and tyrosine.[3] Since fingerprinting will identify many mutant hemoglobins precisely without the need for additional structural analysis, it serves as a quick method of separating new mutants from those previously described. If the abnormal peptide is new, it is eluted from the papers, hydrolyzed with 6N HCl, and then further studied by amino acid analysis. Some investigators use column chromatography to separate the abnormal peptide with subsequent amino acid analysis. The amino acid analyzer determines relative concentrations of specific amino acids. Comparison of these results with the known content of the same peptide from a normal chain will indicate the missing amino acid and its substitution. Sometimes it is impossible to be sure of the point of substitution if two or more of the amino acids are missing in the peptide. Several techniques are available to solve this problem. Edman (stepwise) degradation or enzymes other than trypsin are used. Discussion of these problems and other helpful suggestions can be found in recent reviews.[3,4]

## SPECIFIC TESTS FOR HB S

### Solubility Test

The solubility test distinguishes Hb S from Hbs G, D, and Lepore, which have similar mobilities on cellulose acetate electrophoresis. The solubility test is based on the observation[18] that deoxy Hb S is less soluble in concentrated salt solutions than Hb A and most other hemoglobin mutants except Hb C Harlem. This test is simple to perform, but often yields false results. False positive results may occur when whole blood is used and turbidity due to elevated plasma proteins or lipids is interpreted as precipitated Hb S. False negative readings may occur in individuals with Hb S and anemia and in neonates or young infants in whom the percentage of Hb S is low. Because of the errors associated with the solubility test, it is recommended that citrate agar gel electrophoresis be used to confirm the presence of Hb S when a Hb S-like migrating band is observed on cellulose acetate electrophoresis.

The solubility test reagent is commercially available (Helena Laboratories; Ortho Diagnostics, Inc., Raritan, New Jersey)[19] or may be prepared in the laboratory by mixing a concentrated phosphate buffer with saponin and sodium dithionite.[20] Saponin hemolyses red cells and sodium dithionite deoxygenates oxy Hb S, which is insoluble in the concentrated salt solution.

### Shaking Test

This test is based on the observation that oxy Hb S denatures and precipitates rapidly upon mechanical shaking.[21] It is performed by adding red blood cells in a fragment of a microhematocrit tube to a vial containing 2 ml of 10 mM sodium phosphate buffer, pH 8.0. The vial is placed in a mechanical shaker and shaken at a frequency of 30 to 50 Hz for 2 minutes. Turbidity indicates the presence of Hb S or other mechanically unstable hemoglobins.[22] No false results were observed in a recent study used to identify children with Hb S.[22] The shaking test can also be used to quantitate the amount of Hb S in a hemolysate. Dilute hemolysate is placed in a spectrophotometric cuvette (Capcell, Technical Consulting Services, Southampton, Pennsylvania) and the optical density at 577 nm is measured before and after shaking. After shaking, the cuvettes are centrifuged at 5000 $\times$ g for 5 minutes and the optical density measured. The percentage of hemoglobin remaining in solution is calculated by extrapolating the denaturation curve to $t = 0$. Recently, the quantitative shaking test was used to detect syndromes with Hb S in neonates less than 4 days old and in a 19-week-old abortus with Hb SS disease, and no false results were observed.[23]

Several rare abnormal hemoglobins, such as Hb C Harlem, Hb M Saskatoon ($\beta$63 His→Tyr), Hb Köln ($\beta$98 Val→Met), Hb Leiden ($\beta$6 or 7 Glu→o), Hb Gun Hill ($\beta$91-95 deleted), Hb H, Hb Shepherds Bush ($\beta$74 Gly→Asp), and Hb Zürich ($\beta$63 His→Arg), also precipitate upon forceful shaking.[24] The shaking test is recommended in the study of unstable hemoglobins as an adjunct to the heat and isopropanol stability and the brilliant cresyl blue (BCB) tests. This technique is recommended as a screening procedure for the detection of Hb S, with hemoglobin electrophoresis to be performed later. The shaking test is preferable to the dithionite solubility test as a fast screening test for Hb S because false negative results have not been observed and because additional abnormal hemoglobins can also be detected.

## SPECIFIC TESTS FOR UNSTABLE HEMOGLOBINS

Unstable hemoglobins are mutant hemoglobins in the heterozygous state that precipitate in the red blood cell and produce inclusions. In the presence of a functioning spleen, inclusion bodies are removed from the red cells, frequently resulting in shortened red cell survival.[25] Unstable hemoglobins may be detected by heat or isopropanol precipitation, the presence of intraerythrocytic inclusions, and by forceful shaking. Since unstable hemoglobins tend to have altered oxygen affinity, they may be detected nonspecifically by measuring oxygen affinity and analyzing the oxygen dissociation curve.[26] Some unstable hemoglobins may be associated with the formation of methemoglobin. In addition, methemoglobin is found in patients with abnormal hemoglobins known as M hemoglobins. Methemoglobin may be measured spectrophotometrically.[27]

### Heat Test

One ml of hemolysate is added to an equal volume of 0.1 M TRIS buffer, pH 7.4, and the solution is heated at 50°C for 2 hours.[28] The hemolysate is examined for flocculent precipitate, and the amount determined. In the normal control, the amount of hemoglobin precipitated does not exceed 1%; in the patient with Hb H, methemoglobin, or an unstable hemoglobin, a precipitate of 5% or more may be formed.

### Isopropanol Precipitation

Isopropanol buffer is prepared by mixing 17 ml of isopropanol with 83 ml of 0.1 M TRIS-HCl buffer, pH 7.4. The buffer is stoppered and kept at room temperature. The test is performed by mixing 0.2 ml of fresh 10% hemolysate with 2 ml of isopropanol buffer. The mixture from the patient and a separate mixture from a normal control are incubated in stoppered tubes at 37°C for 40 minutes. In the presence of an unstable hemoglobin, the solution will become cloudy in 5 minutes, and a precipitate will form in 20 minutes. The control tube will remain clear for 40 minutes. Hemoglobin H or methemoglobin, if available, may serve as a positive control. In the presence of an elevated Hb F level, a precipitate may form after 20 minutes of incubation. A positive isopropanol precipitation test should be confirmed with the heat stability test.[29]

## Intraerythrocytic Inclusion Bodies

One drop of fresh anticoagulated peripheral blood is mixed with one drop of a 1% solution of brilliant cresyl blue (BCB) and incubated at room temperature for 24 to 48 hours. The BCB solution is prepared by adding 1 gm of BCB powder to 100 ml citrate-saline, which consists of 0.4 gm of sodium citrate in 100 ml of 0.9% saline. Smears are made and examined with an oil immersion objective for the presence of greenish-blue inclusions.[28] These inclusions are denatured globin precipitated and stained by the supravital redox dye BCB. They are found in the red cells of all patients with Hb H disease and in many individuals with an unstable hemoglobin such as hemoglobins Köln, Gun Hill, Zürich, Philly, or Shepherds Bush.[30]

An occasional red blood cell with fine inclusions is found in Orientals who carry the gene for $\alpha$-thalassemia-1. The BCB solution occasionally fails to precipitate and stain inclusions in known cases of Hb H[30]; therefore, each new preparation should be checked with fresh red blood cells known to contain Hb H. It is also important to differentiate red cells with BCB inclusions from reticulocytes in which the reticulum appears as dark blue filaments.

Methyl violet is a nonredox supravital dye which stains preformed inclusion bodies.[30,31] One drop of blood or marrow is mixed with 4 drops of filtered 0.5% methyl violet in 0.9% NaCl and incubated at room temperature for 10 to 30 minutes. Blood films are prepared from the buffy coat and examined with an oil immersion objective for the presence of inclusions. Typical purple stained chunks, 1 to 3 $\mu$ in diameter, of precipitated $\alpha$ chains or $\beta$ chains are found in the cytoplasm of polychromatophilic and orthochromatic normoblasts in the bone marrow of patients with homozygous $\beta$ thalassemia ($\beta^O/\beta^O$, $\beta^+/\beta^+$, $\delta\beta/\delta\beta$), doubly heterozygous $\delta\beta$ and $\beta$ thalassemia ($\beta^O/\beta^+$, $\beta/\beta^{silent}$, $\beta^O/\delta\beta$, $\beta^+/\delta\beta$), Hb H disease, and heterozygous $\beta$ thalassemia of unusual severity.[32-36] These inclusions may also be seen in unstained red cells by phase contrast microscopy.[34]

The demonstration of methyl violet inclusions in approximately 30% or more of marrow normoblasts is the most accurate, simple, and usually the definitive method of establishing the diagnosis of homozygous or doubly heterozygous $\beta$ thalassemia. In splenectomized patients with homozygous $\beta$ thalassemia, Hb H disease, unstable hemoglobin disease, or heterozygous $\beta$ thalassemia of unusual severity, as many as 30% of the peripheral red cells have inclusions of precipitated hemoglobin.[31] Inclusions are usually not present in the marrows of patients with heterozygous $\beta$ thalassemia, Hb Lepore trait, or sickle $\beta$ thalassemia, but occasionally they may be found in patients with severe forms of these disorders.[32,36]

Patients with glucose-6-phosphate dehydrogenase deficiency who are acutely hemolyzing following exposure to an oxidant (camphor, fava beans, primaquine, and others) may have high percentages of inclusions in the red cells, but these are usually cleared from the circulation in several hours. The newborn infant may have occasional inclusions because of temporarily decreased splenic function.

## LABORATORY DIAGNOSIS OF THE THALASSEMIAS

The thalassemias are characterized by decreased or absent production of normal $\beta$ polypeptide globin chain in $\beta$ thalassemia, normal $\alpha$ chain in $\alpha$ thalassemia and in Hb Constant Spring, and normal $\delta$ and $\beta$ chains in $\delta\beta$ thalassemia, Hb Lepore, and hereditary persistence of fetal hemoglobin. Accurate diagnosis of thalassemia is essential for genetic counseling, since as a result of faulty diagnosis some individuals have refrained from having children. In addition, faulty diagnosis has resulted in some patients with $\beta$ thalassemia of intermediate severity being unnecessarily committed to lifelong transfusion therapy.

The laboratory diagnosis of thalassemia is difficult, and it is necessary that accurate and reproducible procedures be established. These procedures include:

1. A complete blood and reticulocyte count, red cell indices, blood film, serum iron and total iron binding capacity, and free erythrocyte protoporphyrin.

2. Hb electrophoresis, Hb $A_2$ and Hb F quantitations, and a Betke-Kleihauer Hb F stain.

3. Bone marrow aspirate stained for methyl violet inclusions.

4. Globin synthesis and radioactive $\alpha$ chain pool measurements.

Additional procedures that are useful, but not essential, for the diagnosis of the thalassemias include:

5.  Glycine/alanine ratios at position 136 of the γ chain.
6.  An individual with β-thalassemia trait should have at least one parent or sibling with the same trait. Therefore, family studies are most helpful in detecting this condition.

## Hemoglobin A₂

Hemoglobin A$_2$ is a normal minor fraction of the total hemoglobin and is composed of 2 α globin chains and 2 δ chains.

Since an elevated Hb A$_2$ level usually suggests β thalassemia, a host of methods have been developed to quantitate Hb A$_2$. One accurate but time-consuming method determines Hb A$_2$ by elution after starch block hemoglobin electrophoresis with Veronal buffer, pH 8.6.[39,40] A large amount of concentrated hemolysate can be applied to the block and the weakest bands can be easily visualized. The mean Hb A$_2$ value and one standard deviation measured in 22 normal adults and 37 individuals with β-thalassemia trait were 2.60 ± 0.4 and 5.27 ± 0.35, respectively.[41] Use of the starch block for measuring Hb A$_2$ offers advantages. It is possible to elute a variant fraction in its pure state and at a high concentration for quantitation or for further tests. A near neutral pH buffer may be used to isolate the methemoglobin fraction of various Hb Ms.[42]

Another widely established method is the elution of Hb A$_2$ after cellulose acetate electrophoresis at pH 8.4.[2,43] It is technically easy to perform and is inexpensive, but distinct separation between Hbs S and A$_2$ is not always achieved and precision is low with a Hb A$_2$ content less than 1%. The mean Hb A$_2$ value and one standard deviation measured in 30 normal controls and 28 adults with β-thalassemia trait were 2.56 ± 0.31 and 4.6 ± 0.61, respectively.[44] Scanning of cellulose acetate plates by densitometry after hemoglobin electrophoresis and staining yields inconsistent results and is not recommended for use under any circumstances.[44,45] The absorption of dye by the hemoglobin is not consistent, and the wide range of normal values renders analysis by scanning useless for definitive work.

A simple, rapid, and accurate microchromatographic method has been recently described.[46,47] This method uses DE-52 cellulose, Pasteur pipettes, and two buffers. One volume of freshly prepared hemolysate is mixed with 2 volumes of a 0.2 M glycine-0.01% KCN buffer, pH 7.4 ± 0.1. This solution is placed on the column, and Hb A$_2$ is eluted with a 0.2 M glycine-0.01% KCN–0.0175 M NaCl buffer, pH 7.8 ± 0.05. The remaining hemoglobin is eluted with a 0.2 M glycine-0.01% KCN–0.2 M

NaCl buffer, pH 7.4 ± 0.1. The mean Hb $A_2$ value and the range, measured in 99 normal controls and 24 individuals with $\beta$-thalassemia trait, were 2.5 (1.6 to 2.9) and 4.45 (4.1 to 5.4), respectively.[47] Commercially prepared buffers and microcolumns packed with DE-52 cellulose are available (Isolab, Akron Ohio; Helena Laboratories). An additional advantage of the microcolumn method is that capillary blood collected in a microhematocrit tube or on filter paper may be used. Normal and $\beta$-thalassemia trait blood should be included with each Hb $A_2$ measurement as controls. Small aliquots of hemolysate prepared from the blood of a person with high Hb $A_2$ $\beta$-thalassemia trait and from a normal nonthalassemic control may be stored at $-70°C$ or in liquid nitrogen for as long as one year.

Screening hemoglobin electrophoresis on cellulose acetate, pH 8.4, should always precede Hb $A_2$ quantitation for many reasons: first, to detect abnormal bands, such as C, E, O, C Harlem, which would interfere with Hb $A_2$ quantitation; second, to identify Hb $A_2$ mutants which must be considered as part of the total Hb $A_2$ quantitation; third, to identify increased Hb F bands, which may suggest $\delta\beta$ or $\beta$ thalassemia, HPFH, or Hb Lepore; and finally, to detect Hb Lepore and Hb Constant Spring. An elevated Hb $A_2$ usually indicates the presence of $\beta$ thalassemia. A normal Hb $A_2$ in association with genetically-proven $\beta$ thalassemia may be associated with iron deficiency,[48] $\beta$ thalassemia major, $\delta\beta$ thalassemia, or $\alpha\beta$ thalassemia. An increased level of Hb $A_2$ has been reported in pernicious anemia[49] and in $\beta$ chain unstable hemoglobin disorders.[50]

In heterozygotes for hereditary persistence of fetal hemoglobin, or in Hb H disease, Hb $A_2$ may be normal or reduced. Hb $A_2$ is absent in homozygous $\delta\beta$ thalassemia, homozygous Hb Lepore, and homozygous HPFH.

## Hemoglobin F

Hemoglobin F is a normal minor fraction of the total hemoglobin composed of 2 $\alpha$ and 2 $\gamma$ globin chains. In normal adults or in children beyond 5 years, it comprises between 0 and 1.0% of the total hemoglobin when determined by a specific method of alkali denaturation.[51] We use a modification,[2] based on the method of Betke, which is simple and easy to reproduce. This method yields accurate results only when the Hb F level comprises less than 20% of the total. In persons with a Hb F content of 20% or higher, one should use an alternative method of alkali denaturation[2,52,53] or dilute the sample with Hb F free hemolysate and determine Hb F by the Betke method.[54] Densitometric quantitation of Hb F after cellulose acetate hemoglobin electrophoresis and staining yields spurious results and is not recommended for accurate measurement of Hb F.[55] Hb F can also be quantitated by a combination of DEAE-Sephadex, CM-Sephadex chromatography, and amino acid analysis of isoleucine.[56] No matter which method is used, normal and high Hb F controls should be measured concurrently with each batch of Hb F determinations.

Hemoglobin F is elevated in numerous hematologic and genetic disorders, including the hemoglobinopathies and thalassemias. In the majority of patients with homozygous $\beta$ thalassemia who carry the genotype $\beta^+/\beta^+$, $\beta^+/\beta^0$, or $\beta^+/\delta\beta$, Hb F is usually greater than 35% of the total hemoglobin. In approximately half of all the cases with high Hb $A_2$ heterozygous $\beta$ thalassemia, Hb F is increased above the normal value but seldom exceeds 15% of the total. In heterozygous $\delta\beta$ thalassemia and HPFH, the Hb F level may be as high as 35%.

**Betke-Kleihauer Stain for Hb F**    Hemoglobin F does not elute from smears of fresh red cells containing Hb F which are fixed to a slide with methanol and incubated in an acid citrate-phosphate buffer. In contrast, Hb A and mutant hemoglobins do elute when treated similarly.[57,58] A commercial kit is available for the differential staining of Hb F among the red cells (Fetal Hemoglobin Kit, Boehringer Mannheim Corporation, New York). The Hb F differential stain with this kit is simple and yields generally consistent results, but a positive control from a neonate or cord blood and a negative control should be stained concurrently with the test blood smear. A homogeneous distribution of Hb F among the red cells is defined as a variable degree of eosin coloring of almost every red cell in the film. The distribution of Hb F is defined as heterogeneous when 2% or more of the red cells have failed to absorb any eosin dye and are visualized as ghosts. Blood smears from persons with HPFH have a homogeneous distribution of Hb F among the red cells, while those from normal adults have mainly ghosts and those from patients with an elevated Hb F level other than HPFH exhibit a heterogeneous distribution. This technique is of particular help in differentiating Hb S-HPFH from homozygous sickle cell disease. In the latter peripheral films show a heterogeneous distribution of Hb F while patients with Hb S-HPFH have a homogeneous distribution of Hb F.

## Globin Synthesis

The synthesis of polypeptide globin chains is measured in vitro in intact reticulocytes or normoblasts from peripheral blood or bone marrow. A radioactive amino acid such as $^{14}$C-leucine or $^3$H-leucine, 2 to 4 ml of freshly drawn heparinized whole blood or bone marrow, and 4 to 8 mg of dextrose are gently mixed for 2 hours at 37°C. The red cells are washed with isotonic saline and hemolyzed by the addition of 4 volumes of 1 mM $MgCl_2$, gentle mixing for 90 seconds, and restoration of tonicity by adding one volume of 1.5 M KCl to each volume of packed red cells. Heme is removed with acid acetone and globin is separated into $\beta$ and $\alpha$ chains by carboxymethyl cellulose (CM-52) chromatography at pH 6.5 in 8 M urea with a sodium phosphate gradient.

The phosphate gradient may be prepared by using a gradient mixing apparatus consisting of four interconnecting chambers. The chambers are filled with equal volumes of buffers containing 8 M urea, $6 \times 10^{-4}$ M dithiothreitol, and varying concentrations of $Na_2HPO_4$. The respective concentrations of $Na_2HPO_4$ in the four chambers are $2.6 \times 10^{-3}$ M, $1.7 \times 10^{-2}$ M, $1.7 \times 10^{-2}$ M, and $3.2 \times 10^{-2}$ M. Alternatively, the phosphate gradient may be generated by an LKB 11300 Ultragrad Gradient mixer and valve (LKB Instruments, Inc., Rockwell, Maryland).

Absorption at 280 nm and $\beta$ scintillation are measured in aliquots from tubes of the eluted globin peaks. The radioactivity (RA) $\beta/\alpha$ ratio is calculated by summing up the net counts per minute from the tubes of the $\beta$ chain peak and the $\alpha$ chain peak and dividing the former by the latter. Prior to calculation of the specific activity of each globin chain, it is necessary to divide the optical density of the $\beta$ chain by 1.52 and that of the $\gamma$ by 2.00. The specific activity (SA) $\beta/\alpha$ ratio is calculated by dividing the radioactivity counts by the absorbance value for each of the top 3 to 4 tubes from the $\beta$ peak and the $\alpha$ peak. The SA values from the peak tubes of each chain should not vary by more than 5%. The mean SA value for the $\beta$ chain is divided by that of the $\alpha$ chain, yielding the SA $\beta/\alpha$ ratio.[59]

SA $\beta/\alpha$ ratios are more reliable than RA $\beta/\alpha$ ratios because the former exhibit more of a narrow range in heterozygotes for thalassemia and in nonthalassemic controls with low reticulocyte counts.[59] In those with higher reticulocyte counts, the RA $\beta/\alpha$ ratios match the SA ratios in accuracy and reliability. The successful performance of globin synthesis by CM-52 chromatography depends on accurate regulation of pH and ionic conductivity of the phosphate buffers. A detailed summary of the method is found in a recent review.[59]

## $\alpha$ Chain Pool

A small pool of free unattached $\alpha$ chains is present in human normoblasts and reticulocytes. When globin is synthesized by reticulocytes incorporating $^{14}$C-leucine in vitro, newly formed radioactive $\alpha$ chains are diluted into the small pool of free nonradioactive $\alpha$ chains that is present. The fraction of newly formed radioactive $\alpha$ chains that remains in the free $\alpha$ chain pool is dependent on the initial size of the pool; the larger the pool, the greater the fraction of radioactive $\alpha$ chains contained in it at the end of the incubation.

The $\alpha$ chain pool is derived by incubating marrow or peripheral blood with $^{14}$C-leucine for 2 hours at 37°C.[60] A small aliquot of freshly prepared hemolysate is applied to a Sephadex G-100 column at 4°C and is eluted with a 0.1 M phosphate buffer, pH 7.0. The eluate reveals several peaks. The first peak consists of proteins with a molecular weight greater than hemoglobin. The next peak consists of visible hemoglobin which corresponds to hemoglobin tetramers ($\alpha_2\beta_2$, $\alpha_2\alpha_2$, $\alpha_2\delta_2$). The next two radioactive peaks contain mainly $\alpha$ chains and correspond to dimers ($\alpha_2$) and monomers ($\alpha$) of globin, respectively. The tubes containing hemoglobin tetramers are pooled separately from the tubes containing $\alpha$ chain dimers and monomers. Nonradioactive hemoglobin carrier is added to each pool and chromatography on CMC is performed as described in the section on globin synthesis studies.

The relative size of the free $\alpha$ chain pool is calculated from the CMC chromatograms by adding the total radioactivities in the radioactive $\alpha$ chains of the dimer and monomer peaks, correcting for contamination with the radioactive $\beta$ chains, and dividing by the sum of the radioactive $\alpha$ chains in all three peaks. Alpha chain pools can be done on marrow or on peripheral blood rich in reticulocytes. The $\alpha$ chain pool procedure, although complex and costly, provides the most accurate means for the definitive diagnosis of $\alpha$ thalassemia.[14] It is of great value in differentiating hemoglobin disorders or $\beta$ thalassemia in association with $\alpha$ thalassemia from similar disorders without $\alpha$ thalassemia.[61,62]

## Analysis of Glycine at $\gamma^{136}$

Schroeder et al observed that the normal $\gamma$ chain of Hb F is comprised of a mixture of two types of $\gamma$ chains.[63] One type contains glycine ($^G\gamma$) at position 136 and the other contains alanine ($^A\gamma$) at the same position. These two types of $\gamma$ chains are the products of nonallelic structural genes.[63] To determine the glycine to alanine ratio ($^G\gamma/^A\gamma$) at position 136, the $\gamma$ chain is isolated, purified, and cleaved with cyanogen bromide into three peptides. Peptide 3 ($\gamma$CB-3), which contains the C-terminal 13 amino acids of the $\gamma$ chain, including $\gamma^{136}$, is analyzed and the quantity of glycine (at position 136) and alanine (at positions 136, 138 and 140) residues determined. If all $\gamma$CB-3 peptides contain only glycine at position 136, the ratio of glycine to alanine residues measured will be 1:2; only $^G\gamma$ chains are present in this person. If only $^A\gamma$ chains are present, no glycine residues are detected in the analysis of $\gamma$CB-3. Usually a mixture of $^G\gamma$ and $^A\gamma$ are present. At birth $^G\gamma/^A\gamma$ ratio is about 3:1 ($^G\gamma$ of 0.75); in adults the ratio is usually 2:3 ($^G\gamma$ of 0.4). Studies done in duplicate over prolonged periods of time do not vary by more than 0.05 residues of $^G\gamma$ in any particular case.[64,65] The major value of determining $^G\gamma/^A\gamma$ has been in genetic studies of thalassemia and hereditary persistance of fetal hemoglobin.

## REFERENCES

1. Efremov, G.D., and Huisman, T.H.J. The laboratory diagnosis of the hemoglobinopathies. *Clin. Haematol.* 3:527–570, 1974.
2. Weatherall, D.J., and Clegg, J.B. *The Thalassaemia Syndromes.* 2nd Ed. Oxford: Blackwell Scientific Publications, 1972.
3. Lehman, H., and Huntsman, R.G., Editors. *Man's Haemoglobins.* 2nd Ed. Philadelphia: J.B. Lippincott Co., 1974.
4. Winter, W.P., and Rucknagel, D.L. Peptide mapping of hemoglobin. Edited by J.W. King and W.R. Faulkner. In *CRC Critical Review in Clinical Laboratory Science.* Vol. 5. Cleveland: CRC Press, Inc., 1974.
5. Huisman, T.H.J., and Jonxis, J.H.P. *The Hemoglobinopathies — Techniques of Identification.* Edited by M.K. Schwartz. New York: Marcel Dekker, Inc., 1978.
6. Schmidt, R.M., Ed. *Abnormal Haemoglobins and Thalassemic-Diagnostic Aspects.* New York: Academic Press, Inc., 1975.
7. Asakura, T., Minakata, K., Adachi, A., et al. Denatured hemoglobin in sickle erythrocytes. *J. Clin. Invest.* 59:633–640, 1977.
8. Chindavanig, S., and Gummardpetch, R. Separation and quantitation of hemoglobin H and hemoglobin Bart's by electrophoresis on gelantinized cellulose acetate. *Am. J. Clin. Pathol.* 60:458–461, 1973.
9. Schneider, R.G., Hightower, B., Hosty, T.S., et al. Abnormal hemoglobins in a quarter million people. *Blood* 48:629–637, 1976.
10. Pearson, H.A., O'Brien, R.T., McIntosh, S., et al. Routine screening of umbilical cord blood for sickle cell diseases. *JAMA* 227:420–421, 1974.
11. Schroeder, W.A., Huisman, T.H.J., Powars, D., et al. Microchromatography of hemoglobins. IV. An improved procedure for the detection of hemoglobins S and C at birth. *J. Lab. Clin. Med.* 86:528–532, 1975.
12. Schneider, R.G., Hosty, T.S., Tomlin, G., et al. Identification of hemoglobins and hemoglobinopathies by electrophoresis on cellulose acetate plates impregnated with citrate agar. *Clin. Chem.* 20:74–77, 1974.
13. Atwater, J., and Schwartz, E. Separation of hemoglobins. Edited by W.J. Williams, E. Beutler, A.J. Erslev, and R.W. Rundles. In *Hematology.* 2nd Ed. New York: McGraw Hill Book Company, 1977.
14. Friedman, Sh., Atwater, J., Gill, F.M., et al. $\alpha$-Thalassemia in Negro infants. *Pediatr. Res.* 8:955–959, 1974.
15. Schneider, R.G. Differentiation of electrophoretically similar hemoglobins such as S, D, G, and P, or $A_2$, C, E, and O by electrophoresis of the globin chains. *Clin. Chem.* 20:1111–1115, 1974.
16. Chernoff, A.I., and Pettit, N.M. The amino acid composition of hemoglobin. III. A qualitative method for identifying abnormalities of the polypeptide chains of hemoglobin. *Blood* 24:750–756, 1964.
17. Schneider, R.G., and Hightower, B. Structure in relation to behavior of mutant hemoglobins in citrate agar electrophoresis. *Hemoglobin* 1:427–444, 1977.
18. Itano, H.A. Solubilities of naturally occurring mixtures of human hemoglobins. *Arch. Biochem. Biophys.* 47:148–159, 1953.
19. Schmidt, R.M., and Wilson, S. Standardization in detection of abnor-

mal hemoglobins. Solubility tests for hemoglobin S. *JAMA* 225:1225–1230, 1973.

20. Nalbadian, R.M., Nichols, B.M., Camp, F.R., et al. Dithionite tube test—A rapid inexpensive technique for detection of hemoglobin S and non-S sickling hemoglobin. *Clin. Chem.* 17:1028–1031, 1971.

21. Asakura, T., Agarwal, P.L., Relman, D.A., et al. Mechanical instability of the oxy-form of sickle hemoglobin. *Nature* 244:437–438, 1973.

22. Asakura, T., Segal, M., Friedman, Sh., et al. A rapid test for sickle hemoglobin. *JAMA* 233:156–157, 1975.

23. Friedman, Sh., Back, B., Delivoria-Papadopoulos, M., et al. A simple test for detection of sickle hemoglobin in the neonatal period. *Am. J. Clin. Pathol.* 70:85–88, 1978.

24. Vella, F. Mechanical stability of human hemoglobins. *Acta Haematol.* 54:257–260, 1975.

25. White, J.M. The unstable hemoglobin disorders. *Clin. Haematol.* 3:333–356, 1974.

26. Charache, S. Haemoglobins with altered oxygen affinity. *Clin. Haematol.* 3:357–381, 1975.

27. Herzog, P., and Feig, S.A. Methaemoglobinaemia in the newborn infant. *Clin. Haematol.* 7:75–83, 1978.

28. Atwater, J., and Schwartz, E. Tests for Hb H and other unstable hemoglobins. Edited by W.J. Williams, E. Beutler, A.J. Ersley, and R.W. Rundles. In *Hematology.* 2nd Ed. New York: McGraw Hill Book Company, 1977.

29. Carrell, R.W., and Kay, R. A simple method for the detection of unstable haemoglobins. *Br. J. Haematol.* 23:615–619, 1972.

30. Papayannopoulou, T., and Stamatoyannopoulos, G. Stains for inclusion bodies. Edited by J.W. King and W.F. Faulkner. In *CRC Critical Review in Clinical Laboratory Science.* Vol. 5. Cleveland: CRC Press, Inc., 1974.

31. Fessas, Ph. Inclusions of hemoglobin in erythroblasts and erythrocytes of thalassemia. *Blood* 21:21, 1963.

32. Friedman, Sh., Ozsoylu, S., Luddy, R., et al. Heterozygous beta thalassemia of unusual severity. *Br. J. Haematol.* 32:65–77, 1976.

33. Stamatoyannopoulos, G., Fessas, Ph., and Papayannopoulou, T. F-Thalassemia. A study of 31 families with simple heterozygotes and combinations of F-thalassemia with $A_2$ thalassemia. *Am. J. Med.* 47:194–208, 1969.

34. Yatganas, X., and Fessas, Ph. The pattern of hemoglobin precipitation in thalassemia and its significance. *Ann. NY Acad. Sci.* 165:270–286, 1969.

35. Schwartz, E. The silent carrier of beta-thalassemia. *N. Engl. J. Med.* 281:1327–1333, 1969.

36. Stamatoyannopoulos, G., Woodson, R., Papayannopoulou, T., et al. Inclusion body β thalassemia trait. *N. Engl. J. Med.* 290:939–943, 1974.

37. Ingram, V.M. Abnormal human hemoglobins. I. The comparison of normal human and sickle cell haemoglobins by "fingerprinting." *Biochim. Biophys. Acta* 28:539–545, 1958.

38. Baglioni, C. An improved method for the fingerprinting of human hemoglobin. *Biochim. Biophys. Acta* 48:392–396, 1961.

39. Kunkel, H.G., Ceppellini, R., Muller-Eberhard, U., et al. Observations on the minor basic hemoglobin component in the blood of normal individuals and patients with thalassemia. *J. Clin. Invest.* 36:1615–1625, 1955.

40. Gerald, P., and Diamond, L.K. The diagnosis of thalassemia trait by starch block electrophoresis of the hemoglobin. *Blood* 13:61–69, 1958.

41. Huisman, T.H.J. Chromatographic determination of Hb $A_2$. Edited by J.W. King and W.R. Faulkner. In *CRC Critical Review in Clinical Laboratory Science.* Vol. 5. Cleveland: CRC Press, Inc., 1974.

42. Gerald, P., and George, P. Second spectroscopically abnormal

methemoglobin associated with hereditary cyanosis. *Science* 129:393–394, 1959.

43. Marengo-Rowe, A.J. Rapid electrophoresis and quantitation of haemoglobins on cellulose acetate. *J. Clin. Pathol.* 18:790, 1965.

44. Schmidt, R.M., Rucknagel, D.L., and Necheles, T.F. Comparison of methodologies for thalassemia screening by Hb $A_2$ quantitation. *J. Lab. Clin. Med.* 86:873–882, 1975.

45. Shibato, S., Miyaji, T., and Ohba, Y. Evaluation of precision of procedures for estimation of Hb $A_2$ and Hb F in hemolysates. Edited by R.M. Schmidt. In *Abnormal Haemoglobins and Thalassemia-Diagnostic Aspects.* New York: Academic Press, Inc., 1975.

46. Efremov, G.D., Huisman, T.H.J., Wrightstone, R.N., et al. A rapid chromatographic method for the determination of Hb $A_2$. *J. Lab. Clin. Med.* 83:657–664, 1974.

47. Schleider, C.T.H., Mayson, S.M., and Huisman, T.H.J. Further modification of the microchromatographic determination of Hb $A_2$. *Hemoglobin* 1:503–504, 1977.

48. Wasi, P., Disthasongchan, P., and Na-Nakorn, S. Effect of iron deficiency on the levels of hemoglobin $A_2$ and E. *J. Lab. Clin. Med.* 71:85–91, 1968.

49. Josephson, A.M., Masri, M.S., Singer, L., et al. Starch block electrophoretic studies of human hemoglobin solutions. Results in cord blood, thalassemia and other hematologic disorders: Comparison with tiselius electrophoresis. *Blood* 13:543, 1958.

50. Rieder, R.F., Zinkham, W.H., and Holtzman, N.A. Hemoglobin Zürich. Clinical, chemical, and kinetic studies. *Am. J. Med.* 39:4, 1965.

51. Betke, K., Marti, H.R., and Schlicht, I. Estimation of small percentages of foetal haemoglobin. *Nature* 184:1877, 1959.

52. Jonxis, J.H.P., and Visser, H.K.A. Determination of low percentages of foetal haemoglobin in blood of normal children. *Am. J. Dis. Child.* 92:588–589, 1956.

53. Singer, K., Chernoff, A.I., and Singer, L. Studies on abnormal hemoglobins. I. Their demonstration in sickle cell anemia and other hematologic disorders by means of alkali denaturation. *Blood* 6:413–428, 1951.

54. Columbo, B., Kim, B., Perez-Atencis, B., et al. The pattern of fetal haemoglobin disappearance after birth. *Br. J. Haematol.* 32:79–87, 1976.

55. Schmidt, R.M., Brosious, E.M., and Holland, S. Quantitation of fetal hemoglobin by densitometry. *J. Lab. Clin. Med.* 84:740–745, 1974.

56. Schroeder, W.A., Huisman, T.H.J., Shelton, J.R., et al. An improved method for quantitative determination of human fetal hemoglobin. *Anal. Biochem.* 35:235–243, 1970.

57. Betke, K., and Kleihauer, E. Fetaler and Bleibender Blut-tarbstoff in Erythrozyten und Erythroblasten von Menschlichen Feten and Neugeborenen. *Blut* 4:421, 1958.

58. Atwater, J., and Erslev, A.J. Fetal hemoglobin differential staining. Edited by W.J. Williams, E. Beutler, A.J. Erslev, and R.W. Rundles. In *Hematology.* 2nd Ed. New York: McGraw-Hill Book Company, 1977.

59. Schwartz, E. Abnormal globin synthesis in thalassemia red cells. *Semin. Hematol.* 11:549–567, 1974.

60. Gill, F.M., and Schwartz, E. Free $\alpha$ globin pool in human bone marrow. *J. Clin. Invest.* 52:3057–3063. 1973.

61. Kim, H.C., Weierbach, R.G., Friedman, Sh., et al. Globin biosynthesis in sickle cell, Hb SC and Hb C disease. *J. Pediatr.* 91:13–18, 1977.

62. Kim, H.C., Weierbach, R.G., Friedman, Sh., et al. Detection of $\alpha$ or $\beta^0$ thalassemia by studies of globin biosynthesis. *Blood* 49:785–792, 1977.

63. Schroeder, W.A., Huisman, T.H.J., Shelton, J.R., et al. Evidence for multiple structural genes for the $\gamma$ chain of human fetal hemoglobin. *Proc. Nat. Acad. Sci. USA* 60:537–544, 1968.

64. Huisman, T.H.J., Schroeder, W.A., Efremov, G.D., et al. The present status of the heterogeneity of fetal hemoglobin in $\beta$ thalassemia. An attempt to unify some observations in thalassemia and related conditions. *Ann. NY Acad. Sci.* 232:107–124, 1974.

65. Huisman, T.H.J., Miller, A., Cook, L., et al. The molecular heterogeneity of some types of hereditary persistence of fetal hemoglobin (HPFH). Edited by M. Aksoy. In *International Istanbul Symposium on Abnormal Hemoglobins and Thalassemia*. TBTAK, 1975.

# 4 Morphology: Pathophysiology Illustrated*

Fredric T. Serota, M.D.
Natale Tomassini
Klaus Hummeler, M.D.
Elias Schwartz, M.D.

Hemoglobin's structural changes, biochemical properties, and interactions with the red cell membrane are often reflected in the appearance of erythrocytes. Altered shape or size of erythrocytes implies a corresponding molecular change in hemoglobin and enables the observer to anticipate pathophysiology.

Several terms are used routinely to describe the appearance of the peripheral blood smear. Variations in erythrocyte shape and size are termed poikilocytosis and anisocytosis, respectively. Bessis has encouraged the use of names derived from Greek for different types of poikilocytes.[1] Some are commonly used, whereas others may be unfamiliar. For example, an acanthocyte is a spiculated erythrocyte, a codocyte is a "hat form," and a drepanocyte is a sickle cell. The familiar teardrop shape is a dacryocyte, and a crenated cell is an echinocyte. Stomatocytes are mouth-shaped cells. A leptocyte or

*We would like to thank Janet Fithian for editorial assistance and Ruth Cuthbert for typing the manuscript. This work was supported in part by NIH grant AM 16691, NIH Research Training Award 5T32 HL07150, The Cooley's Anemia Fund, and the Tommy Fund.

target cell is thinner than normal due to increased surface/volume ratio. This is the opposite of a spherocyte, a cell with a marked decrease in surface/volume ratio. Since artifacts due to preparation of smears are common, it is necessary to be sure that what appear to be poikilocytes are found distributed throughout a smear in which there are also cells of normal shape.

Anisocytes include macrocytes, mature red cells with diameters greater than 8 $\mu$ and either a normal or increased thickness/diameter ratio. Macrocytes always have a well-defined central depression which distinguishes them from megalocytes. Microcytes have a decreased diameter without a change in the thickness/diameter ratio and with an area of central pallor; they contain lower than normal total amounts of hemoglobin and very often their hemoglobin concentration is below normal as well.

Quantitation of cell size and hemoglobin content is usually performed by automated instruments which determine mean values for cell volume (MCV) and cell hemoglobin concentration (MCHC). Since mean values do not indicate whether several different populations of cells are present, such values may be misleading, especially when there is anisocytosis and poikilocytosis.

In the examination of blood smears it is important to choose smears with a minimum of artifact in order to avoid diagnostic errors. The proper area for study is near the center of a well-made smear, where the cells do not overlap and each red cell has an area of central pallor which fades gradually toward the periphery of the cell. Artifact is present when the area of central pallor appears entirely colorless and is sharply demarcated from the stained peripheral ring of cytoplasm. Red cells along the sides and feather edge of the smear will appear flattened and round, without an area of central pallor. Cells flattened by surface tension rather than pressure during preparation of the smear more clearly demonstrate internal details.

No longer an instrument for morphologic study alone, the electron microscope has become an important tool in the investigation of molecular events. Whereas transmission electron microscopy (TEM) permits study of cellular organelles, scanning electron microscopy (SEM) allows visualization of cell surfaces and shape. The transmission electron microscope has a resolving power of 0.2 nm, the SEM 20 nm, and the light microscope 200 nm. Each system produces its own artifacts with which the experienced microscopist needs to become familiar.

## SICKLE CELL SYNDROMES

Variable percentages of sickled cells are found in air-dried smears from patients with homozygous sickle cell disease. The frequency of

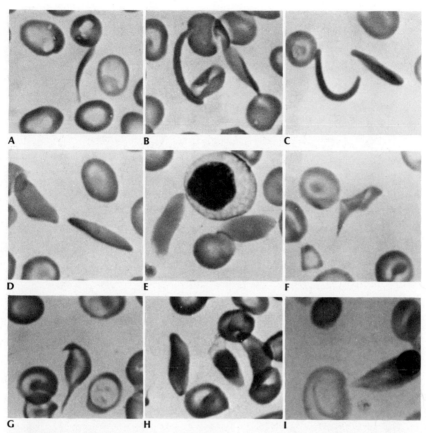

**Figure 4-1.** Homozygous sickle cell disease. Light microscopy of Wright-Stained peripheral blood. **(A–G)** Heterogeneous appearance of sickle forms. **(H)** Dense aggregate of Hb in center of cell. **(I)** Nucleated sickled cell.

sickle forms correlates less with the presence of crisis than with the quantity of Hb F or the presence of a modulating interactive hemoglobinopathy.[2,3,4] Sickle forms vary from fat shapes called "oat cells" to long spindle shapes (Figures 4-1, 4-2). The smear in homozygous sickle cell disease is also characterized by polychromatophilia, target cells, erythrocytes with punctate basophilia, and a leukocytosis with a mild shift to less mature forms. An increase in polychromasia, indicative of the presence of a young red cell population, and increased numbers of nucleated red blood cells may indicate recovery from an aplastic crisis or some other stress on the marrow. Platelets may be increased or normal. Reticulocytes, and occasionally polychromatophilic erythroblasts, usually increased in numbers, may become sickled (Figure 4-1-i). Howell-Jolly bodies, which are small, round remnants of nuclear material located eccentrically, are found in patients who have developed functional asplenia.[5]

78

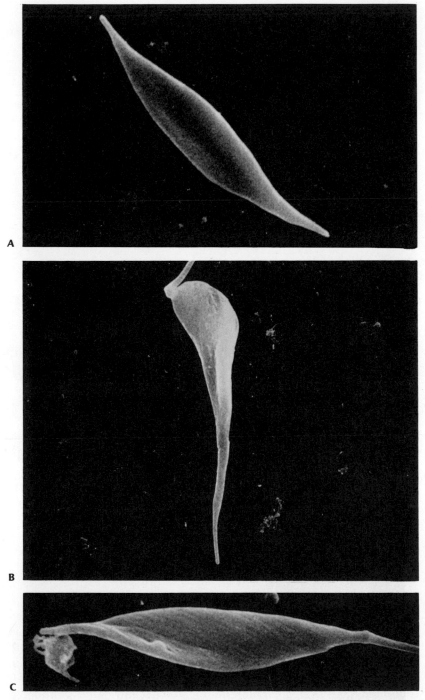

**Figure 4-2.** Homozygous sickle cell disease. Scanning electron microscopy. **(A,B,C)** Pencil forms. **(D,E)** Thicker forms. **(F)** Target forms.

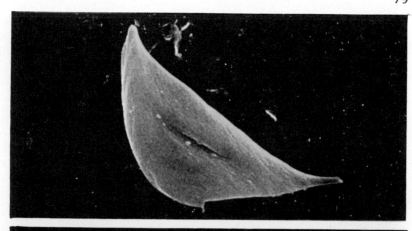

D

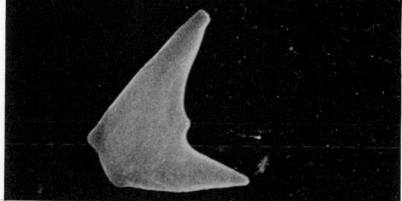

E

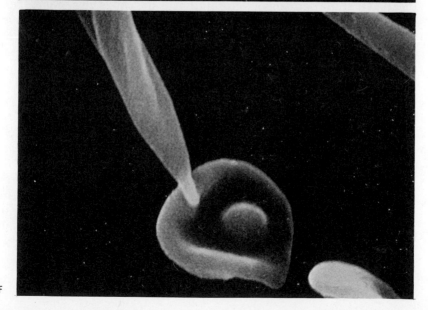

F

It cannot be determined from the appearance of many of the sickle forms on the peripheral blood smear whether or not these cells are irreversibly sickled. Irreversibly sickled cells (ISC) are cells that do not return to the biconcave form even after vigorous oxygenation.

Cells which sickle and unsickle repeatedly in response to the cycle of oxygenation-deoxygenation as the cell circulates eventually become irreversibly sickled. The mechanism of formation of an irreversibly sickled cell (ISC) might be loss of cell membrane material during the course of reoxygenation[6] or the irreversible deformation of the spectrin-actin membrane lattice.[7] Hybrid erythrocytes consisting of membranes from normal cells with Hb S introduced have been shown to sickle under deoxygenation and to become irreversibly sickled after prolonged anoxia.[8] The alterations to the erythrocyte membrane that occur during sickling have recently been extensively reviewed.[9] In addition to the shape transformation, there is increased passive diffusion of sodium and potassium with resultant cellular dehydration and accumulation of calcium. There is also increased association of hemoglobin with erythrocyte membranes.[10]

Although some abnormalities of oxy Hb S due to $\beta^6$ Glu$\rightarrow$Val substitution have been noted, the major pathology is due to the consequences of deoxygenation. Deoxy Hb S polymerizes into very high molecular weight filaments.[11,12,13] These filaments, visible by transmission electron microscopy, associate laterally to form fibers and bundles of fibers which, in vivo, distort the red cell into the characteristic sickle shape (Figure 4-3). The oxygenated ISC retains the sickled shape but demonstrates an amorphous internal structure, indicating that the permanent deformation of the cell is now maintained by membrane rather than by hemoglobin abnormalities. ISCs have been isolated by ultracentrifugation and shown to contain a lesser quantity of Hb F than the average population of cells in the sample, suggesting that Hb F helps prevent formation of ISCs.[14]

The simultaneous presence of hemoglobins other than sickle hemoglobin within the erythrocyte can influence the polymerization of Hb S molecules.[15,16] Increased amounts of Hb F, which is heterogeneously distributed among red cells in homozygous sickle cell disease, inhibit the sickling phenomenon by raising the minimum gelling concentration, the critical hemoglobin concentration at which there is a sudden appearance of high molecular weight Hb S polymers and gelling. The young patient with homozygous sickle cell disease who still retains high levels of Hb F characteristically has a blood smear which exhibits only mild morphologic changes (Figure 4-4). Sickle forms may be difficult to find on the peripheral blood smears of these patients.

In patients heterozygous for both Hb S and $\beta$ thalassemia, the mean cell hemoglobin concentration is low, reducing the capacity of the cell to sickle because the minimum gelling concentration is less readily achieved.[17,18] Sickle forms are less evident on peripheral smears of these patients than on those with Hb SS, but there is hypochromia, anisocytosis, and poikilocytosis (Figure 4-5).

Smears of patients with Hb SC (heterozygotes for both Hb S and Hb C) predominately show target cells and "paper hat" cells, whereas their blood counts reveal normal or close to normal hemoglobin levels. Only rarely are sickle forms found (Figure 4-6). Patients doubly heterozygous for Hb S and the various D hemoglobins exhibit fewer target cells than patients with Hb SC. Patients with SO Arab have a marked anemia and a severe clinical course, correlating with the lower minimum gelling concentration of a mixture of Hb S and Hb O Arab.[19] The severe clinical course is accompanied by major abnormalities of red cell morphology (Figure 4-7).

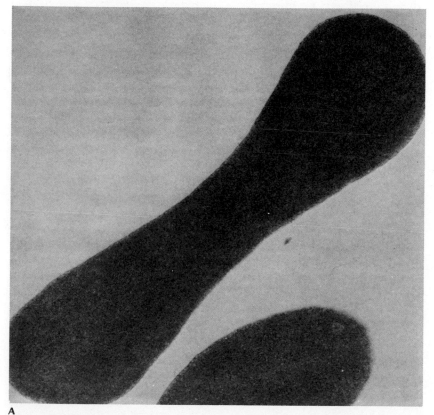

A

**Figure 4-3.** Heparinized peripheral blood, obtained from a patient with Hb SS, was deoxygenated by incubating in nitrogen atmosphere for 30 minutes and then fixed in glutaraldehyde, Transmission electron microscopy. **(A)** Prior to incubation. **(B)** Following deoxygenation. Note formation of polymers of hemoglobin. **(C)** Reoxygenated. ISC is defined after reoxygenation. [By permission from J.F. Bertles and J. Dobler. *Blood* 33:884, 1969.]

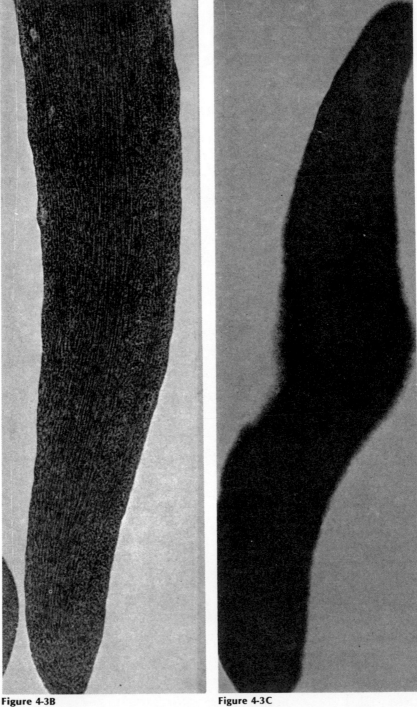

**Figure 4-3B**

**Figure 4-3C**

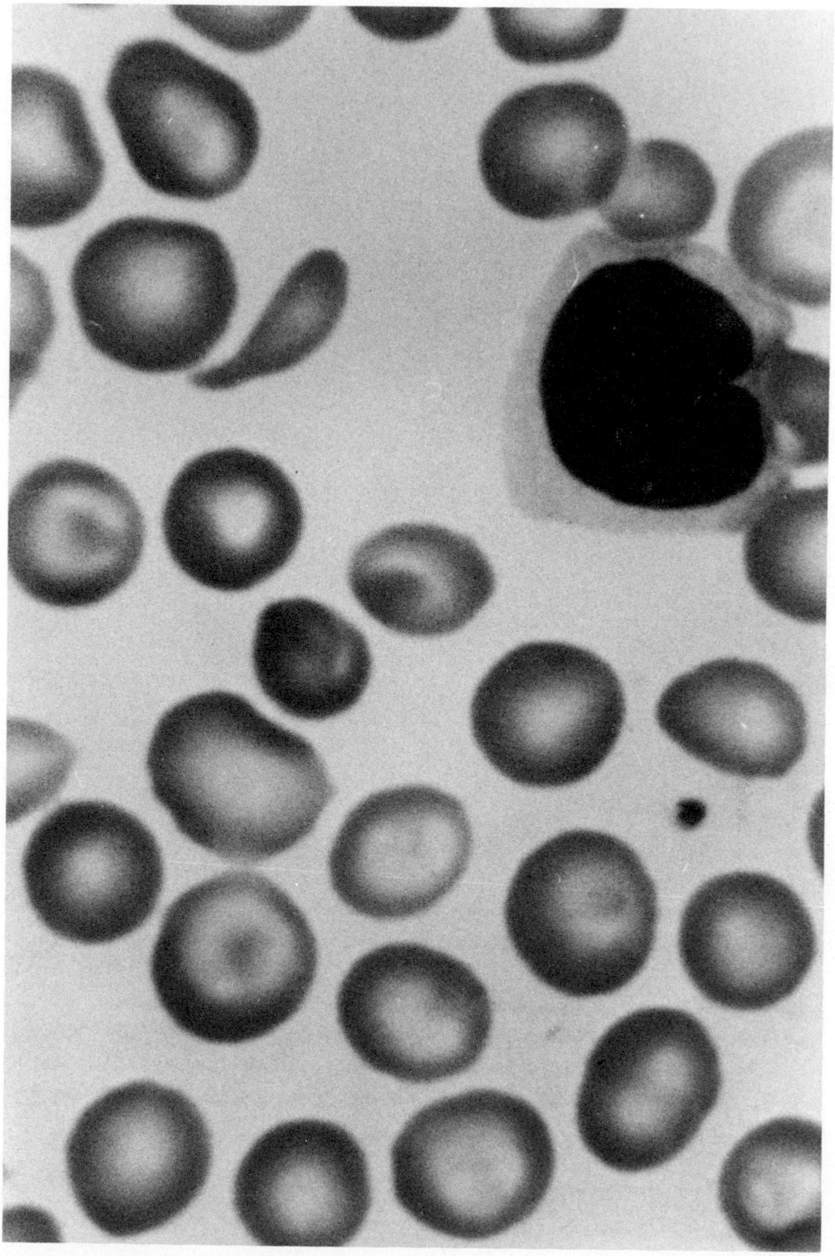

**Figure 4-4.** Homozygous sickle cell disease. Eight-month-old male who presented at age 6 months with hand-foot syndrome. Hb A$_2$ 2.0%, Hb level 9.3 g/dl, Hct 28.7%, reticulocytes 5.0%, WBC 9,000/mm$^3$, MCV 81$\mu^3$, MCHC 32.4%, 1 NRBC/100 WBC, platelets 267,000/mm$^3$, G6PD 1.22 units (deficiency).

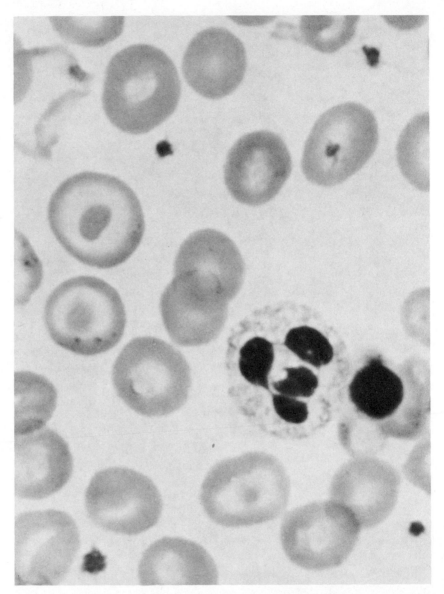

**Figure 4-5.** Hb S-$\beta$ Thalassemia. Four-year-old female who presented with fever and leg pain. Liver palpable 2 cm below and spleen palpable 8 cm below costal margins. Hb 6.8 g/dl, Hct 21.5%, reticulocytes 31.6%, WBC 13,900/mm³ with normal differential. MCV 68$\mu$³, 136 NRBC/100 WBC, Howell-Jolly bodies were evident. Cellulose acetate electrophoresis shows Hb S, Hb F, Hb A. Hb A₂ 3.0%, Hb F 9.7%, Betke-stain heterogeneous distribution of Hb F. Patient's mother has sickle cell trait; father has Hb A₂ 4.3%, Hb F 0.6%, indicating $\beta$-thalassemia trait.

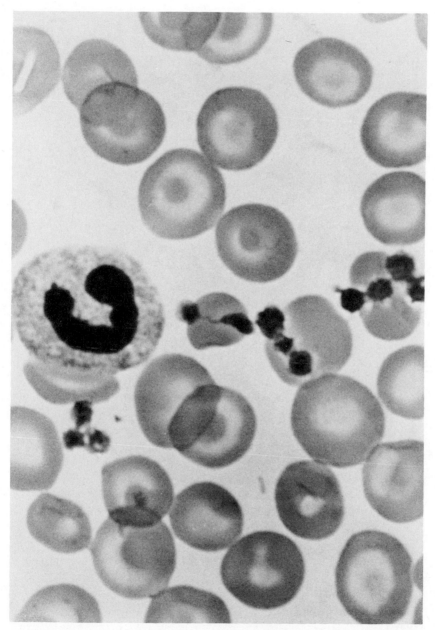

**Figure 4-6.** Hb SC. Fourteen-year-old male hospitalized only twice, both times for epistaxis. The patient has never had a painful crisis. Hb 10.4 g/dl, Hct 30.0%, reticulocytes 2.0%, WBC 7,600/mm³, MCV 80μ³, MCH 27.6μμg, MCHC 34.2%, Hb F 0.4%, Hb C crystals formed on incubation with 3% NaCl.

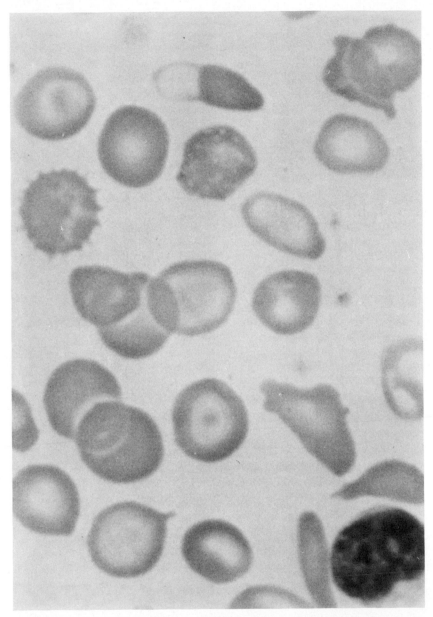

**Figure 4-7.** Hb SO$_{Arab}$. Four-year-old male diagnosed at age 5 months after presenting with hand-foot syndrome. More than 10 hospitalizations and numerous emergency room visits for vaso-occlusive crises since diagnosis. Pneumococcal meningitis at age 1 year. Hb 7.9 g/dl, Hct 26.2%, reticulocytes 7.6%, WBC 14,200/mm³ with normal differential, MCV 83$\mu^3$, MCH 27.8$\mu\mu$g, MCHC 33.2%, Hb F 4.2%.

In patients with sickle cell trait, sickle cells are not found on the routine peripheral blood smear. Erythrocytes from these patients can be made to sickle only if placed under extreme hypoxic stress or when incubated with a reducing agent such as sodium metabisulfite, the classical method of demonstrating the presence of Hb S.

## HEMOGLOBINS C, D, AND E

The presence of Hb C ($\beta^6$ Glu→Lys) within the erythrocyte is characterized by target cells on the peripheral smear. Target cells, normally deformable and therefore not threatened by fragmentation, are also characteristic of liver disease. In liver disease, however, there is a relative increase in cell membrane in relation to cell content, and the cell has increased osmotic resistance.[20] In Hb C disease (Figure 4-8) targets may form because of the tendency of Hb C to aggregate into precipitates or crystals as the cells dry on a glass slide.[21] In fact, a wet preparation fails to show targets, and the area/volume ratio has been shown to be normal.

Several variants of a hemoglobin which comigrates with Hb S when electrophoresis is run at alkaline pH have been named with the prefix D followed by the locale where they were discovered—Hb D Punjab, Hb D Ivan, Hb D Ibadan. None of these hemoglobins sickles, although they can interact with Hb S. Hb D Punjab is the most commonly encountered. Patients with homozygous Hb D have normal hemoglobin values with no evidence of hemolysis on the peripheral blood smear, although leptocytes are evident.[22]

Hemoglobin E is a very common hemoglobin variant in Southeast Asia. Patients with Hb E trait (Hb AE) have no hematologic abnormalities. The erythrocyte morphology of patients homozygous for Hb E is characterized by target cells (Figure 4-9). Patients who are doubly heterozygous for Hb E and $\beta$ thalassemia have an anemia which is variable in its severity, but generally more severe than in patients with Hb S-$\beta$ thalassemia.[23,24]

## $\beta$ THALASSEMIA

Few peripheral blood smears are as dramatic as those of patients with homozygous $\beta$ thalassemia, also called Cooley's anemia (Figure 4-10). Poorly hemoglobinized normoblasts (which are increased following splenectomy), marked hypochromia, microcytosis, poikilocytosis,

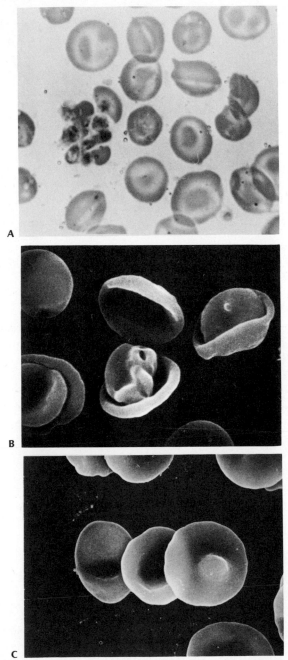

**Figure 4-8.** Hb CC. Three-year-old male. **(A)** Hb 10.6 g/dl, Hct 33.2%, reticulocytes 2.4%, MCV 68$\mu^3$, MCH 22.1$\mu\mu$g, MCHC 32.3%, Hb F 1.0%. Hb C crystals formed in 3% salt. **(B)** Scanning electron micrographs of target cells, demonstrating Hb C crystals. **(C)** SEM of erythrocytes from patient with chronic active hepatitis, demonstrating target cells formed due to acquired increase in membrane.

and anisocytosis are evident. Polychromasia is less than might be expected, because of markedly ineffective erythropoiesis. Basophilic stippling, an artifact which occurs during drying of the smear, is caused by aggregation of ribosomes, sometimes associated with mitochondria and siderosomes.[25] Some of the variation in size and shape of red cells is lost following splenectomy. Because of the intense hemolysis and increased nucleic acid turnover, some patients who do not receive folic acid supplements develop megaloblastic changes.

Ultrastructural and light microscopy evidence suggests that as a result of unbalanced globin synthesis in the thalassemia syndromes the excess globin chains precipitate.[26] The precipitate probably predisposes the cell to rigidity and premature destruction. In wet preparations $\alpha$ chain inclusions in $\beta$ thalassemia appear to be pulled out or pitted by reticuloendothelial cells in the spleen, thus producing teardrop forms.[27] Inclusions are found free within splenic pulp. It is

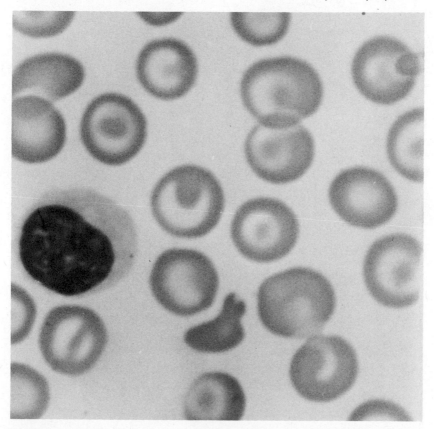

**Figure 4-9.** Hb EE. Ten-year-old oriental female found to have low indices on CBC obtained as part of routine physical examination. Hb 11.5 g/dl, Hct 36.2%, reticulocytes 0.5%, WBC 11,900/mm³, RBC 584 × 10⁶/mm³, MCV 62μ³, MCH 19.9μμg, MCHC 32.1%, Hb F 5%.

90

not known why the teardrop shape becomes permanent. Prolonged stretching may result in loss of deformability.

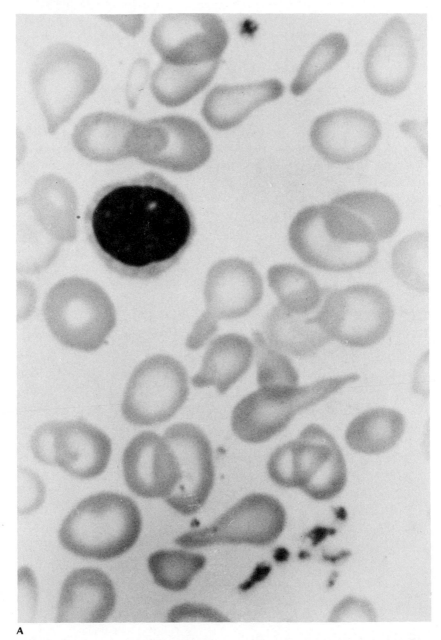

A

**Figure 4-10.** Homozygous β Thalassemia. **(A)** Ten-year-old male of Albanian descent not requiring transfusion support. Minimal facial changes. Spleen palpable 8 cm below left costal margin. Hb 6.1 g/dl, Hct 23%, RBC 3.87 × 10⁶/mm³, WBC 14,400/mm³, 3 NRBC/100 WBC, reticulocytes 7.1%, MCV 59.5μ³, MCH 15.7μμg, MCHC 26.5%, Hb A₂, 4.8%, Hb F

Heinz bodies, which are inclusions of precipitated denatured hemoglobin, are not visible on the routine peripheral blood smear of these patients. After splenectomy, inclusions become apparent on smears stained with supravital dyes or examined with the transmission

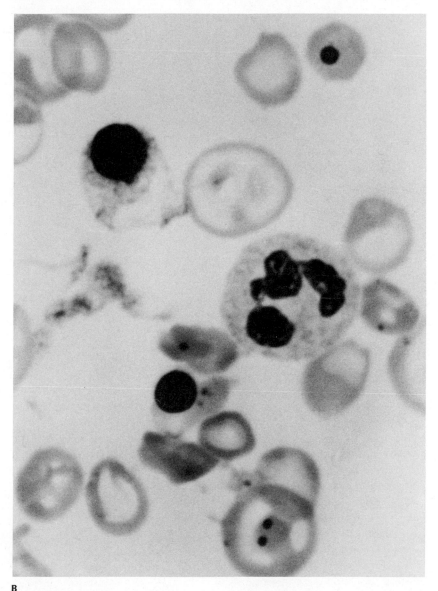

**B**

6.2%. (B) Twenty-two-year-old female, initially diagnosed at 3 years of age after presenting with anemia and hepatosplenomegaly. She has not required transfusion therapy since splenectomy at age 7 years. Hb 7.8 g/dl, Hct 25.3%, reticulocytes 9.2%, MCV 88$\mu^3$, MCH 27.5$\mu\mu$g, MCHC 30.8%, 540 NRBC/100 WBC, reticulocytes 10.4%, WBC 12,900/mm³, Hb A$_2$ 4.8%, Hb F 50.3%.

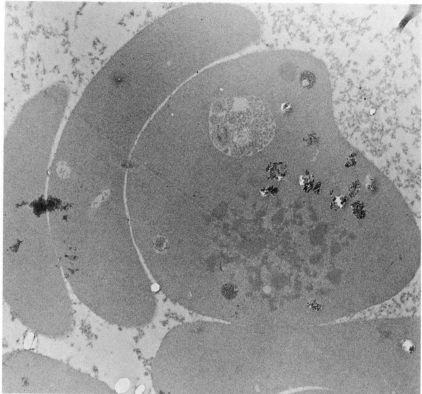

**Figure 4-11.** Heinz Bodies. Transmission electron microscopy. The dense inclusions contain excess iron, while the lighter inclusions are precipitated hemoglobin.

electron microscope (Figure 4-11). There is some correlation between severity of disease and Heinz body formation, for Heinz bodies are a reflection of the underlying imbalance in globin synthesis in the thalassemia syndromes.[28]

Electron microscopic examination of the erythrocyte in β thalassemia also demonstrates increased amounts of ferritin, as well as iron-loaded mitochondria (Figure 4-12). It should be noted that the MCV and MCHC are low despite the hypersideremia, probably because of the unbalanced globin synthesis.

The morphology of β-thalassemia trait is that of mild hypochromia and microcytosis, slight anisocytosis and poikilocytosis, and occasional basophilic stippling (Figure 4-13). In fact, on morphologic grounds alone this type of smear is difficult to distinguish from that of a patient with iron deficiency. A definite diagnosis can usually be made by considering the smear in relation to the patient's ethnic background, serum iron and iron binding capacity, free erythrocyte protoporphyrin (FEP), Hb $A_2$, and Hb F.

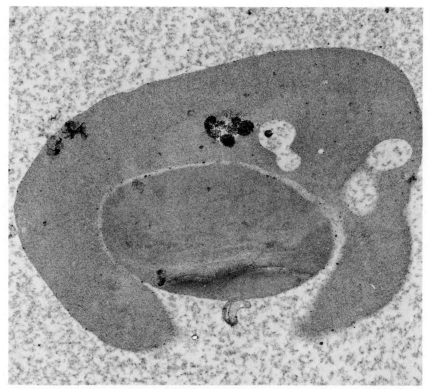

**Figure 4-12.**  Ultrastructure of iron overload. Transmission electron microscopy. Increased amounts of ferritin as well as iron-loaded mitochondria are apparent.

Heterozygous β thalassemia of unusual severity has been reported.[29] These patients have a diversity of clinical expression and the peripheral smear exhibits marked anisocytosis, poikilocytosis, target cells, polychromasia, and nucleated red blood cells (Figure 4-14). As might be anticipated from these findings, unbalanced globin synthesis was found both in bone marrow and peripheral blood reticulocytes.

## α THALASSEMIA

The peripheral blood smear from an hydropic infant homozygous for α thalassemia demonstrates large numbers of nucleated red blood cells and extreme poikilocytosis associated with the absence of production of α chains (Figure 4-15).

Patients with Hb H disease have smears that are characterized by hypochromia, microcytosis, poikilocytosis, targeting, and polychromasia (Figure 4-16). Because of a relative decrease in α chain synthesis, heme-containing $\beta$ chain tetramers (Hb H) are formed. These tetramers are easily oxidized, precipitate, and are pitted by the spleen. Inclusions are visible in the peripheral blood red cells postsplenectomy. Because Hb H is relatively stable in comparison with free $\alpha$ chains, the ineffec-

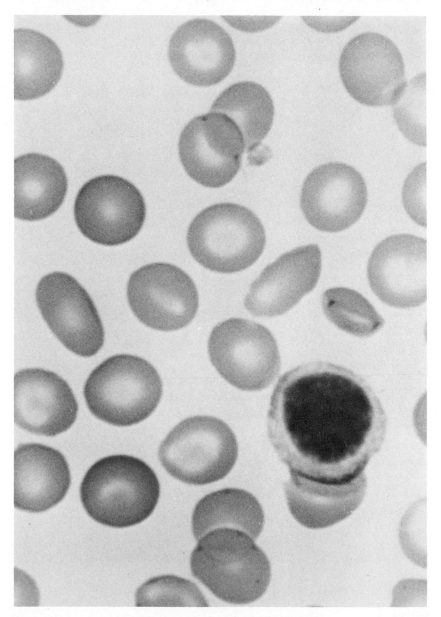

**Figure 4-13.** Heterozygous $\beta$ thalassemia. Father of patient with Cooley's anemia. Hb 15.2 g/dl, Hct 44.7%, RBC 6.99 × 10⁶/mm³, MCV 65μ³, MCH 21.5μμg, MCHC 33.6%, reticulocytes 2.2%, platelets 360,000/mm³, Hb A₂ 4.8%, Hb F 0.8%.

tive erythropoiesis, which is found in homozygous $\beta$ thalassemia due to the destruction of young cells with excess, unstable $\alpha$ chain, is not a prominent feature of Hb H disease.[30]

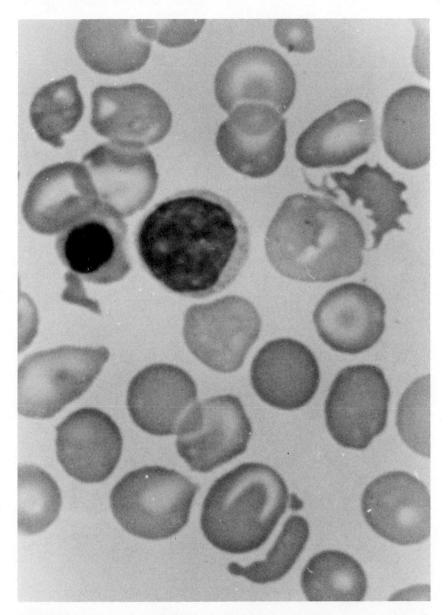

**Figure 4-14.** Heterozygous $\beta$ thalassemia of unusual severity. Forty-seven-year-old male of English-German extraction first found anemic at age 30 years during routine physical examination. Following splenectomy at age 39 years, general well-being improved. Hb 11.0 g/dl, Hct 36.0%, 18 NRBC/100 WBC, MCV 70$\mu^3$, MCH 90.0$\mu\mu$g, MCHC 29.0%, Hb A$_2$ 5.3%, Hb F 3.2%. Peripheral blood $\beta/\alpha$ 0.80, free radioactive $\alpha$ chain pool 58.4%.

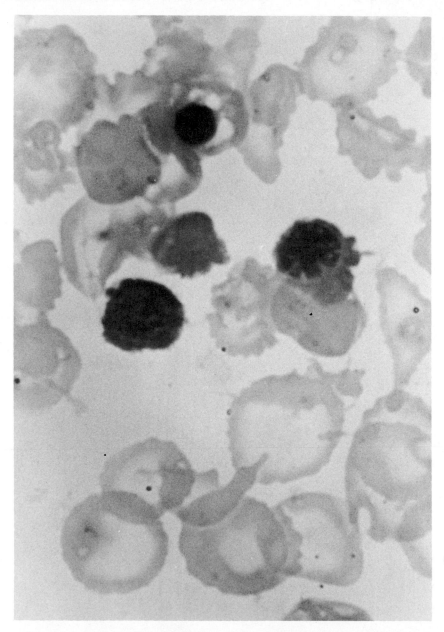

**Figure 4-15.** Homozygous α thalassemia. Chinese infant product of 34-week gestation complicated by toxemia, polyhydramnios, falling maternal platelet count, and fibrinogen. Baby was hydropic, with massive ascites and hepatosplenomegaly, and survived only a few minutes. Placenta was large and hydropic. The following data were obtained on cord blood: Hb 6.4 g/dl, WBC 118,900mm³ (uncorrected), 605 NRBC/25WBC, MCV 113μ³, MCH 27.2μμg, MCHC 24.2%. Cellulose acetate electrophoresis demonstrated Hb Bart's, Hb Portland, and some Hb H. Albumin 1.1 g/dl. Peripheral blood α/β ratios: father 0.78, mother 0.80, baby—no radioactivity incorporated into α chain.

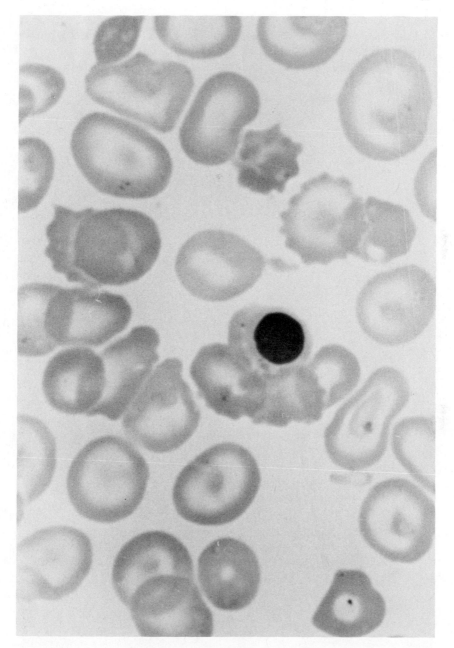

**Figure 4-16.** Hemoglobin H Constant Spring disease. Two-year-old Vietnamese male with enlarged liver (5 cm below RCM) and spleen (11 cm below LCM). Height and weight below third percentile on American growth charts. Hb 6.5 g/dl, Hct 24.2%, reticulocytes 23.6%, MCV 79$\mu^3$, MCH 21.7$\mu\mu$g, MCHC 27.0%, Hb F 2.6%. Cellulose acetate electrophoresis shows Hb H, Hb Constant Spring, and Hb Bart's. Cr[51] erythrocyte survival, t½ = 7.5 days; excessive splenic sequestration demonstrated by surface counting.

98

In α-thalassemia-1 trait there is mild microcytosis and hypochromia with only some anisocytosis and poikilocytosis without anemia (Figure 4-17). Alpha-thalassemia-1 trait can be distinguished from β-thalassemia trait by the presence of normal levels of Hb $A_2$ and

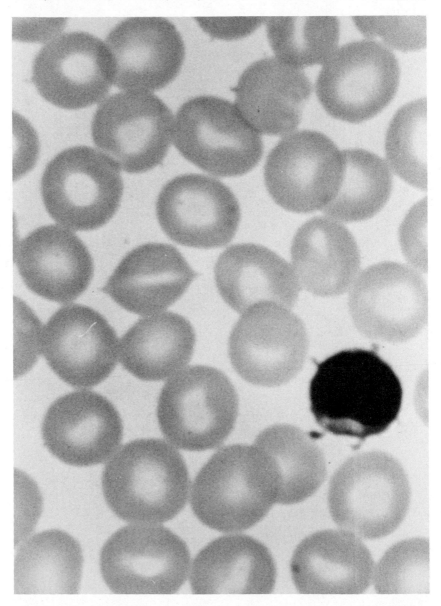

**Figure 4-17.** α-Thalassemia trait. Three-year-old black male found to have Hb Bart's 3.6% by neonatal screening. No medical problems. Hb 10.7 g/dl, Hct 32.7%, RBC 4.82 × $10^6$/mm³, reticulocytes 3.0%, MCV 70μ³, MCH 22.4μμg, MCHC 32.0%, BCB preparation negative for inclusions. Hb $A_2$ 1.6%, Hb F 0.3%.

Hb F and by a reduced rate of $\alpha$ chain synthesis in reticulocytes.[31] The hematologic findings in patients with heterozygous $\alpha$-thalassemia-2 are minimally abnormal or normal,[32] and it is impossible to distinguish $\alpha$-thalassemia-2 trait on morphologic findings. Diagnosis must be inferred from family study.

## HEREDITARY PERSISTENCE OF FETAL HEMOGLOBIN

Hereditary persistence of fetal hemoglobin (HPFH) denotes a group of inherited conditions in which increased amounts of fetal hemoglobin continue to be synthesized throughout life. In homogeneous, or pancellular, HPFH, almost every erythrocyte contains Hb F. In heterogeneous, or heterocellular, HPFH, less than 50% of erythrocytes in the heterozygote contain Hb F.[33] Furthermore, the pancellular form can be subdivided into individuals with absence of $\beta$ and $\alpha$ chain synthesis or only $\beta$ chain production cis to the HPFH mutation and also according to the relative expression of $\gamma^G$ and $\gamma^A$ genes.[34,35]

The peripheral smear of patients with Hb A-HPFH is normal with occasional target cells. Smears of patients with Hb S-HPFH may be slightly abnormal with occasional target cells and variations in red cell size and shape, without sickle forms (Figure 4-18). The uncommon

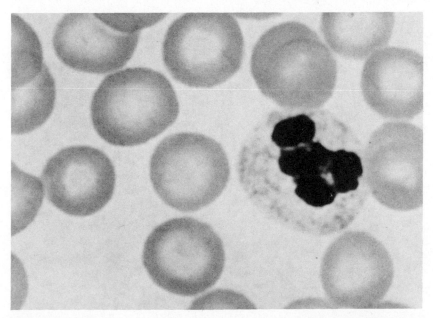

**Figure 4-18.** Hb S-HPFH. Asymptomatic cousin of previous patient, diagnosed through family study. Cellulose acetate electrophoresis Hb SF. Hb F 35.7%, Hb $A_2$ 1.8%.

black patient homozygous for HPFH has slightly low MCH and MCV values and red cell changes similar to those found in heterozygous $\beta$ thalassemia. These patients have decreased $\gamma/\alpha$ globin synthesis ratios. Patients with heterozygous (pancellular) HPFH have Hb F in greater than 99% of red cells, although in varying amounts per cell (Figure 4-19).

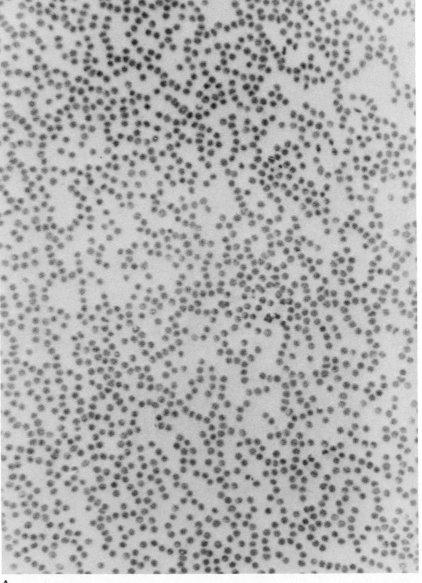

A

**Figure 4-19.** HPFH. **(A)** Pancellular distribution of Hb A. Demonstrated by the Betke technique. **(B)** Heterocellular distribution of Hb F in a patient with aplastic anemia.

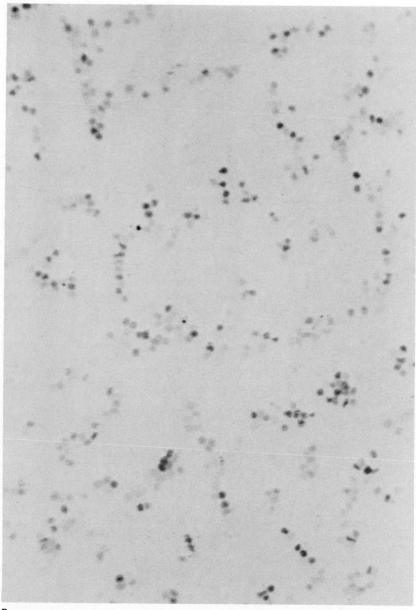

B

## REFERENCES

1. Bessis, M. *Blood Smears Reinterpreted.* Berlin: Springer-Verlag, 1977, p. 63.
2. Serjeant, G.R., Serjeant, B.E., and Milner, P.F. The irreversibly sickled cell: A determinant of haemolysis in sickle cell anemia. *Br. J. Haematol.* 17:527–533, 1969.

3. McCormack, M.K., Bresson, V.L., and Serjeant, G.R. Fetal hemoglobin and the irreversibly sickled cell in sickle cell disease. *J. Pediatr.* 85:435, 1974.

4. Rieber, E.E., Veliz, G., and Pollack, S. Red cells in sickle cell crisis: Observations on the pathophysiology of crisis. *Blood* 49:967–979, 1977.

5. Pearson, H.A., Spencer, R.P., and Cornelius, E.A. Functional asplenia in sickle-cell anemia. *N. Engl. J. Med.* 281:923–926, 1969.

6. Radilla, F., Bromberg, P.A., and Jensen, W.N. The sickle-unsickle cycle: A cause of cell fragmentation leading to permanently deformed cells. *Blood* 41:653–660, 1973.

7. Lux, S.E., John, K.M., and Karnovsky, M. Irreversible deformation of the spectrin-actin lattice in irreversibly sickled cells. *J. Clin. Invest.* 58:955–963, 1976.

8. Clark, M.R., and Shohet, S.B. Hybrid erythrocytes for membrane studies in sickle cell disease. *Blood* 47:121–131, 1976.

9. Palek, J. Red cell membrane injury in sickle cell anemia. *Br. J. Haematol.* 35:1–9, 1977.

10. Asakura, T., Minakata, K., Adachi, K., et al. Denatured hemoglobin in sickle erythrocytes. *J. Clin. Invest.* 59:633–640, 1977.

11. May, A., and Huehns, E.R. The mechanism and prevention of sickling. *Br. Med. Bull.* 32:223–233, 1976.

12. Grasso, J.A., Sullivan, A.L., and Sullivan, L.W. Ultrastructural studies of bone marrow in sickle cell anemia. I. The structure of sickled erythrocytes and reticulocytes and their phagocytic destruction. *Br. J. Haematol.* 31:135–148, 1975.

13. Grasso, J.A., Sullivan, A.L., and Sullivan, L.W. Ultrastructural studies of bone marrow in sickle cell anemia. II. The morphology of erythropoietic cells and their response to deoxygenation in vitro. *Br. J. Haematol.* 31:381–389, 1975.

14. Bertles, J.F., and Milner, P.F.A. Irreversibly sickled erythrocytes: A consequence of the heterogeneous distribution of hemoglobin types in sickle cell anemia. *J. Clin. Invest.* 47:1731–1741, 1968.

15. Bookchin, R.M., and Nagel, R.I.L. Ligand-induced conformational dependence of hemoglobin in sickling interactions. *J. Mol. Biol.* 60:263–270, 1971.

16. Moffat, K. Gelation of sickle cell hemoglobin: Effects of hybrid tetramer formation in hemoglobin mixtures. *Science* 185:274–277, 1974.

17. Serjeant, G.R., and Serjeant, B.E. A comparison of erythrocyte characteristics in sickle cell syndromes in Jamaica. *Br. J. Haematol.* 23:205–213, 1972.

18. Bookchin, R.M., and Nagel, R.L. Interactions between human hemoglobins: Sickling and related phenomena. *Semin. Hematol.* 11:577–595, 1974.

19. Milner, P.R., Miller, C., et al. Hemoglobin $O_{Arab}$ in four Negro families and its interaction with hemoglobin S and hemoglobin C. *N. Engl. J. Med.* 283:1417–1425, 1970.

20. Cooper, R.A., and Jandl, J.H. Bile salts and cholesterol in the pathogenesis of target cells in obstructive jaundice. *J. Clin. Invest.* 47:809–822, 1968.

21. Charache, S., Conley, C.L., Waugh, D.F., et al. Pathogenesis of hemolytic anemia in homozygous hemoglobin C disease. *J. Clin. Invest.* 46:1795–1811, 1967.

22. Ozsoylu, S. Homozygous hemoglobin D-Punjab. *Acta Haematol. (Basel)* 43:353–359, 1970.

23. Sturgeon, P., Itano, H.A., and Bergren, W.R. Clinical manifestations of

inherited abnormal hemoglobins. II. Interaction of hemoglobin E and thalassemia trait. *Blood* 10:396–404, 1955.

24. Chernoff, A.I., Minnich, V., Nakorn, S.N., et al. Studies of hemoglobin E. I. The clinical, hematologic, and genetic characteristics of the hemoglobin E syndromes. *J. Lab. Clin. Med.* 47:455–489, 1956.

25. Jensen, W.N., Moreno, G.D., and Bessis, M. An electron microscopic description of basophilic stippling in red cells. *Blood* 25:933–943, 1965.

26. Polliack, A., and Rachimilewitz, E.A. Ultrastructural studies in β thalassemia major. *Br. J. Haematol.* 24:319–326, 1973.

27. Nathan, D.G. Thalassemia. *N. Engl. J. Med.* 286:586–594, 1972.

28. Yataganas, X., and Fessas, P. The pattern of hemoglobin precipitation in thalassemia and its significance. *Ann. NY Acad. Sci.* 165:270–287, 1969.

29. Friedman, S., Ozsoylu, S., Luddy, R., et al. Heterozygous beta thalassemia of unusual severity. *Br. J. Haematol.* 32:65–77, 1976.

30. Gabozda, T.G., Nathan, D.G., and Gardner, F.H. The metabolism of the individual $C^{14}$-labeled hemoglobins in patients with H thalassemia, with observations on radiochromate binding to the hemoglobins during red cell survival. *J. Clin. Invest.* 44:315–325, 1965.

31. Walford, D.M. α-Thalassemia in the United Kingdom. *Br. J. Haematol.* 35:347–350, 1977.

32. Wasi, P. Is the human globin α-chain locus duplicated? *Br. J. Haematol.* 24:267–273, 1973.

33. Boyer, S.H., Margolet, L., Boyer, M.L., et al. Inheritance of F cell frequency in heterocellular hereditary persistence of fetal hemoglobin: An example of allelic exclusion. *Am. J. Hum. Genet.* 29:256–271, 1977.

34. Huisman, T.H.J., Schroeder, W.A., Efremov, G.D., et al. The present status of the heterogeneity of fetal hemoglobin in β thalassemia: An attempt to unify some observations in thalassemia and related conditions. *Ann. NY Acad. Sci.* 232:107–124, 1974.

35. Weatherall, D.J., and Clegg, J.B. Hereditary persistence of fetal hemoglobin. *Br. J. Haematol.* 29:191–198, 1975.

36. Friedman, S., Schwartz, E., Aherns, E., et al. Variations of globin chain synthesis in hereditary persistance of fetal hemoglobin. *Br. J. Haematol.* 32:357–364, 1976.

# 5 Sickle Cell Screening, Counseling, and Education*

Bertram H. Lubin, M.D.
William C. Mentzer, Jr., M.D.
Winfred Wang, M.D.
Julian R. Davis, Jr., M.D.

Technologic advances have increased the capability of early diagnosis of genetic disease and have facilitated the widespread development of genetic screening programs. Those programs in which clear-cut goals have been established prior to screening have been the most successful. In such programs, patients with disease have been detected and treated, preventing morbidity and mortality; carriers at risk of having children with genetic disease have been identified and counseled regarding the various reproductive options available to them; and education of both lay and professional groups has increased awareness of many genetic conditions.[1]

Screening programs for sickle hemoglobin are gradually moving closer to the optimal model just described, but the process has been

*We are grateful for the advice and assistance of members of the sickle cell staffs at Children's Hospital of the East Bay (Della Simpson, Sarah Nelson, David Nelson, Klara Kleman, and Elmirie Robinson) and at San Francisco General Hospital (Terry Tschopp, Cathi Sullivan, Theresa Payne, Cathy Wallace, and Tony Gill). This work was supported by contract HSM 240-76-0033 from the Sickle Cell Disease Program, Bureau of Community Health Services, and NHLB1 grants 1 KO4 HL00086 and 1 RO1 HL20985.

difficult and has left permanent scars. Initial mass screening efforts to detect sickle hemoglobin created social, ethical, political, and legal problems.[2] Lacking clear-cut goals, some programs confused screening for sickle cell trait with screening for sickle cell disease, and sickle cell trait was projected as a health hazard. In some instances screening was performed without consent, counseling, or education. Inadequate awareness of the sickling disorders existed throughout the professional and lay community. Several states, in response to political pressure, passed legislation making sickle cell screening mandatory. As a consequence of these and other problems, carriers of sickle cell trait suffered unnecessary psychological stress and felt stigmatized.[3]

Although some inadequacies remain, efforts on the part of local, state, and federal groups to improve the quality of sickle cell programs have for the most part been effective.[4] Technologic advances, such as cord blood screening and intrauterine diagnosis, together with improved therapeutic measures for specific complications of sickle cell disease, have greatly increased the desirability of providing programs for sickle cell diagnosis, counseling, and education.

Several years ago, the Bureau of Community Health Services, in the Department of Health, Education, and Welfare, became interested in developing guidelines for such programs.[5] As participants in this project, during the past five years we have established an institutional-based program with a large outreach component. In this chapter, we will use the experience gained in this program to illustrate principles of screening (with an emphasis on cord blood screening), counseling, and education, which are applicable to programs for detecting sickle cell disease as well as other hemoglobinopathies, including thalassemia. To assist in counseling and to provide a balanced perspective on certain controversial publications, a comprehensive review of the literature of the medical implications of sickle cell trait has been included.

## GENERAL GUIDELINES

In the development of any screening program, the first step is to establish clearly the specific objectives of the program.

### Goals

The goals of our sickle cell program are:

1. To detect patients with sickle cell disease prior to the onset of complications and to provide a program for comprehensive medical care, counseling, and education.

2.  To detect carriers of hemoglobin traits who are at risk of having children with sickle cell disease and to provide genetic counseling so that the significance of these traits can be fully understood.
3.  To develop and implement education programs that will increase awareness and understanding of sickle cell disease and trait in the lay and professional community.
4.  To incorporate sickle cell screening into comprehensive medical care and include procedures which will identify other causes of anemia.

## Target Population

When the primary purpose of screening is to detect patients with sickle cell disease, the ideal target population is the black newborn. Because almost all deliveries occur in a hospital, it is theoretically possible to screen every newborn at risk. One out of 250 black newborns will have a clinically significant hemoglobinopathy. Early diagnosis alerts the physician and family prior to the onset of symptoms, and prompt, sensitive counseling helps the family cope with the disease. Education of physicians and families may be effective in preventing some of the early morbidity and mortality from the disease. Discovery of sickle trait in a newborn infant will identify families who may be at risk of producing a homozygous offspring in subsequent pregnancies. If such parents elect to be screened, couples at risk may be identified and counseled during their reproductive years. We also recommend screening pregnant black women and all black patients undergoing anesthesia or other potentially hypoxic experiences as the milder forms of sickle cell disease, such as Hb SC disease or Hb S-$\beta$ thalassemia, occasionally escape detection until late childhood or even adulthood.[6]

When the goal is to detect heterozygosity for an abnormal hemoglobin, the optimal groups to screen are adolescents and adults of childbearing age, in order to provide accurate information for genetic counseling. Screening procedures should be capable of detecting sickle cell trait, Hb C trait, and $\beta$-thalassemia trait, as any of these $\beta$ chain abnormalities, when inherited in combination with sickle cell trait, will result in a clinically significant sickling disorder. Programs initiated in secondary schools, adolescent clinics, and family planning clinics have been the most successful. When an index case has been identified in any of the target populations, screening should be offered to other family members.

**Informed Consent**

Sickle cell screening must be voluntary, and an individual who does not wish to be screened should never be denied medical care or other services. Informed consent should be obtained in writing prior to screening, and consent forms should not be signed until the person being tested has an understanding of the significance of the test. The consent form must be written in understandable terms and contain the following information: the purpose of testing, the potential benefits and risks, the right to withdraw from the testing program at any time, the right to receive testing results and a copy of the consent form, and the conditions under which the information can be released.[7]

It has been argued that informed consent should not be required for cord blood screening since the screening procedure causes no harm or discomfort to mother or infant and the main purpose for screening is to detect disease. As there are absolutely no medical implications of sickle cell trait for the newborn and the emotional impact of the diagnosis on the family may be pronounced, we recommend that informed consent be obtained prior to cord blood screening.

**Confidentiality**

An appropriate record-keeping system must not only provide ready access to screening information by authorized individuals but also, simultaneously, maintain the rights to confidentiality of those screened. One way of achieving this is to assign each person an identification number that is used for laboratory specimens and counseling records. Information is recorded and filed under the name of the client only in a single centralized location where release can be controlled.

**Notification**

Persons found to have sickle cell trait are notified by mail that the test has been completed and that a counselor is available to discuss the results. The results are not indicated in the notification letter, as we have found that people are less anxious and benefit more from counseling when the counselor informs them directly. When a newborn with sickle cell trait is identified, the parents are notified that the hemoglobin electrophoresis results can be obtained from their physician or from a counselor in the sickle cell program. The anxiety level of the parents and the rapport between the health provider and the family determines the optimal time for discussion of the results.

All clients with normal hemoglobin electrophoresis are notified by mail.

When a diagnosis of sickle cell disease has been made, the patient or his/her parents are promptly contacted and told that test results are available and should be discussed in the clinic. After confirmation of the diagnosis and counseling of the family, the patient may continue to receive medical care in the sickle cell program or be followed by the family physician, with support from the sickle cell program when necessary.

## Community Participation

Community members, either in an advisory capacity or as active participants in community-oriented screening and education programs, are essential participants of a screening program. An effective relationship between the community and screening program involves a commitment to a joint educational process. This process will enable members of the screening program to understand community needs while members of the community can be informed of the medical and technical aspects of the program. Together, both groups can discuss the social, ethical, and legal implications of screening and can develop program objectives and administrative guidelines which will enhance the success of the project.

## Comprehensive Care

The most effective sickle cell screening, counseling, and education programs are those which have been incorporated into comprehensive care programs. The combined program does not require centralization of all program activities within a hospital setting, but does require a working relationship based upon mutual respect between medical facilities and community organizations. Duplication of effort, lack of follow-up, inadequate testing procedures, and failure to recognize other health care priorities are all likely to occur in the absence of a comprehensive approach.

## LABORATORY METHODS

Our approach to the laboratory analysis of abnormal hemoglobins closely follows the guidelines of the Center for Disease Control.[8] The initial screening test for a qualitative hemoglobin abnormality should be electrophoresis on cellulose acetate at alkaline pH. A solubility test should be carried out on all specimens containing hemoglobin migrating in the position of Hb S.[9] The shake test, described by Asakura and his coworkers, which measures the solubility of oxy, rather than deoxy, hemoglobin may also be utilized to distinguish Hb S from other abnormal hemoglobins.[10] The screening method we prefer for cord blood samples is hemoglobin electrophoresis on both cellulose acetate at pH 8.4 and citrate agar at pH 6.4.

Repeat testing at age 3 to 6 months is recommended for newborns with patterns suggesting sickle cell or Hb C trait. All infants with findings suggesting clinically important disorders should be evaluated further as soon as possible. Sickle cell anemia (Hb SS) cannot be easily distinguished from Hb S-$\beta$ thalassemia or Hb S hereditary persistence of fetal hemoglobin in the newborn. Family and follow-up studies are needed to confirm the diagnosis.

## Microcytosis

The widespread availability of electronic particle counters has made the determination of red cell size the best initial screening test for thalassemia currently available.[11] Large numbers of blood samples can be processed quickly and cheaply. Capillary blood can be used, if necessary. In adults with uncomplicated $\beta$-thalassemia trait, the MCV is less than 80, the lower limit of normal. The same appears to be the case in $\alpha$-thalassemia trait. The normal lower limit of red cell size in infants and children is different than that in adults, due to the developmental microcytosis characteristic of younger individuals. The lower threshold for the normal MCV is 70 in children from 6 months to 2 years of age, 74 in children from 2 to 6 years of age, 76 in children 6 to 12 years of age, and 78 in children from 12 to 18 years of age.[12] In children, an added advantage to the use of red cell size as the initial screening procedure for thalassemia is that other important causes of microcytosis, such as iron deficiency or lead poisoning, will also be detected. In the San Francisco Bay area population we have screened, approximately 27% of children and 29% of adults have microcytic red cells. Of these, 1.4% have $\alpha$-thalassemia trait (based on studies of cord blood) and 2.0% have $\beta$-thalassemia trait.

Once preliminary screening has identified the presence of microcytosis, additional tests are required to specify its cause. The usual diagnostic dilemma is the differentiation of iron deficiency from thalassemia trait. If appropriate instrumentation is available, preliminary data suggest that a red cell size distribution plot or Price-Jones curve may serve to distinguish the two conditions.[13] A variety of discriminant functions, based upon the routine blood counts obtained from the electronic particle counter, have also been developed to assist in the differentiation of iron deficiency from thalassemia trait (Table 5-1).[14] In cases uncomplicated by other factors, such as pregnancy, coexistent illness, and the like, each of the indices appears to be about 80% to 90% effective. Such results are not sufficiently accurate for use in genetic counseling, but they may be quite helpful in the selection of the most appropriate battery of tests for confirmation of a diagnosis.

**Table 5-1**
**Differentiation of Iron Deficiency from Thalassemia Trait Using Routine Blood Counts**

| Index | Characteristic Score | |
|---|---|---|
| | Thalassemia | Iron Deficiency |
| $\dfrac{MCV}{RBC}$[15] | < 13 | > 14 |
| $\dfrac{MCH}{RBC}$[16] | < 4.4 | > 4.4 |
| $(MCV)^2$ MCH[17] | < 1530 | ? |
| MCV-(5 × Hb)-RBC-3.4[18] | (−) | (+) |

Determination of the free erythrocyte protoporphyrin (FEP) is another useful laboratory approach to differentiate the causes of microcytosis.[12] The red cell FEP is elevated in disorders affecting heme synthesis, such as iron deficiency or lead poisoning, and is normal in abnormalities of globin synthesis, such as thalassemia. Using a micro extraction procedure, Stockman and his coworkers showed that iron deficiency could be distinguished from $\beta$-thalassemia trait with an accuracy greater than 90%.[19] Koenig was 100% successful in distinguishing a small group of $\alpha$-thalassemia trait carriers from other individuals with iron deficiency.[20] A recently developed hematofluorometer utilizes front face fluorimetry to measure FEP levels directly on one to two drops of whole blood without the need for extraction or other chemical manipulation. The entire procedure requires no more than 30 seconds and thus lends itself to large scale screening efforts. The instrument has proven its utility in screening for lead poisoning[21] and, in our preliminary experience, it seems equally promising in the evaluation of microcytic blood samples for the presence of iron deficiency or thalassemia trait.

The definitive diagnosis of $\beta$-thalassemia trait requires quantitative determination of Hb $A_2$ and Hb F in suspect blood specimens. Because these procedures are relatively expensive and time-consuming, the various screening maneuvers previously discussed are of particular value in limiting the number of samples requiring additional testing. Alpha thalassemia is most readily recognized in the newborn period by the presence of Hb Bart's and microcytic red cells; by 6 months of age, Hb Bart's disappears and the hemoglobin electrophoresis thereafter is completely normal. Definitive diagnosis of α-thalassemia trait requires in vitro studies of globin chain synthesis or other procedures of similar complexity. The abnormality can be strongly suspected wherever familial microcytosis unresponsive to a therapeutic trial of iron is present.

## RESULTS OF CORD BLOOD SCREENING

The incidence of positive findings when cord blood specimens are screened for hemoglobinopathies varies greatly with the population surveyed (Table 5-2).[22-29] In the four surveys that were limited to black newborns, the overall incidence of abnormal hemoglobins was approximately 12%. In surveys primarily composed of other ethnic groups in the United States or England the incidence of abnormal hemoglobins was much lower (0.5% to 2.0%).

**Table 5-2**
**Cord Blood Hemoglobinopathy Screening Results**

| Location | No | Race | FA (nl) | FAS | FAC | FA Bart's | FS | FSC | FS(A) |
|---|---|---|---|---|---|---|---|---|---|
| Galveston[26] | 9224 | Black | 86.6 | 6.1 | 1.6 | 4.5 | 0.13 | 0.07 | 0.05 |
| New Haven[24] | 756 | Black | 86.9 | 8.1 | 2.1 | 1.8 | 0.79 | 0.13 | 0.1 |
| Houston[28] | 7500 | Black | 88.4 | 6.7 | 2.2 | 2.2 | 0.12 | 0.03 | — |
| Los Angeles[27] | 1205 | Black | 89.6 | 8.1 | 1.9 | — | 0.25 | 0.08 | — |
| Buffalo[23] | 2435 | 5–10% Black | 99.1 | 0.58 | 0.12 | — | | | |
| Manchester, Eng.[29] | 7691 | 3% Black | 99.4 | 0.38 | 0.09 | 0.07 | | | |
| Los Angeles[27] | 8048 | Spanish | 99.5 | 0.37 | 0.09 | — | | | |
| Los Angeles[27] | 1148 | Other | 98.0 | 1.31 | 0.61 | — | | | |
| Galveston[26] | 7006 | White | 98.9 | 0.06 | 0.06 | 0.86 | | | |

In the San Francisco Bay area, 1000 cord blood samples a month are obtained from nine hospitals (Table 5-3). The racial composition of the screened population is approximately 32% black, 12% Asian, and 56% white. Clinically significant hemoglobinopathies (SS, SC, β-S thalassemia, CC) have been identified in 28 black newborns, with an incidence of 1:250 in blacks. Several unusual heterozygous hemoglobinopathies of no clinical significance were identified in white newborns, and $\alpha$-thalassemia trait was frequently found in Asian newborns. The total cost of cord blood hemoglobinopathy screening, including materials, technical, and clerical effort, was approximately $3.50 per newborn. At present, therefore, the cost to detect a clinically significant hemoglobinopathy is $2625 per case; if screening were limited to blacks, the cost would fall to $875.

**Table 5-3**
**San Francisco Bay Area Cord Blood Screening Results (3/74–11/77)**

| Hgb pattern | Adult genotype | No. | Incidence (%) All ethnic groups | Blacks* |
|---|---|---|---|---|
| FA (normal) | AA | 21,424 | 95.0 | 88.0 |
| FAS | AS | 540 | 2.4 | 7.5 |
| FAC | AC | 195 | 0.86 | 2.7 |
| FS | SS (or S-$\beta^0$ thal) | 14 | 0.062 | 0.19 |
| FSC | SC | 7 | 0.031 | 0.10 |
| FSA | S-$\beta^+$ thal | 1 | 0.004 | 0.014 |
| FC | CC | 6 | 0.027 | 0.083 |
| FA Bart's | $\alpha$ thal trait | 307 | 1.4 | |
| FAS Bart's | AS-$\alpha$ thal | 7 | 0.031 | |
| FAC Bart's | AC-$\alpha$ thal | 2 | 0.009 | |
| FA Variant | — | 42 | 0.002 | |
| | | 22,545† | 100.0 | 100.0 |

*Estimated
† $\sim$ 7200 black

# GENETIC COUNSELING

Counseling is best conducted on an individual basis by a single counselor interacting with one client or family at a time. Doctors (for example, pediatric hematologists), nurse practitioners, lay genetic counselors, or social workers may be the most effective counselors, depending upon the needs of a particular client.

A prospective lay genetic counselor should first successfully complete a training program and thereafter participate in continuing education programs on genetic counseling for hemoglobinopathies. Necessary expert consultants should always be available for this counselor. Although lay genetic counselors have not been utilized extensively for genetic screening programs other than those dealing with sickle hemoglobinopathies, their acceptance by the community, their sensitivity to special problems of black counselees, and their ability to transmit information effectively would make them a valuable asset to many genetic screening programs that focus on other disorders. A lay genetic counselor is usually responsible for counseling individuals with sickle cell trait, Hb C trait, and $\beta$-thalassemia trait. The counselor may also be involved in discussions with sickle cell disease patients in conjunction with other members of the counseling team.

Detailed guidelines are available that describe appropriate counseling for individuals with Hb S, Hb C, and $\beta$-thalassemia trait.[5,30,31] Pamphlets, visual aids, and movies are widely available and are used to augment the counseling process. Clients benefit from written information which can be taken home for study and further reference. Specific biologic, genetic, and medical information should be reviewed, but it is also essential to deal with the psychosocial impact of the diagnosis on the patient. A counseling checklist will help prevent omission of important information during counseling, but the counselor must recognize that the direction of the counseling session should be determined by the counselee, who should feel free to address what he/she considers to be the most important questions first. Problems with self-concept resulting from the diagnosis of sickle cell trait should be identified and discussed. Misconceptions concerning the medical implications of sickle cell trait should be corrected. Counseling should be informative, not directive, and should be presented in a manner that encourages the counselee to be an active participant.

The risk of having a child with sickle cell disease should be clearly presented and the options for couples at risk reviewed. These include: (1) acceptance of the 1 in 4 risk of sickle cell disease associated with each pregnancy, (2) early termination of any unplanned pregnancy by abortion, (3) avoidance of all pregnancies by use of birth control techniques, (4) artificial insemination by a noncarrier donor, and (5) prenatal diagnosis and selective abortion of fetuses with proven sickle cell disease.[32] The last alternative, which requires intrauterine diagnosis, must be carefully explained and the advantages and disadvantages discussed. The couple being counseled should understand that the counselor's only interest is to provide information which can be used to plan a course of action.

When $\alpha$-thalassemia trait is diagnosed in a newborn, parents should be informed that this condition is associated with very mild anemia and microcytosis, and that $\alpha$-thalassemia trait is occasionally confused with iron deficiency. There is little impetus to provide genetic counseling to blacks with $\alpha$-thalassemia trait since hydrops fetalis, the disorder associated with homozygous $\alpha$ thalassemia in Orientals, has not been described in blacks and Hb H disease is uncommon.

## EDUCATION

A concerted effort to focus public attention on sickle cell disease has occurred during the last seven years. Workers in the field have been impressed by the lack of knowledge of these disorders in the general public and in the population at risk.[33,34] It is not surprising, therefore, that misconceptions about sickle cell disease have steadily spread. Physicians have been no exception. In a study by Kellon and Butler, many physicians were unaware of rare complications of sickle cell trait; others felt that sickle cell trait could be responsible for major complications.[35] Twenty percent of the physicians questioned felt that it was difficult to distinguish sickle cell trait from disease. Of the physicians who elected to do genetic counseling, 50% were unaware of the interaction between sickle cell trait and $\beta$-thalassemia trait.[35] All of these misconceptions clearly point out the importance of education in a sickle cell program.

Benefits may accrue from education regarding hemoglobin disorders directed toward any segment of the population. The major thrust in our program is directed toward (1) children in school settings at primary and secondary levels, (2) adults of childbearing age in the population at risk, (3) medical professionals and allied health personnel, and (4) personnel of public service agencies. It is beyond the scope of this chapter to provide an education manual for sickle cell disease; the topic is addressed comprehensively by a recent Department of Health, Education and Welfare publication.[5]

Several basic points should be included in most education programs:

1. The differences between sickle cell trait and disease.
2. An explanation of the origin and persistence of the sickle gene in the affected population.
3. A discussion of the genetics of sickle cell disease.
4. Treatment — medical, psychological, educational — present and future.
5. The availability of screening and counseling.

This agenda should be modified depending on the audience addressed.

Schools are natural settings in which to introduce concepts about sickle cell disease. Appropriate education units can be devised for children ages 8 through 12 and for adolescents through age 18. Programs have been developed in which sickle cell disease is discussed in the context of general science and health instruction. Groundwork is set by lessons on the structure and function of the human body — its circulatory system and the form and physiologic role of red blood cells.

Concepts about variability among different human population groups (their languages, physical appearance, and diseases which affect them, including genetic disorders) can be taught as an introduction to the fact that sickle cell disease occurs most often among blacks. Finally, the genetic aspects of sickle hemoglobinopathies can be incorporated readily into the teaching of elementary genetic concepts related to plants and animals. Other human diseases with a genetic basis may be covered in the same study unit.

Programs designed for teenagers should emphasize both the genetic aspects of sickle hemoglobinopathies and the concepts of probability. Older children are better equipped to understand probability, and the prospects of marriage and childbearing are real. Furthermore, the significance of sickle hemoglobinopathies to black adolescents can be appreciated best in the broader context of "planning for the future." To adolescents in general, and to minority teenagers in particular, planning is an alien concept. Among many teenagers, there is a global feeling of powerlessness, whether it is related to jobs or to having children — "Things just happen." The notion that one has a choice or can make informed decisions must be communicated, and questions related to sickle hemoglobinopathies made part of that framework. Similar approaches have been used in many general adolescent and family planning clinics, both excellent settings in which to provide sickle cell education.

An education program should be developed for the school health team,[36] incorporating basic facts about sickle cell disease and trait. Early signs of vaso-occlusive crises should be familiar to this team, as students who have sickle cell anemia may require the health team's support. The school health team should participate in the development of education programs, home bound or hospital based, for patients with prolonged illness. Recreational activities, although normal for many sickle cell patients, may have to be modified for others. In addition, the school health team can encourage special interest projects on sickle cell disease that will help patients cope with peer pressure.

Individuals of childbearing age are the primary target group among adult audiences. Adults may be reached through health education programs on the job, in community groups, such as churches, civic and social organizations, or in health settings, such as clinics (general medical, prenatal, family planning) and doctors' offices.

Medical and other health service personnel must be adequately informed about sickle cell disease and trait. Methods of diagnosis, treatment, and counseling should be incorporated into programs of continuing medical education. Quality assurance programs will help measure quality of medical care for patients with sickle cell disease and provide a baseline to begin education efforts. Education programs on sickle cell disease and trait for physicians and other health workers have been successfully organized by sickle cell organizations, post-graduate programs of hospitals, and local medical societies. Health professional schools must evaluate and update programs of medical genetics, including materials on sickle cell disease. Other public service personnel should also be informed about sickle cell disease. This group includes personnel of social service and vocational rehabilitation agencies who play key roles in providing a variety of support services for sickle cell patients. Many health departments and voluntary sickle cell organizations have conducted in-service training for these groups.

There is now a wealth of material available to the lay and professional publics on sickle cell disease. Numerous private and public organizations, including the federal government, have produced or sponsored a vast array of pamphlets, brochures, books, and audio-visual materials. Comprehensive lists and critiques of available materials may be obtained from the Sickle Cell Disease Division of the Health Services Administration.[37]

## EVALUATION

Evaluation of sickle cell screening programs usually has been based upon laboratory results. Since the major value of screening for hemoglobin traits is to be able to inform individuals about potential risks to their children, the validity of screening efforts should be judged by the effectiveness with which this information has been transmitted.[38] Unfortunately, the acquisition of knowledge from genetic counseling, when documented, has been poor.[39] Long-range studies of the impact of genetic counseling in sickle cell programs have not been performed. The success of counseling should be judged by the counselee's understanding and retention of information and not by the counselee's reproductive decisions.

Evaluation of the impact of education programs has also been incomplete. Numerous groups have made use of tests administered both before and after an education session to assess what audiences have learned; however, larger questions regarding how such programs affect behavior remain unanswered.

## SICKLE CELL TRAIT

An understanding of the nature of sickle cell trait is essential to provide accurate counseling to affected individuals and appropriate education to the community. The readiness of employers or insurance companies to respond to possible adverse effects of a genetic trait with discriminatory employment practices or selective increases in insurance rates makes it of the utmost importance to separate myth from reality clearly in analyzing any hypothetical effects of sickle cell trait on morbidity or mortality.

A number of observations attest to the benign nature of sickle trait in nearly all affected individuals. Unlike homozygotes with sickle cell disease, sickle trait carriers are not anemic and exhibit no abnormalities of red cell morphology. In the United States, there is no reduction in the frequency of the trait with advancing years, and thus no discernible influence on longevity.[40] In fact, in malarious regions of the world, possession of the sickle trait may actually increase longevity by providing partial protection from the lethal consequences of falciparum malaria.[41] The frequency of sickle trait in professional football players and track athletes is the same as that found in the general population.[42] No untoward effects were noted by sickle cell trait carriers who competed in the Mexico City Olympic Games at an altitude of 7000 feet.[43] Thus, at least in well-conditioned athletes, extreme physical exertion, even at high altitude, seems completely innocuous for sickle cell heterozygotes. The frequency of pyelonephritis during pregnancy is roughly twofold greater in females with sickle trait than in blacks with a normal hemoglobin genotype[44]; however, there are no other discernible adverse effects of sickle cell trait during pregnancy on either mother or fetus.[44,45,46] On the contrary, there is evidence in malarious regions of the world that both male and female sickle cell heterozygotes exhibit increased fertility.[47]

Although these observations are reassuring, they do not establish that the sickle trait is totally harmless under all circumstances. These conclusions have been challenged. Sporadic examples of infarctive episodes resembling those typical of sickle cell disease have also been reported in sickle cell trait. As in sickle cell disease, these episodes of infarction may involve virtually any organ system.[48,49] Rarely, there have been reports of sudden death in individuals with sickle trait in whom obvious causes of death other than the hemoglobinopathy could not be discovered.[50] By and large, most such reports do not establish a clear cause-and-effect relationship between sickle trait and infarction. Often, the frequency of the type of infarction in the normal black population is either unknown or is similar to that reported for sickle heterozygotes.[51] Furthermore, particularly in earlier reports, a rigorous hematologic documentation of the true hemoglobin genotype is lacking and some patients may have had sickle thalassemia or another clinically more severe hemoglobinopathy. In addition, when a careful search is made, another plausible cause for the described abnormality can often be found. For example, Nagpal and his associates[52] recently described seven sickle cell trait patients who exhibited vasoproliferative retinopathy indistinguishable from that characteristic of sickle cell disease; however, in all seven there was some evidence of an associated systemic disease, such as diabetes or syphilis. Although only conjectural at this point, it remains possible that sickle trait, in an unknown way, may interact with a coexistent systemic disease to increase the likelihood of certain manifestations of the disease.[52]

The rarity of apparent clinical manifestations of sickle cell trait suggests that unusual conditions are required for their appearance. This is in keeping with in vitro observations on sickle trait blood which indicate that sickling cannot be induced unless the $PO_2$ is reduced to about 15 mm Hg, a level incompatible with life.[49] Physical conditions in certain organs, however, may allow sickling even of Hb AS red cells. For example, in the kidney, acidosis, hypertonicity, and hypoxia may combine to initiate sickling.[53] Renal manifestations of sickling, such as hyposthenuria and hematuria, are relatively common in sickle trait. As many as 70% of affected individuals exhibit hyposthenuria.[53] Approximately 4% of heterozygotes will have at least one episode of gross hematuria during their lifetime.[49] However, it should be emphasized that such episodes are rarely, if ever, fatal and usually occur in young adults rather than in children. Their chief importance lies in the need to distinguish them from more serious causes of hematuria.

The possibility that flying might be dangerous to individuals with sickle trait was raised in the 1940's and 1950's by a series of case reports, 23 in all, describing splenic infarction during flight in unpressurized aircraft. However, two of these subjects were not studied by hemoglobin electrophoresis and, of the remainder, seven actually had either Hb SC disease or Hb S-$\beta$ thalassemia, and eight had negative or equivocal sickle preparations. Thus, only six patients actually fulfilled the basic laboratory criteria for the diagnosis of sickle trait.[51] The incidence of sickle trait in black combat pilots during World War II was no different than that of the general population of blacks, suggesting that possession of the trait placed them at no particular disadvantage.[51] A recent report from Ghana describes three military pilots belatedly found to have the sickle trait after logging hundreds of hours of flying time in both pressurized and unpressurized aircraft, at altitudes that at times exceeded 10,000 feet, without incident.[54] Clearly, exposure to such altitudes need not be injurious to sickle cell heterozygotes. Since most commercial air travel takes place in pressurized aircraft where the effective cabin altitude is equivalent, at most, to a ground elevation of 7000 to 8000 feet, there would seem to be no particular hazard involved for sickle trait carriers. In fact, sickling episodes are said never to have been reported in sickle heterozygotes traveling in pressurized aircraft.[43]

General anesthesia, if attended by hypoxia, represents another potential hazard for sickle cell trait carriers. Although several individual case reports describe infarction and even death associated with general anesthesia, surveys of larger numbers of patients have failed to establish a clear-cut special risk of anesthesia for sickle heterozygotes.[51,55,56] Nevertheless, as would be true for any patient, it is important to stress avoidance of hypoxia during procedures requiring anesthesia. Mountain climbing and scuba diving are other situations where the risk of hypoxia is present, but there is no recorded information about the experiences of sickle trait individuals with these particular stresses.

## REFERENCES

1. Lappe, M., Gustafson, J.M., and Roblin, R. Ethical and social issues in screening for genetic disease. *N. Engl. J. Med.* 286:1129, 1972.

2. Powledge, T.M. Genetic screening as a political and social development. *Birth Defects* 10:25, 1974.

3. Whitten, C.F. Sickle-cell programming—An imperiled promise. *N. Engl. J. Med.* 288:318, 1973.

4. California State Senate Bill No. 240, 1977.

5. Department of Health, Education, and Welfare. *Model Protocols for Sickle Cell Counseling and Education.* DHEW Publication No. (HSA) 77-5122. Washington, Department of Health, Education and Welfare, April 5, 1977.

6. Giorgio, A.J., and Boggs, D.R. Large scale screening for hemoglobinopathies, utilizing electrophoresis. *Am. J. Public Health* 64:993–994, 1974.

7. California State Ad Hoc Sickle Cell Advisory Committee, 1977.

8. Schmidt, R.M. Laboratory diagnosis of hemoglobinopathies. *JAMA* 224:1276–1280, 1973.

9. Schmidt, R.M., and Wilson, S.M. Standardization in detection of abnormal hemoglobins. *JAMA* 225:1225–1230, 1973.

10. Asakura, T., Segal, M.E., and Schwartz, E. A rapid test for sickle hemoglobin. *JAMA* 233:156–157, 1975.

11. Pearson, H.A., O'Brien, R.T., and McIntosh, S. Screening for thalassemia trait by electronic measurement of mean corpuscular volume. *N. Engl. J. Med.* 288:351–353, 1973.

12. Dallman, P.R. New approaches to screening for iron deficiency. *J. Pediatr.* 90:678–681, 1977.

13. Cazzavillan, M., Barbui, T., Franchi, F., et al. Comparison of Price-Jones curves obtained with an electronic corpuscle counter in normal subjects and in patients with thalassemia and iron deficiency. *Haemotologia (Budap)* 7:333–337, 1973.

14. Klee, G.G., Fairbanks, V.F., Pierre, R.V., et al. Routine erythrocyte measurements in diagnosis of iron-deficiency anemia and thalassemia minor. *Am. J. Clin. Pathol.* 66:870, 1976.

15. Mentzer, W.C. Differentiation of iron deficiency from thalassemia trait. *Lancet* April 21, 1973, p. 882.

16. Srivastava, P.C., and Bevington, J.M. Iron deficiency and/or thalassemia trait. *Lancet* April 14, 1973, p. 832.

17. Shine, I., and Lal, S. A strategy to detect thalassemia minor. *Lancet* March 26, 1977, pp. 693–694.

18. England, J.M., and Fraser, P.M. Differentiation of iron deficiency from thalassemia trait by routine blood-count. *Lancet* March 3, 1973, pp. 449–452.

19. Stockman, J.A., Weiner, L.S., Simon, G.E., et al. The measurement of free erythrocyte porphyrin (FEP) as a simple means of distinguishing iron deficiency from beta-thalassemia trait in subjects with microcytosis. *J. Lab. Clin. Med.* 85:113–119, 1975.

20. Koenig, H.M., Lightsey, A.L., and Schanberger, J.E. The micromeasurement of free erythrocyte protoporphyrin as a means of differentiating alpha thalassemia trait from iron deficiency anemia. *J. Pediatr.* 86:539–541, 1975.

21. Klein, R., Usher, P., and Madigan, P. Experience with a direct reading dedicated fluorometer for determination of erythrocyte protoporphyrin. *Pediatr. Res.* 10:720–721, 1976.

22. Huntsman, R.G., Metters, J.S., and Yawson, G.I. The diagnosis of sickle cell disease in the newborn infant. *J. Pediatr.* 80:279, 1972.

23. Garrick, M.D., Dembure, P., and Guthrie, R. Sickle cell anemia and other hemoglobinopathies. *N. Engl. J. Med.* 288:1265, 1973.

24. Pearson, H.A., O'Brien, R.T., McIntosh, S., et al. Routine screening of umbilical cord blood for sickle cell diseases. *JAMA* 227:420, 1974.

25. Schneider, R.G., Hosty, T.S., Tomlin, G., et al. Identification of hemoglobins and hemoglobinopathies by electrophoresis on cellulose acetate plates impregnated with citrate agar. *Clin. Chem.* 20:74, 1974.

26. Schneider, R.G., Haggard, M.E., Gustavson, L.P., et al. Genetic haemoglobin abnormalities in about 9000 black and 7000 white newborns. *Br. J. Haematol.* 28:515, 1974.

27. Powars, D., Schroeder, W.A., and White, L. Rapid diagnosis of sickle cell disease at birth by microcolumn chromatography. *Pediatrics* 55:630, 1975.

28. Sexauer, C.L., Graham, H.L., Starling, K.A., et al. A test for abnormal hemoglobins in umbilical cord blood. *Am. J. Dis. Child.* 130:805, 1976.

29. Evans, L.I.K., and Blair, V.M. Neonatal screening for haemoglobinopathy. *Arch. Dis. Child.* 51:127, 1976.

30. Headings, V., and Fielding, J. Guidelines for counseling young adults with sickle cell trait. *Am. J. Public Health* 65:819, 1975.

31. Schmidt, R.M. Hemoglobinopathy screening: Approaches to diagnosis, education and counseling. *Am. J. Public Health* 64:799, 1974.

32. Scott, R.B., and Castro, O.C. *Screening for Early Diagnosis of Abnormal Hemoglobins.* Washington, D.C.: Howard University, Center for Sickle Cell Disease, 1977.

33. Lane, J.C., and Scott, R.B. Awareness of sickle cell anemia among Negroes in Richmond, Virginia. *Public Health Rep.* 84:949, 1969.

34. Binder, R.A., and Jones, S.R. Prevalence and awareness of sickle cell hemoglobin in a military population. *JAMA* 214:909–911, 1970.

35. Kellon, D.B., and Butler, E. Physician attitudes about sickle cell disease and sickle cell trait. *JAMA* 227:71, 1974.

36. Walker, J.E. What the school health team should know about sickle cell anemia. *J. Sch. Health* 45:149, 1975.

37. Sickle Cell Disease Program, Bureau of Community Health Services, Rockville, Maryland.

38. Leonard, C.O., Chase, G.A., and Childs, B. Genetic counseling: A consumer's view. *N. Engl. J. Med.* 287:433, 1972.

39. Hecht, F., and Halmes, L.B. What we don't know about genetic counseling. *N. Engl. J. Med.* 287:433, 1972.

40. Petrakis, N.L., Wiesenfeld, S.L., Sams, B.J., et al. Prevalence of sickle-cell trait and glucose-6-phosphate dehydrogenase deficiency. *N. Engl. J. Med.* 282:767–770, 1970.

41. Luzzatto, L., Nwachuku-Jarrett, E.S., and Reddy, S. Increased sickling of parasitised erythrocytes as mechanism of resistance against malaria in the sickle-cell trait. *Lancet* February 14, 1970, pp. 319–321.

42. Petrakis, N.L. Sickle-cell disease. *Lancet* December 7, 1974, pp. 1368–1369.

43. Green, R.L., Huntsman, R.G., and Serjeant, G.R. The sickle-cell and altitude. *Br. Med. J.* 4:593–595, 1971.

44. Whalley, P.J., Pritchard, J.A., and Richards, J.R. Sickle cell trait and pregnancy. *JAMA* 186:1132–1135, 1953.

45. Pearson, H.A., and Vaughan, E.O. Lack of influence of sickle cell trait on fertility and successful pregnancy. *Am. J. Obstet. Gynecol.* 105:203–205, 1969.

46. DeLamerens, S.A., Lopez-Duran, A., and Morrison, J.C. The offspring of patients with hemoglobin S gene. *South. Med. J.* 65:537–539, 1972.

47. Eaton, J.W., and Mucha, J.I. Increased fertility in males with the sickle cell trait? *Nature* 231:456–457, 1971.

48. Smith, W.B., Mentzer, W.C., and Dallman, P.R. Identifying and counseling patients with sickle trait. *Calif. Med.* 119:1–7, 1973.

49. Harris, J.W., and Kellermeyer, R.W. *The Red Cell.* 2nd Ed. Cambridge: Harvard University Press, 1970, pp. 168–202.

50. Jones, S.R., Binder, R.A., and Donowho, E.M. Sudden death in sickle cell trait. *N. Engl. J. Med.* 282:323–325, 1970.

51. Bristow, L.R. The myth of sickle cell trait. *West. J. Med.* 121:77–82, 1974.

52. Nagpal, K.C., Asdourian, G.K., Patrianakos, D., et al. Proliferative retinopathy in sickle cell trait. *Arch. Intern. Med.* 137:325, 328, 1977.

53. Harrow, B.R., Sloane, J.A., and Liebman, N.C. Roentgenologic demonstration of renal papillary necrosis in sickle-cell trait. *N. Engl. J. Med.* 969–976, 1963.

54. Djabanor, F.F.T. Three military pilots with the sickle-cell trait. *Trop. Doct.* 7:3–5, 1977.

55. McCurdy, P.R., Sickle cell trait. *Am. Fam. Physician* 10:141–146, 1974.

56. Atlas, S.A., The sickle cell trait and surgical complications. *JAMA* 229:1078–1080, 1974.

# 6 Prenatal Diagnosis of Hemoglobinopathies*

Blanche P. Alter, M.D.

Detection of hemoglobinopathies during intrauterine develop-ment is now possible because of the clinical application of research involving the biochemistry and molecular biology of hemoglobin regulation. The techniques that are available for the evaluation of hemoglobin and globin chain synthesis in very small amounts of material have made it possible to document the types and relative amounts of hemoglobin produced by normal human fetuses and to demonstrate the in utero expression of hemoglobinopathies. In addi-tion, obstetricians have developed methods for the acquisition of fetal

*Prenatal diagnosis of hemoglobinopathies is a reality because of the zeal and foresight of Dr. David G. Nathan. I am grateful to him for his support and enthusiasm. I am indebted to my colleagues who provided samples of fetal blood from the cases reported here: Drs. C. Bernadette Modell, Denys Fairweather, John C. Hobbins, Maurice J. Mahoney, Fredric D. Frigoletto, Tracy B. Perry, and Ronald J. Benzie. A vital impetus to this field has come from the work of Drs. Y.W. Kan and M.S. Golbus, and Ms. A.M. Dozy. Excellent technical assistance was provided by Ms. R.G. Gorer, J.B. Metzger, and A.S. Sherman. The work was supported by NIH grant AM-15322, National Foundation-March of Dimes grant 1-277, and NIH Career Development Award HL-00177.

blood during pregnancy. However, since small samples of placental blood are often contaminated with maternal red cells, it has been necessary to develop methods using several properties which distinguish fetal from adult erythrocytes to enrich such samples for their fetal component.

The hemoglobinopathies that have been evaluated include sickle cell disorders and $\beta$ and $\alpha$ thalassemias. Although the course of sickle cell disease varies, it is associated with significant morbidity and increased early mortality; some families wish to have children who do not have the condition. Homozygous $\beta$ thalassemia (thalassemia major, Cooley's anemia) generally has more marked morbidity and significant mortality by early adulthood. The outlook for these patients is improving with the advent of programs for frequent transfusions and iron chelation; nevertheless, many families still do not wish to have affected children. Infants with homozygous $\alpha$ thalassemia (Hb Bart's $(\gamma_4)$, hydrops fetalis) do not survive; they are usually stillborn at 30 to 36 weeks gestation. Unfortunately, approximately half of the mothers develop toxemia when carrying such infants.[1] Thus, prenatal detection of this condition would also be useful.

## HEMOGLOBIN DEVELOPMENT

Intrauterine detection of hemoglobinopathies is based on information about the hemoglobin types and amounts found in normal human development. The hemoglobins are composed of tetramers of various globin chains, each the product of a different globin structural gene (Figure 6-1). The gene (or genes) for $\alpha$ chains is located on chromosome 16[2]; it is probable that the embryonic $\alpha$-like gene, $\zeta$, is also on that chromosome. The non-$\alpha$ genes, $\gamma$, $\delta$, and $\beta$, are on chromosome 11,[3] and $\epsilon$ is presumably syntenic to those genes.

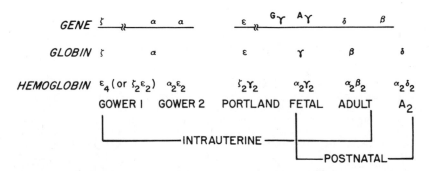

**Figure 6-1.** Hemoglobins during human development. The order of the genes on the non-$\alpha$ chromosome is probably $\gamma$, $\delta$, $\beta$.

The first hemoglobins produced by human fetuses are the embryonic proteins, Gower 1 and Gower 2.[4] Gower 1 was initially thought to be $\varepsilon_4$. Recently it was suggested that Gower 1 is actually $\zeta_2\varepsilon_2$,[5] although this conclusion is not shared by all.[6] Gower 2 is $\alpha_2\varepsilon_2$. Hemoglobin Portland, $\zeta_2\gamma_2$, is a third embryonic hemoglobin.[7-9] The proportion of these embryonic hemoglobins decreases by ten weeks. The predominant hemoglobin during the rest of intrauterine development is fetal hemoglobin ($\alpha_2\gamma_2$), although small amounts of adult hemoglobin ($\alpha_2\beta_2$) also begin to accumulate. Shortly after birth adult hemoglobin predominates and the minor adult tetramer, Hb $A_2$ ($\alpha_2\delta_2$), appears. The time course of the appearances and disappearances of the relevant globin chains, which was derived from electrophoreses of hemoglobins or globin chains, is shown in Figure 6-2.

A more sensitive method for the analysis of hemoglobin development involves the measurement of incorporation of radioactive amino acids into newly synthesized globin chains by erythroblasts and reticulocytes. This allows analysis of very tiny samples of material. With these methods, several groups have detected the synthesis of Hb A, or of $\beta$ chains, in very early fetuses: 5 weeks,[10] 6 weeks,[11] 7 weeks,[12] 11 weeks,[13] and 13 weeks.[14] In addition, the expression of the gene for sickle globin, $\beta^s$, has also been detected during in utero development.[10,15,16,17]

Two groups of investigators suggested that the biosynthetic techniques mentioned above could be employed to establish the

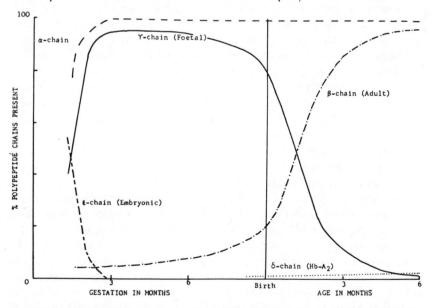

**Figure 6-2.** Development of human hemoglobin chains. [From E.R. Huehns et al.[4]]

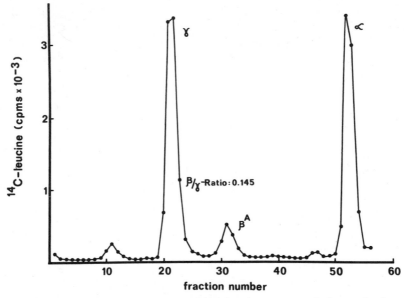

**Figure 6-3.** CM-cellulose chromatogram of globin from a 20-week fetus. Blood was labeled with $^{14}$C-leucine.

precise pattern of hemoglobin or globin synthesis in fetuses of various gestational ages and could then be used for the prenatal detection of hemoglobinopathies. Hollenberg et al[18] separated hemoglobin tetramers by ion exchange chromatography. Kan et al[16] were concerned about the possibility of subunit exchange and therefore chose to employ globin chain analysis in urea on carboxymethylcellulose columns (Figure 6-3), a method first described by Clegg et al.[19] The non-$\alpha$ chains, $\gamma$ (of fetal hemoglobin) and $\beta$ (of adult hemoglobin), are clearly separated. With this system, the $\beta^s$ chains of sickle hemoglobin would appear between the normal $\beta$ and the $\alpha$ chains. The production of $\beta$ chains rises during gestation, while there is a reciprocal fall of $\gamma$ chain synthesis. Figure 6-4 shows the correlation of the $\beta/\gamma$ synthetic ratio with gestational age in blood obtained from 40 normal fetuses at 5 to 23 weeks gestation.[20] A similar correlation of percent Hb A synthesis was obtained by Kazazian and Woodhead.[12]

In utero detection of $\beta$ thalassemia requires demonstration of total absence of $\beta$ chain synthesis ($\beta^0$ thalassemia) or of a marked reduction in the small amount of $\beta$ chain seen in normal fetuses ($\beta^+$ thalassemia). Chang et al[21] studied blood obtained from abortuses from pregnancies terminated because the fetuses were known to be at risk for $\beta$ thalassemia. In two cases, the $\beta/\gamma$ ratios were approximately half the value expected for each gestational age, while in one fetus the ratio was close to zero. The former were presumed to have had $\beta$-thalassemia trait, while the latter was thought to be homozygous for $\beta$

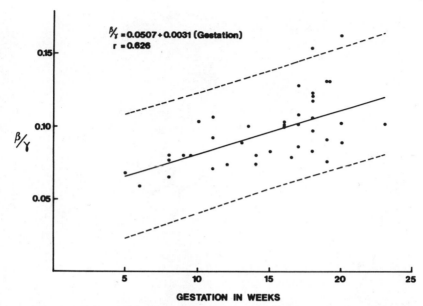

**Figure 6-4.** Correlation of β/γ synthetic ratios and gestational ages. ●: synthetic ratio in each of 40 normal fetuses. —: mean, and –: 95% confidence interval, derived by linear regression analysis by the least squares method.

thalassemia. The β-thalassemia genes were expressed in utero and could be detected by the methods employed.

## TECHNIQUES FOR OBTAINING FETAL BLOOD

Since it had been shown that fetal blood could be used to distinguish normal fetuses from those with hemoglobinopathies, techniques were sought for obtaining fetal blood during ongoing pregnancies. Frigoletto[16] had suggested that fetal blood could be obtained from the placenta during the midtrimester. The practicality of this suggestion was confirmed by Kan and his coworkers,[22,23] who aspirated fetal blood by transabdominal insertion of a needle into the anterior placenta.

Subsequently, Valenti[24] described the use of an instrument, now called a fetoscope, to obtain fetal blood under direct visualization. Hobbins and Mahoney[25,26] adapted a Dyonics arthroscope (Dyonics Instrument Co., Woburn, Massachusetts) by the addition of a sidearm cannula through which a long 27-gauge needle can be passed to perform a placental venipuncture. Hobbins and Mahoney,[25,26] Patrick et al,[27] and Benzie and Doran[28] demonstrated the usefulness of this instrument for fetal blood sampling.

The procedure is as follows: Ultrasound examination is employed to determine the gestational age of the fetus according to the

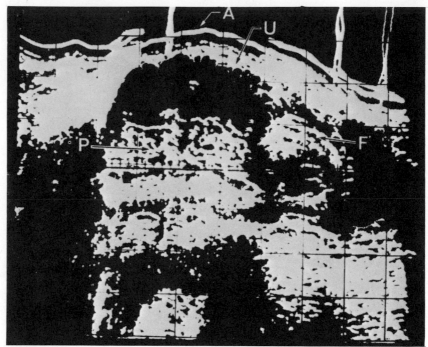

**Figure 6-5.** Ultrasound pattern at 20 weeks gestation. A. Maternal abdominal wall. U. Uterine wall. P. Placenta. F. Fetus. [Photograph by courtesy of John C. Hobbins, M.D.]

biparietal diameter[29] and to locate the placenta. Figure 6-5 shows such an ultrasound pattern, in which the placenta is posterior. Figure 6-6 shows the performance of fetoscopy. The fetus and placenta are observed directly and a fetal blood vessel is located on the surface of the placenta. The needle in the fetoscope sidearm is used to perform a fetal vessel venipuncture. A small sample of fetal blood is obtained mixed in amniotic fluid. Such samples often contain pure fetal blood, although at times there is a mixture of fetal and maternal cells. Chang et al[31] demonstrated that samples obtained in this way could be used for studies of globin chain synthesis. The amount of fetal blood loss from fetoscopy was less than 5% of the fetal blood volume in most cases.[26] This method can be used to obtain blood from anterior placentas[32] as well as posterior ones.

## ENRICHMENT FOR FETAL BLOOD

### Maternal Transfusion

Blood samples obtained by placental aspiration or by fetoscopy do not always contain pure fetal cells, since fetal vessels are small

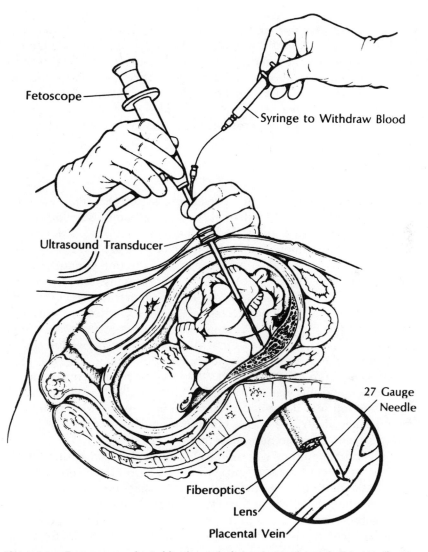

Fetoscope

Syringe to Withdraw Blood

Ultrasound Transducer

27 Gauge
Needle

Fiberoptics

Lens

Placental Vein

**Figure 6-6.** Fetoscopy to obtain blood sample from placental vessel. [From Nadler.[30]]

compared to the maternal lacunae in the placenta. Several approaches have been used with such mixed specimens. In the first place, fetal reticulocytes are as much as 50- to 500-fold more active than blood from a normal adult in the biosynthesis of globin.[10] However, the reticulocyte counts of pregnant women with sickle or thalassemia traits are higher than those of normal pregnant women,[33,34,35] which to some extent cancels the biosynthetic advantage.

In practice, samples of mixed fetal-maternal blood which contain more than 50% fetal cells can be used without any enrichment procedures. Because some samples have less than 50% fetal cells, Modell[36] pointed out that the maternal reticulocytes can be suppressed by transfusion of the mother 7 to 14 days before the planned fetal blood sampling. The mother is given sufficient packed red cells to raise her hemoglobin above 14 g/dl; four units are required usually. In order to decrease the risks for hepatitis or cytomegalovirus, frozen blood or white-cell-free blood more than four days old is used. With this method, accurate diagnoses have been made on samples with less than 5% fetal cells.[36]

## Mathematical Techniques

In another approach to correction of mixed fetal-maternal samples, described by Cividalli et al,[10] placental samples are diluted in known proportions of pure maternal blood, incubations are done, and the $\beta/\gamma$ ratios determined. The $\beta/\gamma$ ratios are plotted against $1 + b$, where b is the ratio of maternal to placental cells. The line connecting the points is extrapolated to $(1 + b) = 0$, which represents the $\beta/\gamma$ ratio of pure fetal blood. Figure 6-7 shows a study in which the mixed placental sample had 6% fetal blood. Placental blood was mixed at one part placental to one part maternal, and one placental to three maternal. The $\beta/\gamma$ ratio rose as the maternal $\beta$ chain synthesis became more prominent in the mixtures. The extrapolation is shown; the corrected $\beta/\gamma$ ratio was zero. This fetus was thought to have homozygous $\beta$ thalassemia; and this was confirmed at abortion. Mathematical proof of this method was described by the authors,[10] who pointed out the method failed if $\beta/\gamma$ was above 0.5 in the placental sample or if this ratio was below 5 in the pure maternal blood.

Still another method was used by Chang et al,[21] who evaluated the $\beta/\gamma$ ratios of placental and of pure maternal blood from separate but identical incubations. The specific activity (counts per minute per mg) of each globin chain was determined, and the maternal contribution was thereby subtracted. Use of this method required a mixed placental sample sufficiently large ($> 5$ mg) to analyze by chromatography without the addition of carrier protein. This method assumes the identity of intracellular leucine pools and leucine transport mechanisms in fetal and maternal red cells. This assumption may not be valid, since fetal and adult erythrocytes are very different in size (mean cell volume 140 $\mu^3$ versus 80 $\mu^3$) and hemoglobin content (mean cell hemoglobin 44 pg versus 34 pg).[37] Thus, the specific activity of intracellular leucine may differ in the two cell types.

## Immunologic Techniques

In addition to the mathematical techniques described above, fetal and adult cells can be separated by immunologic means. Fetal cells have i antigen on their membranes, while adult cells have I. Kan et al[38] used antiserum to i to agglutinate fetal cells. Artificial mixtures of 5% or 10% fetal cells were enriched to 30% to 85%. Recovery of fetal

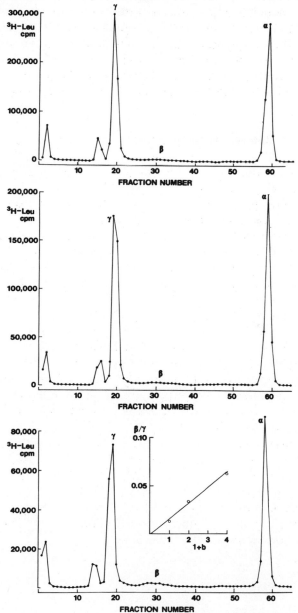

**Figure 6-7.** CM-cellulose chromatograms of globin from a 17-week fetus. Placental blood which was 6% fetal (top panel) was diluted in one part (middle panel) and three parts (bottom panel) maternal blood. Incubations were in ³H-leucine. Insert shows β/γ versus 1 + b. Extrapolation indicates homozygous β-thalassemia in the fetus.

cells was approximately 25%. However, anti-i is a weak agglutinating agent at 20°C and cross-reacts with adult cells at lower temperatures. Samples with less than 5% fetal cells fail to provide reliable fetal cell recovery or enrichment. Kan has reported some success with samples containing at least 5% fetal cells.[39] Goossens et al[40] took the opposite approach. They used anti-I to agglutinate adult cells and were able to enrich from 1% to 5% fetal blood up to 30% to 50% fetal cells; the recovery was not stated. Thus, fetal and maternal reticulocytes may be separated because of differences in their membrane antigens.

## Hemolysis of Maternal Reticulocytes

Fetal and adult erythrocytes also differ in their content of carbonic anhydrase, which can be employed for differential hemolysis. Fetal cells have low activities of this enzyme, and the small activity that is present can be further inhibited by acetazolamide. When cells are incubated in $NH_4Cl$ and $NH_4HCO_3$, adult cells take up $CO_2$ and produce $HCO_3^-$, which is exchanged for $Cl^-$. $NH_3$ enters the cell, becomes $NH_4^+$, and is trapped by the $Cl^-$. Water then enters the cell, which eventually bursts. In the absence of carbonic anhydrase, as in fetal cells, this production of $HCO_3^-$ occurs very slowly. Fetal cells are therefore relatively resistant to this type of hemolysis. This method of differential osmotic hemolysis was described by Boyer et al[41] and termed the Ørskov effect, after the chemist who originally proposed the mechanism. Alter et al[42] utilized this method and enriched mixed fetal-adult samples that were only 2.5% fetal by several hundred-fold. Therefore, selective hemolysis of maternal reticulocytes provides another method for dealing with placental samples in which the fetal component is below 5%.

Thus, many approaches have been taken to solve the problem of mixed fetal-maternal blood samples. These are based on mathematical, biochemical, and immunologic principles. Use of some of these, alone or in combination, may obviate the need for suppression of maternal reticulocytes by transfusion. However, the most important approach is obstetric. If a good sample of fetal blood can be obtained, cell separation techniques become unnecessary.

## CLINICAL APPLICATION

More than 500 cases have now been studied for hemoglobinopathies in ongoing pregnancies. The largest numbers of cases have been evaluated in San Francisco,[39,43-46] and in Boston, London, and New Haven.[20,36,47,48] The most active centers now are Athens and

Sardinia, Italy. A few cases have been studied in Israel,[49] and centers are being established in Melbourne, Munich, and Paris. Most of the fetuses studied so far have been at risk for $\beta$ thalassemia, although 10% of the studies have been for sickle cell disorders. Samples have been obtained by fetoscopy and by placental aspiration. The relative yield of fetal blood is higher with fetoscopy (Figure 6-8), but pure fetal blood can be obtained with either method. When placental aspiration is used, the fetal percentage is similar whether the placenta is anterior or posterior.[39,46] Fetoscopy also can be used for anterior or posterior placentas, although it is easier in the latter situation.

In the reported cases, several of the methods discussed above were employed to deal with impure samples. The Boston-New Haven-London collaborative cases have had corrected $\beta/\gamma$ ratios determined by mathematical methods (extrapolation and specific activity), while the San Francisco group has utilized agglutination with anti-i. In 54 cases that we have analyzed, 40 mothers received prior transfusions to suppress reticulocyte globin synthesis. In retrospect, this was helpful in 15, in whom the best samples contained less than 50% fetal blood. Data were also corrected by specific activity and/or extrapolation methods, in order to provide accurate diagnoses. In 24 cases reported by the San Francisco group,[46] seven samples were enriched for fetal cells by selective agglutination with anti-i. This represents a similar proportion of cases. The San Francisco group also introduced the use of

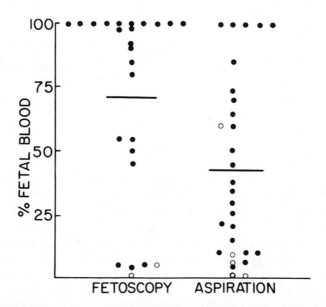

**Figure 6-8.** Percent fetal blood obtained by fetoscopy and by placental aspiration. ●: adequate samples. O: inadequate samples, in cases where mothers were not transfused, or in one case with laboratory technical problems.

the Coulter particle size analyzer (Coulter Electronics Co., Hialeah, Florida). This instrument provides immediate determination of the proportion of fetal cells in a sample, since fetal cells are larger than maternal cells. Despite all these procedures, nondiagnostic samples have been obtained in several cases (7 out of 54 cases in our series, 3 out of 29 cases reported by Kan[39]). Future research must develop methods for handling very small and impure samples.

Examples of CMC-chromatograms of globin from a normal fetus, from one with sickle trait, and from one with sickle cell disease are shown in Figure 6-9. All samples contained pure fetal blood. In the normal 21-week fetus (Figure 6-9, top), the $\beta/\gamma$ synthetic ratio was 0.10, within the normal limits. In the study from an 18-week fetus shown in the middle panel, $\beta^A/\gamma$ was 0.056 and $\beta^S/\gamma$ was 0.047; thus, this fetus had sickle cell trait. In two other fetuses with sickle trait (one studied in utero and one studied following spontaneous abortion), $\beta^A/\gamma$ was 0.026 and 0.062, and $\beta^S/\gamma$ was 0.017 and 0.035. In all cases of sickle trait studied by us or others, $\beta^A$ or Hb A synthesis has exceeded that of $\beta^S$ or Hb S. This feature distinguishes such fetuses from those with sickle/thalassemia.[50] The bottom panel of Figure 6-9 depicts the study of a 19-week fetus with sickle cell disease; $\beta^S/\gamma$ was 0.057, and there was no $\beta^A$ synthesis. In two other fetuses who were homozygous for $\beta^S$, $\beta^S/\gamma$ was 0.054 and 0.076. Two cases reported by Kan et al[39,45] had $\beta^S/\gamma$ ratios of 0.05 and 0.07. These ratios are less than the $\beta/\gamma$ values expected for normal fetuses at similar gestational ages. The low proportion of $\beta^S$ could be due to decreased synthesis of that $\beta$ chain or to increased $\beta^S$ proteolysis.

In the two large series reported in the literature,[20,46] 11 fetuses were studied because they were at risk for sickle cell disease or sickle/thalassemia. Adequate samples were obtained in eight. Two of those had sickle trait. Five were diagnosed prenatally as sickle cell disease and were confirmed at abortion. In one case, the prenatal impression was sickle trait, but the infant turned out to have the disease. There were multiple technical problems with that assay,[47] which subsequently have been corrected.

Many more cases have been evaluated because of the risk for thalassemia (Figure 6-10). The top panel is the same normal fetus as shown in Figure 6-9. The middle panel represents the study of a sample with 99% fetal blood from a 19-week fetus; $\beta/\gamma = 0.043$, which indicates that this fetus had $\beta$-thalassemia trait. The bottom panel shows the study of 6% fetal blood, obtained at 17 weeks. This is the same case for which the extrapolation data are shown in Figure 6-7. The uncorrected $\beta/\gamma$ ratio was 0.013; it corrected to zero by extrapolation, as well as by the specific activity method. This mother had been

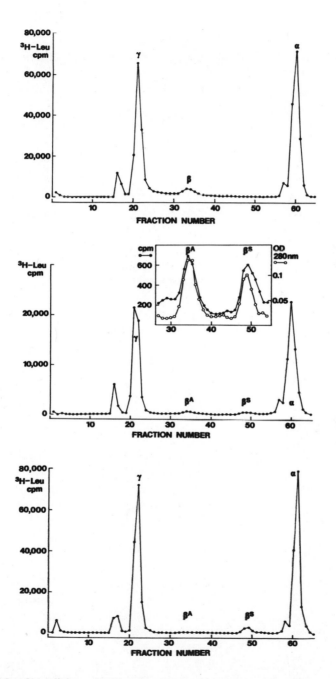

**Figure 6-9.** CM-cellulose chromatograms from three fetuses. All samples were 100% fetal blood. ●: ³H-leucine counts per minute. O: $A_{280}$ of carrier globin. Top: normal. Middle: sickle trait. Bottom: sickle cell disease.

transfused previously, which significantly reduced globin chain synthesis by her reticulocytes. The fetus was diagnosed as homozygous for β thalassemia.

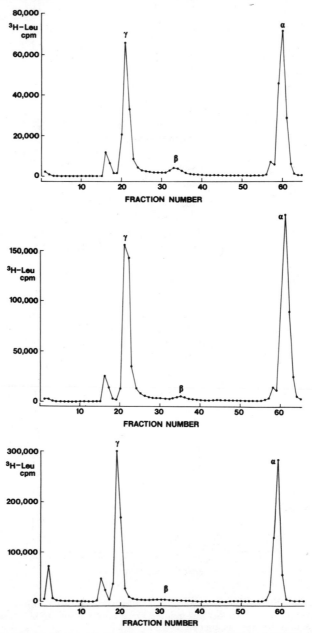

**Figure 6-10.** CM-cellulose chromatograms from three fetuses. Samples labeled with ³H-leucine. Top: normal. Middle: β-thalassemia trait. Bottom: homozygous β thalassemia.

Figures 6-11 and 6-12 summarize the $\beta/\gamma$ ratios in 41 fetuses at risk for $\beta$ thalassemia and compare them with normal values. Final diagnoses are not available in six cases not yet delivered and two in which follow-up is incomplete. Final diagnoses are determined by a combination of blood counts, hemoglobin electrophoreses, and globin chain synthesis studies at birth and in the first year. Studies of chain synthesis at birth do not reliably define $\beta$-thalassemia trait.[51] Twelve fetuses were shown later to have normal $\beta$ chain production. In eleven, the prenatal $\beta/\gamma$ ratios were within the 95% confidence interval determined previously for normal fetuses. One case was below this range. In the twelve studies of fetuses who turned out to have $\beta$-thalassemia trait, eight $\beta/\gamma$ ratios were below normal, while four were in the normal range. However, only one of those was high normal, while the others were in a range which defines the overlap between normal and trait. When the one very high value is excluded, the mean $\beta/\gamma$ ratio for $\beta$-thalassemia trait is $0.0595 \pm 0.0364$. Since the normal mean $\beta/\gamma$ ratio at 16 to 23 weeks is $0.1094 \pm 0.0452$ (2 SD), the values do indeed overlap. However, this distinction is not important. Although the precise prenatal diagnosis is intellectually satisfying, there is no clinical relevance to identification of a fetus as normal compared to $\beta$-thalassemia trait.

On the other hand, it is very important to distinguish fetuses with homozygous $\beta$ thalassemia from those with $\beta$-thalassemia trait. This may be difficult, if the type of thalassemia is $\beta^+$. Five of our cases were diagnosed as homozygotes. The corrected $\beta/\gamma$ ratios were all below 0.025. In most, it was not possible to determine whether they were at risk for $\beta^+$ or $\beta^0$ thalassemia. When possible, confirmation of hematologic status was sought in blood from the abortuses, by electrophoresis on cellulose acetate and on citrate agar, and by globin chain synthesis studies in pure fetal blood. Actual $\beta/\gamma$ values will vary from one laboratory to another, because of slight differences in the column separation methods. The choice of $\beta/\gamma$ ratio below which homozygous thalassemia is diagnosed thus depends on the laboratory involved. In addition, a large number of cases must be collected before the definitive distinction between $\beta^+$-thalassemia homozygotes and $\beta^0$ heterozygotes will be known. Kan et al[46] have reported four homozygotes; there was no $\beta$ chain production in any of them.

Although prenatal testing has focused on $\beta$-chain hemoglobinopathies, the same methods can be used for $\alpha$ chain disorders. One of the cases that was homozygous for the sickle $\beta$ gene was heterozygous for $\alpha^{G-Philadelphia}$,[47] which was readily detected on the CMC columns. Two of the cases at risk for $\beta$ thalassemia turned out to have normal $\beta$-chain production, but had $\alpha$-thalassemia trait. The one with $\alpha$-thalassemia-1 was diagnosed in utero because $(\beta + \gamma)/\alpha = 1.3$,[48] while the one with the milder condition, $\alpha$-thalassemia-2, was not diagnosed

138

until birth.[20] In both families, further investigation by globin chain synthesis studies revealed that one parent had both β- and α-thalassemia traits, while the other had only β-thalassemia trait. Homozygous α thalassemia would be readily detected prenatally, since there would be no production of α chains. However, this diagnosis can also be made in utero by molecular hybridization of fibroblast DNA.

Table 6-1 summarizes 54 cases in which globin chain analyses were performed on samples obtained in New Haven, London, Boston,

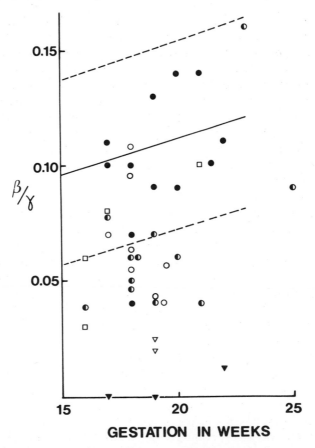

**Figure 6-11.** Correlation of prenatal β/γ synthetic ratios with final diagnoses, where available. Prenatal β/γ ratios are shown for 41 fetuses at risk for β thalassemia. Final diagnoses were determined following abortion, birth, or at intervals during infancy, and were based on globin chain synthesis, hemoglobin electrophoresis, and Coulter counts. —: mean, and –: 95% confidence interval for β/γ ratio in normal fetuses, from Fig. 4. ●: normal infant. ◐: β-thalassemia trait abortus or infant. ▼: homozygous β-thalassemia abortus. ▽: probable homozygous β-thalassemia abortus, no confirmation available. □: fetal loss or elective abortion, no confirmation available. ○: not yet born, or born but no confirmation available.

Montreal, and Toronto. Twenty-five were done by fetoscopy and 29 by placental aspiration. An adequate sample was defined as one with 5% to 50% fetal blood in a case where the mother had been transfused, or with above 50% fetal blood whether or not transfusion had been used. One sample with 60% fetal cells could not be evaluated because of laboratory problems. In all, 23 out of 25 (92%) of the fetoscopy samples and 24 out of the 29 (83%) of the aspiration samples were analyzable. Kan[39] reported 26 out of 29 (89%) useful samples.

There were seven fetal losses following the procedures, and three women had amniotic fluid leakage. Two losses followed fetoscopy: one intrauterine fetal death occurred due to bleeding, and one spontaneous abortion occurred due to an incompetent cervix four weeks after fetoscopy. Five losses followed placental aspiration: one woman went into labor four days after an unsuccessful attempt at placental

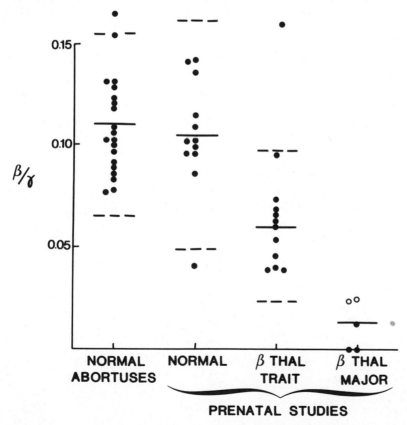

**Figure 6-12.** Prenatal β/γ ratios in normal and thalassemic fetuses. ●: diagnosis established at abortion or in infancy. O: confirmation not available. —: mean, and –: two standard deviations, using data from cases in which the diagnosis was established. (The single very high value in β-thalassemia trait was excluded.)

aspiration; two losses were due to fetal bleeding; one woman developed amnionitis; and there was one abortion of a macerated fetus due to undetermined causes. The overall fetal loss rate was 13%, which is similar to the rate reported by Kan et al.[39,46] The loss rate associated with fetal blood sampling exceeds the 3% midtrimester abortion rate found in the control and experimental groups by the combined Amniocentesis Study.[52] The loss rate associated with attempts to obtain fetal blood is declining in large unpublished series in which the obstetricians are gaining experience. The current loss rate is 9%. Ultrasound is used simultaneously to provide direct guidance. The quality of samples is monitored with the Coulter channelyzer, and sampling ceases as soon as an adequate specimen is obtained. The precise proportion of fetal blood is determined later with the acid elution stain.[53] Although the fetoscope has a larger diameter (2.7 mm) than the 20-gauge needle used for placental aspiration, the advantages of direct visualization outweigh the theoretical hazards of the larger needle. This instrument has also been used for safe visualization of fetuses at risk for physical anomalies[54,55] and to obtain fetal blood in cases at risk for Duchenne muscular dystrophy.[56]

As discussed above (Table 6-1), in our sample of 54 cases, eight fetuses were at risk for sickle cell disease. We were able to evaluate six. Three were predicted to be homozygous, while the fourth was

**Table 6-1**
**Prenatal Diagnosis of Hemoglobinopathies**

|  | Fetoscopy | Aspiration | Total |
|---|---|---|---|
| Total cases | 25 | 29 | 54 |
| Fetal loss | 2 | 5 | 7 |
| Analyzable samples | 23 | 24 | 47 |
| Percent fetal cells | 71 | 43 | 56 |
| Sickle disorders | 6 | 2 | 8 |
| Analyzable samples | 6 | 0 | 6 |
| Homozygosity—established | 3 | 0 | 3 |
| —missed, born | 1 | 0 | 1 |
| Born—sickle trait | 2 | 0 | 2 |
| Thalassemia | 19 | 27 | 46 |
| Analyzable samples | 17 | 24 | 41 |
| Homozygosity—established | 1 | 4 | 5 |
| Born—beta thalassemia trait | 5 | 6 | 11 |
| —alpha thalassemia trait | 0 | 2 | 2 |
| —normal | 3 | 7 | 10 |
| —diagnosis unknown | 1 | 1 | 2 |
| Still pregnant | 5 | 1 | 6 |

diagnosed at birth. Two had sickle trait. Forty-six cases were studied for thalassemia. Samples were adequate in 41. Five fetuses were homozygous for $\beta$ thalassemia, 11 were heterozygous, and ten completely normal. Two had normal $\beta$ chain synthesis, but turned out to have a $\alpha$-thaslasemia trait. Two have not completed postnatal evaluation, and six pregnancies continue.

Due to a combination of fetal losses, elective abortions, or inadequate specimens, only 42 of our total of 54 cases were suitable for evaluation. Data are available in 34, either at birth or at abortion for homozygosity. Of the nine homozygotes, eight were diagnosed in utero. The remaining 25 were correctly predicted to be free of the disease for which they were at risk.

Thus, prenatal diagnosis of $\beta$-chain hemoglobinopathies is becoming reliable. Failure to obtain adequate samples, fetal loss, and technical laboratory problems[47] are declining as experience grows. The procedure remains cumbersome, time-consuming, and expensive, but it is considered a feasible approach for certain families who understand the problems and who wish to have children who are not afflicted with $\beta$-chain hemoglobinopathies.

## FIBROBLASTS

An alternative approach to the prenatal detection of hemoglobinopathies would be to use fetal amniotic fibroblasts rather than fetal blood. Several attempts have been made to elicit hemoglobin synthesis by fibroblasts fused with heterologous erythroid cells. When hybrid cell lines are formed, all hemoglobin synthesis is extinguished.[57,58,59] When the heterokaryons (the multinucleate cells formed immediately after fusion) are examined, the only hemoglobin produced is coded by the erythroblast partner in the fusion.[60-63] Human amniotic fibroblasts do not contain detectable globin messenger RNA,[63] although this possibility has been suggested in studies of chick fibroblasts.[64] Thus, fibroblasts do not currently provide a diagnostic tool for studies which require expression of globin genes.

Certain hemoglobinopathies are associated with the deletion of globin genes, and fibroblasts can be employed to detect those disorders. Alpha genes are deleted in $\alpha$ thalassemia,[65,66] and $\delta$ and $\beta$ genes are absent in $\delta\beta$ thalassemia.[67] Kan and associates have shown that molecular hybridization of DNA obtained from amniotic fibroblasts can be used for the prenatal detection of $\alpha$-thalassemia disorders.[68,69] Amniotic fluid is obtained at 15 weeks gestation, and the fibroblasts grown in tissue culture until > $3 \times 10^8$ cells are obtained (usually 5 to 6 weeks). The DNA is extracted and hybridized with highly purified radioactive $\alpha$ complementary DNA. These studies are complex and technically difficult. It is a tribute to the expertise of Kan's group to have accomplished them.

More recently deletion of gene fragments in homozygous $\delta\beta$ thalassemia[70,71] and in homozygous $\alpha$ thalassemia[71,72] has been demonstrated using restriction endonuclease mapping techniques. These methods are more sensitive than liquid hybridization and may be performed on samples of fetal fibroblasts from amniotic fluid. Although these analyses can be performed only in very specialized laboratories, the fibroblasts can be easily obtained in many places and shipped to the laboratory from anywhere in the world. If sufficient cells are not available by 20 weeks gestation, fetal blood sampling could be employed. Therefore, more than one diagnostic method can be utilized for the $\alpha$ chain abnormalities.

Kan and Dozy[73] have now applied restriction endonuclease mapping techniques to the prenatal diagnosis of sickle cell disease. They have described[74] a specific polymorphism in the $\beta$ globin DNA map which was associated with many cases of sickle cell disease. The frequency of the association of this polymorphism with the $\beta^s$ gene was approximately 80%. DNA from fetal amniotic fibroblasts was then obtained in a case at risk for sickle cell disease. Sickle trait was diagnosed, based on the detection of normal and abnormal $\beta$ DNA fragments. This diagnosis was confirmed by study of globin synthesis in fetal blood obtained at the same time. Thus, many fetuses at risk for sickle cell disease may be studied by amniocentesis, without the added risk of fetal blood sampling.

## CONCLUSIONS

Several techniques are available for the examination of fetuses at risk for hemoglobinopathies. The procedures are not entirely free from the risks of fetal loss, failure to obtain adequate specimens, or diagnostic error, nor are the methods sufficiently simple to be readily available to all who want or need them. The first women studied were already pregnant and had sought terminations because of the 25% risk of an affected child. More recently, pregnancies have been begun because of the availability of the test. These couples have required careful counseling, because these studies must still be regarded as research procedures.

Several of the cases have resided in the United States and England, although some have traveled to those centers from great distances. The largest numbers have come from Italy and Greece. Centers are now being established in those areas, because their needs far outweigh those of the United States and England.

The social, ethical, and political aspects of the prenatal diagnosis of hemoglobinopathies have been reviewed extensively elsewhere.[75,76,77] Despite any mitigating circumstances, the decision to have a prenatal test should be made by the couple who is involved. Many couples have chosen to prevent all pregnancies. Another alternative is now possible. Guidance must be provided by geneticists, obstetricians, and hematologists. The tests must be simplified and improved, in order to increase the safety, reliability, and availability. These approaches are not only feasible, but they are desired by the parents who are directly involved.

## REFERENCES

1. Wasi, P., Na-Nakorn, S., Pootrakul, S., et al. Alpha- and beta-thalassemia in Thailand. *Ann. NY Acad. Sci.* 165:60–82, 1969.
2. Deisseroth, A., Nienhuis, A., Turner, P., et al. Localization of the human α-globin structural gene to chromosome 16 in somatic cell hybrids by molecular hybridization assay. *Cell* 12:205–218, 1977.
3. Deisseroth, A., Nienhuis, A., Lawrence, J., et al. Chromosomal localization of human β globin gene on human chromosome 11 in somatic cell hybrids. *Proc. Natl. Acad. Sci. USA* 75:1456–1460, 1978.
4. Huehns, E.R., Dance, N., Beaven, G.H., et al. Human embryonic hemoglobins. *Cold Spring Harbor Symp. Quant. Biol.* 29:327–331, 1964.
5. Huehns, E.R., and Farooqui, A.M. Oxygen dissociation properties of human embryonic red cells. *Nature* 254:335–337, 1975.
6. Kamuzora, H., and Lehmann, H. Human embryonic haemoglobins including a comparison by homology of the human ζ and α chains. *Nature* 256:511–513, 1975.
7. Kaltsoya, A., Fessas, P., and Stavropoulos, A. Hemoglobins of early human embryonic development. *Science* 153:1417–1418, 1966.
8. Capp, G.L., Rigas, D.A., and Jones, R.T. Evidence for a new haemoglobin chain (ζ-chain). *Nature* 228:278–280, 1970.
9. Kamuzora, H., Jones, R.T., and Lehmann, H. The ζ-chain, an α-like chain of human embryonic haemoglobin. *FEBS Lett.* 46:195–199, 1974.
10. Cividalli, G., Nathan, D.G., Kan, Y.W., et al. Relation of beta to gamma synthesis during the first trimester: An approach to prenatal diagnosis of thalassemia. *Pediatr. Res.* 8:553–560, 1974.
11. Basch, R.S. Hemoglobin synthesis in short-term cultures of human fetal hematopoietic tissues. *Blood* 39:530–541, 1972.
12. Kazazian, H.H., Jr., and Woodhead, A.P. Hemoglobin A synthesis in the developing fetus. *N. Engl. J. Med.* 289:58–62, 1973.
13. Shchory, M., and Weatherall, D.J. Haemoglobin synthesis in human fetal liver maintained in short-term tissue culture. *Br. J. Haematol.* 30:9–20, 1975.
14. Wood, W.G., and Weatherall, D.J. Haemoglobin synthesis during human foetal development. *Nature* 244:162–165, 1973.
15. Pataryas, H.A., and Stamatoyannopoulos, G. Hemoglobins in human fetuses: Evidence for adult hemoglobin production after the 11th gestational week. *Blood* 39:688–696, 1972.

144

16. Kan, Y.W., Dozy, A.M., Alter, B.P., et al. Detection of the sickle gene in the human fetus. Potential for intrauterine diagnosis of sickle-cell anemia. *N. Engl. J. Med.* 287:1–5, 1972.

17. Kazazian, H.H., Jr., Kaback, M.M., Woodhead, A.P., et al. Further studies on the antenatal detection of sickle cell anemia and other hemoglobinopathies. *Adv. Exp. Med. Biol.* 28:337–346, 1972.

18. Hollenberg, M.D., Kaback, M.M., and Kazazian, H.H., Jr. Adult hemoglobin synthesis by reticulocytes from the human fetus at midtrimester. *Science* 174:698–702, 1971.

19. Clegg, J.B., Naughton, M.A., and Weatherall, D.J. Abnormal human haemoglobins: Separation and characterization of the α and β chains by chromatography, and the determinations of two new variants, Hb Chesapeake and Hb J (Bangkok). *J. Mol. Biol.* 19:91–108, 1966.

20. Alter, B.P., and Nathan, D.G. Antenatal diagnosis of haematologic disorders—"1978." *Clin. Haematol.* 7:195–216, 1978.

21. Chang, H., Modell, C.B., Alter, B.P., et al. Expression of the β-thalassemia gene in the first trimester fetus. *Proc. Natl. Acad. Sci. USA* 72:3633–3637, 1975.

22. Kan, Y.W., Valenti, C., Guidotti, R., et al. Fetal blood-sampling in utero. *Lancet* 1:79–80, 1974.

23. Golbus, M.S., Kan, Y.W., and Naglich-Craig, M. Fetal blood sampling in midtrimester pregnancies. *Am. J. Obstet. Gynecol.* 124:653–655, 1976.

24. Valenti, C. Antenatal detection of hemoglobinopathies. A preliminary report. *Am. J. Obstet. Gynecol.* 115:851–853, 1973.

25. Hobbins, J.C., and Mahoney, M.J. In utero diagnosis of hemoglobinopathies. Technic for obtaining fetal blood. *N. Engl. J. Med.* 290:1065–1067, 1974.

26. Hobbins, J.C., and Mahoney, M.J. Fetal blood drawing. *Lancet* 2:107–109, 1975.

27. Patrick, J.E., Perry, T.B., and Kinch, R.A.H. Fetoscopy and fetal blood sampling: A percutaneous approach. *Am. J. Obstet. Gynecol.* 119:539–542, 1974.

28. Benzie, R.J., and Doran, T.A. The "fetoscope"—a new clinical tool for prenatal genetic diagnosis. *Am. J. Obstet. Gynecol.* 121:460–464, 1975.

29. Campbell, S. The assessment of fetal development by diagnostic ultrasound. *Clin. Perinatol.* 1:507–525, 1974.

30. Nadler, H.L. Prenatal diagnosis of inborn defects: A status report. *Hosp. Prac.* 6:41–51, 1975.

31. Chang, H., Hobbins, J.C., Cividalli, G., et al. In utero diagnosis of hemoglobinopathies. Hemoglobin synthesis in fetal red cells. *N. Engl. J. Med.* 290:1067–1068, 1974.

32. Benzie, R.J., and Pirani, B.B.K. Fetoscopy and anterior placentas. *N. Engl. J. Med.* 296:573, 1977.

33. Pritchard, J.A., and Adams, R.H. Erythrocyte production and destruction during pregnancy. *Am. J. Obstet. Gynecol.* 79:750–757, 1960.

34. Schuman, J.E., Tanser, C.L., Peloquin, R., et al. The erythropoietic response to pregnancy in β-thalassemia minor. *Br. J. Haematol.* 25:249–260, 1973.

35. Traill, L.M. Reticulocytes in healthy pregnancy. *Med. J. Aust.* 2:205–206, 1975.

36. Alter, B.P., Modell, C.B., Fairweather, D., et al. Prenatal diagnosis of hemoglobinopathies. A review of 15 cases. *N. Engl. J. Med.* 295:1437–1443, 1976.

37. Oski, F.A., and Naiman, J.L. Disorders of red cell metabolism. In

*Hematologic Problems in the Newborn.* 2nd Ed. Philadelphia: W.B. Saunders Co., 1972.

38. Kan, Y.W., Nathan, D.G., Cividalli, G., et al. Concentration of fetal red blood cells from a mixture of maternal and fetal blood by anti-i serum — An aid to prenatal diagnosis of hemoglobinopathies. *Blood* 43:411–415, 1974.

39. Kan, Y.W. Prenatal diagnosis of hemoglobin disorders. *Prog. Hematol.* 10:91–104, 1977.

40. Goossens, M., Beuzard, Y., and Rosa, J. Problemes biochimiques poses par le diagnostic antenatal des hemoglobinopathies. Edited by A. Boué. In *Prenatal Diagnosis.* Paris: Les Colloques de l'Institut National de la Santé et de la Recherche Médicale, 1976.

41. Boyer, S.H., Noyes, A.N., and Boyer, M.L. Enrichment of erythrocytes of fetal origin from adult-fetal blood mixtures via selective hemolysis of adult blood cells: An aid to antenatal diagnosis of hemoglobinopathies. *Blood* 47:883–897, 1976.

42. Alter, B.P., Metzger, J.B., Yock, P.G., et al. Selective hemolysis of adult red blood cells: An aid to prenatal diagnosis of hemoglobinopathies. *Blood* 53:279–287, 1979.

43. Kan, Y.W., Golbus, M.S., Klein, P., et al. Successful application of prenatal diagnosis in a pregnancy at risk for homozygous β-thalassemia. *N. Engl. J. Med.* 292:1096–1099, 1975.

44. Kan, Y.W., Golbus, M.S., and Trecartin, R. Prenatal diagnosis of homozygous β-thalassaemia. *Lancet* 2:790–792, 1975.

45. Kan, Y.W., Golbus, M.S., and Trecartin, R. Prenatal diagnosis of sickle-cell anemia. *N. Engl. J. Med.* 294:1039, 1976.

46. Kan, Y.W., Trecartin, R.F., Golbus, M.S:, et al. Prenatal diagnosis of β-thalassaemia and sickle-cell anaemia. Experience with 24 cases. *Lancet* 1:269–271, 1977.

47. Alter, B.P., Friedman, S., Hobbins, J.C., et al. Prenatal diagnosis of sickle-cell anemia and alpha G-Philadelphia. *N. Engl. J. Med.* 294:1040–1041, 1976.

48. Alter, B.P., Nathan, D.G., Modell, C.B., et al. Prenatal diagnosis of hemoglobinopathies: Detection of α-thalassemia trait and of sickle cell disease *in utero. Hemoglobin* 1:395–400, 1977.

49. Cividalli, G.G., Antebi, S., Klein, R., et al. Prenatal diagnosis of heterozygous β-thalassemia. *Isr. J. Med. Sci.* 12:1313–1315, 1976.

50. Kazazian, H.H., Jr., and Woodhead, A.P. Adult hemoglobin synthesis in the human fetus. *Ann. NY Acad. Sci.* 241:691–698, 1974.

51. Alter, B.P. Beta thalassaemia trait: Imprecision of diagnosis at birth. *Br. J. Haematol.* 38:323–327, 1978.

52. NICHD National Registry for Amniocentesis Study Group. Midtrimester amniocentesis for prenatal diagnosis. Safety and accuracy. *JAMA* 236:1471–1476, 1976.

53. Kleihauer, E., Braun, H., and Betke, K. Demonstration von fetalem Hämoglobin in den Erythrocyten eines Blutausstrichs. *Klin. Wochenschr.* 35:637–638, 1957.

54. Benzie, R.J., Malone, R.M., Miskin, M., et al. Prenatal diagnosis by fetoscopy with subsequent normal delivery — A report of a case. *Am. J. Obstet. Gynecol.* 126:287–288, 1976.

55. Mahoney, M.J., and Hobbins, J.C. Prenatal diagnosis of chondroectodermal dysplasia (Ellis-van Creveld syndrome) with fetoscopy and ultrasound. *N. Engl. J. Med.* 297:258–260, 1977.

56. Mahoney, M.J., Haseltine, F.P., Hobbins, J.C., et al. Prenatal diagnosis of Duchenne's muscular dystrophy. *N. Engl. J. Med.* 297:968–973, 1977.

57. Orkin, S.H., Harosi, F.I., and Leder, P. Differentiation in erythroleukemic cells and their somatic hybrids. *Proc. Natl. Acad. Sci. USA* 72:98–102, 1975.

58. Deisseroth, A., Burk, R., Picciano, D., et al. Hemoglobin synthesis in somatic cell hybrids: Globin gene expression in hybrids between mouse erythroleukemia and human marrow cells or fibroblasts. *Proc. Natl. Acad. Sci. USA* 72:1102–1106, 1975.

59. Deisseroth, A., Velez, R., Burk, R.D., et al. Extinction of globin gene expression in human fibroblast × mouse erythroleukemia cell hybrids. *Somatic Cell Genet.* 2:373–384, 1976.

60. Alter, B.P., and Ingram, V.M. Globin synthesis in fibroblasts fused with erythroblasts. I. Avian fibroblasts. *Somatic Cell Genet.* 1:165–186, 1975.

61. Davis, T.J., and Harris, H. Haemoglobin synthesis in fused cells. *J. Cell Sci.* 18:207–216, 1975.

62. Citkowitz, E., Riggs, M.G., and Ingram, V.M. Globin synthesis in fibroblasts fused with erythroblasts. II. Human fibroblasts. *Somatic Cell Genet.* 1:323–333, 1975.

63. Alter, B.P., Goff, S.C., Hillman, D.G., et al. Production of mouse globin in heterokaryons of mouse erythroleukemia cells and human fibroblasts. *J. Cell Sci.* 26:347–357, 1977.

64. Humphries, S., Windass, J., and Williamson, R. Mouse globin gene expression in erythroid and non-erythroid tissues. *Cell* 7:267–277, 1976.

65. Ottolenghi, S., Lanyon, W.G., Paul, J., et al. Gene deletion as the cause of α-thalassaemia. *Nature* 251:389–392, 1974.

66. Taylor, J.M., Dozy, A., Kan, Y.W., et al. Genetic lesion in homozygous α-thalassaemia (hydrops fetalis). *Nature* 251:392–393, 1974.

67. Ottolenghi, S., Comi, P., Giglioni, B., et al. δβ-Thalassemia is due to a gene deletion. *Cell* 9:71–80, 1976.

68. Kan, Y.W., Golbus, M.S., and Dozy, A.M. Prenatal diagnosis of α-thalassemia. Clinical application of molecular hybridization. *N. Engl. J. Med.* 295:1165–1167, 1976.

69. Koenig, H.M., Vedvick, T.S., Dozy, A.M., et al. Prenatal diagnosis of hemoglobin-H disease. *J. Pediatr.* 92:278–281, 1978.

70. Mears, J.G., Ramirez, F., Leibowitz, D., et al. Changes in restricted human cellular DNA fragments containing globin gene sequences in thalassemias and related disorders. *Proc. Natl. Acad. Sci. USA* 1222–1226, 1978.

71. Orkin, S.H., Alter, B.P., Altay, C., et al. Application of endonuclease mapping to the analysis and prenatal diagnosis of thalassemias caused by globin-gene deletion. *N. Engl. J. Med.* 299:166–172, 1978.

72. Surrey, S., Chambers, J.S., Muni, D., et al. Restriction endonuclease analysis of human globin genes in cellular DNA. *Biochem. Biophys. Res. Commun.* 83:1125–1131, 1978.

73. Kan, Y.W., and Dozy, A.M. Antenatal diagnosis of sickle-cell anaemia by D.N.A. analysis of amniotic-fluid cells. *Lancet* 2:910–912, 1978.

74. Kan, Y.W., and Dozy, A.M. Polymorphism of DNA sequence adjacent to human β-globin structural gene: Relationship to sickle mutation. *Proc. Natl. Acad. Sci. USA* 75:5631–5635, 1978.

75. Alter, B.P., Kan, Y.W., Frigoletto, F.D., et al. The antenatal diagnosis of the haemoglobinopathies. *Clin. Haematol.* 3:509–526, 1974.

76. Nathan, D.G., Alter, B.P., and Frigoletto, F.D. Antenatal diagnosis of hemoglobinopathies: Social and technical considerations. *Semin. Hematol.* 12:305–321, 1975.

77. Nathan, D.G., and Alter, B.P. Antenatal diagnosis of the haemoglobinopathies. *Br. J. Haematol.* 31:143–154, 1975.

7   # The Unstable Hemoglobins, Hemoglobins M, and Hemoglobins with Altered Oxygen Affinity*

Denis R. Miller, M.D.

Structural alterations of human hemoglobin producing increased lability of hemoglobin molecules result in a congenital hemolytic syndrome defined as unstable hemoglobin disease (UHD). Specific amino acid substitutions or deletions in the $\alpha$ or $\beta$ chains of the hemoglobin molecule have been identified in over 70 unstable variants. These result in clinical expression varying from a severe, transfusion-dependent hemolytic anemia to states unassociated with clinical signs and symptoms of hemolysis. Our current knowledge of the three-dimensional structure of hemoglobin permits us to predict the effects of an amino acid substitution on hemoglobin stability and function. The unstable hemoglobin hemolytic anemias are fascinating experiments of nature and have provided us with a much clearer understanding of normal hemoglobin structure and function.

*This work was supported in part by NIH grant RR47 and the Children's Blood Foundation, Inc.

This chapter will review the clinical and laboratory features, treatment, molecular pathology, and mechanisms of hemolysis in UHD, particularly with regard to the pediatric age group.

## Historical Perspective

The history of UHD research reflects the transition in hematology research from descriptive morphology to sophisticated studies of molecular pathology. Intracellular Heinz bodies or precipitated denatured hemoglobin were first identified by supravital staining in 1890. Their presence was thought to be associated with direct toxic exposure of erythrocytes, but the pathogenesis of hemoglobin precipitation was incompletely understood. It is now apparent that Heinz bodies may also result from metabolic defects of enzymes in or related to the pentose phosphate shunt (e.g., G6PD, GSH peroxidase, GSH synthetase), from imbalanced globin chain synthesis (thalassemia syndromes), or from structural abnormalities of the hemoglobin molecule. In 1952 Cathie[1] described the first patient with "congenital Heinz body hemolytic anemia" in whom inclusion bodies were noted only after splenectomy. Lange and Ackeroyd[2] suggested that the dark urine ("dipyrroluria") accompanying the disorder was the result of mesobilifuscin and abnormal heme catabolism, and Schmid and colleagues[3] first proposed that the disorder was familial. In 1960 Scott and coworkers[4] found an electrophoretically abnormal but unclassifiable hemoglobin in patients with Heinz body hemolytic anemia. Hemoglobin Zürich ($\beta$63 His→Arg)[5] was the first documented hemoglobinopathy associated with Heinz body formation following exposure to sulfonamides. Thus, these early studies indicated that the disorder was congenital, familial, and associated with a structural anomaly of hemoglobin.

The link between Heinz body formation and hemoglobin instability was provided by the studies of Grimes and coworkers,[6,7] who described the simple and clinically indispensible heat stability test. Through classic techniques of hemoglobin and chain separation and isolation, hybridization, and amino acid analysis, Hutchison et al[8] and Carrell and coworkers[9] characterized Hb Köln ($\beta$98 Val→Met), the most common unstable hemoglobinopathy. Subsequently, other unstable hemoglobins were identified. Utilizing the elegant pacesetting studies of Perutz and colleagues,[10,11] investigators have been able to relate structural defects to abnormalities of function[12] and stability. Recent attention has been directed to oxidative denaturation of hemoglobin and the hemolytic process itself.[13,14]

**Classification and Molecular Pathology of UHD**

Unstable hemoglobin hemolytic anemias may be classified either clinically, according to the severity of the anemia, or structurally, according to either the specific location of the defect (Table 7-1) or the effect of the anomaly on hemoglobin stability. The latter is most useful in relating structure, function, and stability. The stability of normal hemoglobin depends upon four major factors: (1) the maintenance of $\alpha$-helix conformation, (2) the strength and adequacy of heme-globin binding, (3), the exclusion of water and polar residues from the hydrophobic interior of the molecule, and (4) the integrity of interchain ($\alpha_1\beta_1$, $\alpha_1\beta_2$ subunits) contacts. Chain elongation at the carboxy-terminal end of the $\beta$ chain (Hb Cranston) is a less common cause of instability. Alterations in any of these functions caused by amino acid substitutions or deletions weaken the tertiary and quarternary structure of the molecule and result in heme-globin dissociation, chain unfolding and dissociation, oxidation of heme, and its eventual precipitation and denaturation into Heinz bodies. Clinical symptoms and severity will be determined by the location of the lesion and the importance of that site in controlling molecular stability. Alterations in subunit contacts which control the stability and conformation of the hemoglobin molecule during oxygenation and deoxygenation may affect oxygen affinity as well as stability. Hb Köln is an excellent case in point. The position $\beta^{98}$ not only is important for heme-globin binding but is also one of the 19 $\alpha_1\beta_2$ contact points. A substitution here results in an unstable molecule with increased oxygen affinity. Specific unstable hemoglobins associated with these four structural alterations are listed in Table 7-2.

Some key points are readily apparent:

(1) Proline cannot enter into an $\alpha$-helix, and its insertion in portions of the molecule which are usually helical causes instability. In eight variants (Table 7-2, I) proline is substituted for leucine, reflecting an adenine→guanine transition in the DNA codon (GAA→GGA) which is transcribed as a uracil→cytosine shift in RNA (CUU→CCU).

(2) Twenty-one amino acids in the $\beta$ chain and 19 in the $\alpha$ chain are involved in heme-globin binding. Segments DC, E, EF, F, and FG are in most intimate contact with heme, and substitutions involving these important contact points will weaken the tertiary configuration of hemoglobin, since heme stabilizes the globin chains and prevents unfolding. All but three of the amino acids involved in heme-globin binding are invariant in all normal vertebrate hemoglobins. Figure 7-1 shows the heme pocket surrounded by these contact amino acids. Unstable hemoglobin disease occurs with every substitution. The physical-chemical basis for weakened binding is shown in Figure 7-2,

**Table 7-1**
**The Unstable Hemoglobins**

| Residue and helical number | Amino acid substitution | Name | Oxygen affinity | Severity* |
|---|---|---|---|---|
| α Chain variants[10] | | | | |
| 43(CE1) | Phe→Val | Torino | ↓ | Moderate |
| 47(CE5) | Asp→His | Hasharon | N | Mild |
| | Asp→Asn | Arya | — | — |
| 53(E2) | Ala→Asp | J. Rovigo | — | — |
| 80(F1) | Leu→Arg | Ann Arbor | — | Mild |
| 84(F5) | Ser→Arg | Etobicoke | ↑ | Mild |
| 94(G1) | Asp→Tyr | Setif | ↑ | Mild |
| 112(G19) | His→Gln | Dakar | — | — |
| | His→Asp | Hopkins-2 | ↑ | — |
| 136(H19) | Leu→Pro | Bibba | — | Severe |
| β Chain variants[53] | | | | |
| 14(A11) | Leu→Arg | Sögn | | None |
| | Leu→Pro | Saki | N | — |
| 15(A12) | Trp→Arg | Belfast | ↑ | Moderate |
| 20(B2) | Val→Asp | Strasbourg | — | — |
| 24(B6) | Gly→Arg | Riverdale-Bronx | — | Moderate |
| | Gly→Val | Savannah | — | Severe |
| | Gly→Asp | Moscva | ↓ | — |
| 26(B8) | Glu→Val | Henri Mondor | — | — |
| 27(B9) | Ala→Asp | Volga, Drenthe | — | — |
| 28(B10) | Leu→Gln | St. Louis | ↑ | Moderate |
| | Leu→Pro | Genova | ↑ | Severe |
| 30(B12) | Arg→Ser | Tacoma | ↑ | Mild |
| 32(B14) | Leu→Pro | Perth, Abe Lincoln | Normal | Severe |
| | Leu→Arg | Castilla | ↑ | — |
| 35(C1) | Tyr→Phe | Philly | — | Mild |
| 41(C7) | Phe→Tyr | Meguon | — | — |
| 42(CD1) | Phe→Ser | Hammersmith (Chiba) | ↓ | Severe |
| | Phe→Leu | Louisville (Bucuresti) | ↓ | Moderate |
| 48(CD7) | Leu→Arg | Okaloosa | ↓ | — |
| 51(D2) | Pro→Arg | Willamette | ↑ | — |
| 62(E6) | Ala→Pro | Duarte | ↑ | Mild |
| 63(E7) | His→Arg | Zürich | ↑ | Mild |
| | His→Pro | Bicetre | ↑ | Mild |
| 64(E8) | Gly→Asp | J. Calabria (J. Bari) | — | — |
| 66(E10) | Lys→Glu | I. Toulouse | Normal | Mild |
| 67(E11) | Val→Asp | Bristol | ↓ | Severe |
| | Val→Ala | Sydney | — | Mild |
| 70(E14) | Ala→Asp | Seattle | ↓ | Moderate |

**Table 7-1** *(continued)*

| Residue and helical number | Amino acid substitution | Name | Oxygen affinity | Severity* |
|---|---|---|---|---|
| 71(E15) | Phe→Ser | Christchurch | — | — |
| 74(E18) | Gly→Asp | Shepherds Bush | ↑ | Mild |
| 75(E19) | Leu→Pro | Atlanta | — | — |
| 81(EF5) | Leu→Arg | Baylor | ↑ | — |
| 85(F1) | Phe→Ser | Bryn Mawr (Buenos Aires) | ↑ | Mild |
| 88(F4) | Leu→Arg | Boräs | — | Moderate |
| | Leu→Pro | Santa Ana | — | Moderate |
| 91(F7) | Leu→Pro | Sabine | — | Moderate |
| | Leu→Arg | Caribbean | ↓ | — |
| 92(F8) | His→Gln | Istanbul (St. Etienne) | ↑ | Moderate |
| 98(FG5) | Val→Met | Köln (Ube 1) | ↑ | Moderate |
| | Val→Gly | Nottingham | ↑ | Severe |
| | Val→Ala | Djelfa | ↑ | Mild |
| 101(G3) | Glu→Gln | Rush | — | Moderate |
| 104(G6) | Arg→Ser | Camperdown | — | — |
| 106(G8) | Leu→Pro | Southampton (Casper) | ↑ | Severe |
| 107(G9) | Gly→Arg | Burke | ↓ | — |
| 111(G13) | Val→Phe | Peterborough | ↓ | Mild |
| 115(G17) | Ala→Pro | Madrid | — | Severe |
| 119(GH2) | Gly→Asp | Fannin-Lubbock | — | — |
| 124(H2) | Pro→Arg | Khartoum | — | Mild |
| 130(H8) | Tyr→Asp | Wien | — | Moderate |
| 135(H13) | Ala→Pro | Altdorf | — | — |
| 136(H14) | Gly→Asp | Hope | ↓ | Mild |
| 141(H19) | Leu→Arg | Olmsted | — | Severe |

$\beta$ Chain variants with deleted residues[11]

| Residue and helical number | Amino acid substitution | Name | Oxygen affinity | Severity* |
|---|---|---|---|---|
| $\beta^{6or7}$(A3 or 4) | Glu→O | Leiden | sl↓ | Mild |
| $\beta^{23}$(B5) | Val→O | Freiburg | ↑ | Mild |
| $\beta^{42-44}$(CD1-3) | (Phe-Glu-Ser)→O | Niteroi | ↓ | — |
| $\beta^{43or45}$(CD2-4) | (Glu-Ser-Phe)→O | | | |
| $\beta^{56-59}$(D7-E3) | (Gly-Asn-Pro-Lys)→O | Tochigi | — | — |
| $\beta^{74-75}$(E18-19) | (Gly-Leu)→O | St. Antoine | Normal | Moderate |
| $\beta^{87}$(F3) | Thr→O | Tours | ↑ | Mild |
| $\beta^{91-95}$(F7-FG2) | (Leu-His-Cys-Asp-Lys)→O | Gun Hill | ↑ | Mild |
| $\beta^{131}$(H9) | Glu→O | Leslie | — | — |
| $\beta^{141}$(H19) | Leu→O | Coventry | — | — |

*Severity: Mild, Hgb. 12 to 14 gm/dl
   Moderate, Hgb. 9 to 11 gm/dl
   Severe, < 9.0 gm/dl
   —, not reported

154

with Hb Köln as an example. Normally, valine ($\beta^{98}$) forms a contact with heme at FG5. In Hb Köln disease, methionine, a much larger amino acid, distorts the heme pocket and weakens the bond between heme and globin. In Hb Hammersmith, serine is too small to bridge the

**Table 7-2**
**Structural Classification of Unstable Hemoglobins**

| Unstable hemoglobin | Residue (helical number) | Substitution |
|---|---|---|
| I. Interference with $\alpha$-helix conformation | | |
| Bibba | $\alpha^{136}$(H19) | Leu→Pro |
| Saki | $\beta^{14}$(A11) | Leu→Pro |
| Genoa | $\beta^{28}$(B10) | Leu→Pro |
| Abraham Lincoln | $\beta^{32}$(B14) | Leu→Pro |
| Atlanta | $\beta^{75}$(E19) | Leu→Pro |
| Santa Ana | $\beta^{88}$(F4) | Leu→Pro |
| Sabine | $\beta^{91}$(F7) | Leu→Pro |
| Casper | $\beta^{106}$(G8) | Leu→Pro |
| II. Defective heme binding | | |
| Hammersmith | $\beta^{42}$(CD1) | Phe*→Ser |
| Zürich | $\beta^{63}$(E7) | His*→Arg |
| Bushwick | $\beta^{74}$(E18) | Gly→Val |
| Sabine | $\beta^{88}$(F4) | Leu*→Pro |
| Santa Ana | $\beta^{19}$(F7) | Leu→Pro |
| St. Etienne | $\beta^{92}$(F8) | His*→Glu |
| Gun Hill | $\beta^{91-95}$(F7-FG2) | deletion |
| Köln | $\beta^{98}$(FG5) | Val→Met |
| III. Insertion of polar residues into hydrophobic interior | | |
| Riverdale | $\beta^{6}$(B4) | Gly→Arg |
| Zürich | $\beta^{63}$(E7) | His→Arg |
| Bristol | $\beta^{67}$(E11) | Val→Asp |
| Borås | $\beta^{88}$(F4) | Leu→Arg |
| Wien | $\beta^{130}$(H8) | Tyr→Asp |
| Olmsted | $\beta^{141}$(H19) | Leu→Arg |
| Ann Arbor | $\alpha^{80}$(F1) | Leu→Arg |
| IV. Interference with interchain (subunit) contacts | | |
| $\alpha_1\beta_1$ Contact | | |
| Tacoma | $\beta^{30}$(B12) | Arg→Ser |
| Philly | $\beta^{35}$(C1) | Tyr→Phe |
| $\alpha_1\beta_2$ Contact | | |
| Köln | $\beta^{98}$(FG5) | Val→Met |
| Rush | $\beta^{101}$(G3) | Glu→Gln |
| Kansas | $\beta^{102}$(G4) | Asn→Thr |
| Richmond | $\beta^{102}$(G4) | Asn→Lys |

*Invariant in all hemoglobin chains.

required 5Å gap between globin and heme, breaking the contact with resultant heme-loss.

(3) Water must be excluded from the hydrophobic heme pocket if the molecule is to remain stable. If water gains entry to this area by the

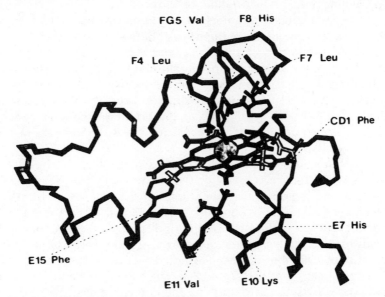

**Figure 7-1.** Segments of the globin chain surrounding the heme group. None of the heme-contact amino acids is shown. Substitutions at each contact point are associated with an unstable hemoglobin hemolytic anemia. [From J.M. White.³²]

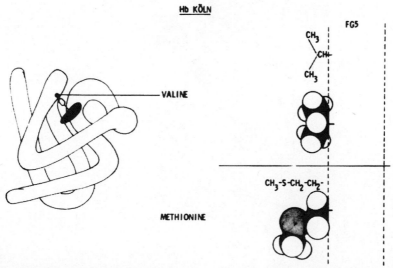

**Figure 7-2.** Molecular pathology of Hb Köln disease. Normally, valine occupies position FG5 and forms a heme-contact. Methionine, which replaces it, is much larger, due to its sulfur group, and distorts the heme pocket. [From J.M. White.³²]

substitution of a polar for a nonpolar residue, ferroheme ($Fe^{2+}$) is easily oxidized to ferriheme ($Fe^{3+}$) and a superoxide radical is generated, setting into motion a series of oxidative hemolytic mechanisms. The substitutions in the unstable hemoglobins listed in Table 7-2, III are all to arginine, a polar, hydrophilic residue.

(4) Hemoglobin tetramers are held together by contacts between the $\alpha$ and $\beta$ chains. Stronger bonds exist between the $\alpha_1\beta_1$ (and $\alpha_2\beta_2$) contact points than between the $\alpha_1\beta_2$ (and $\alpha_2\beta_1$) contacts. If, because of substitution, the $\alpha_1\beta_1$ contact is weakened, $\alpha_1\beta_1$ dimers will dissociate into unstable $\alpha$ and $\beta$ monomers. Substitutions of $\alpha_1\beta_2$ contacts result in dissociation of tetramers into $\alpha\beta$ dimers. Thus, the substitution in Hb Philly ($\beta35$ Tyr→Phe) involves $C_1$, an important $\alpha_1\beta_1$ contact, and results in dissociation of subunits and is associated with moderate hemolysis (Table 7-2, IV).

(5) Deletions of one or more amino acids at any of the above key points will alter the stability of the molecule (Table 7-1). To date 11 unstable hemoglobins with deletions have been described. All are $\beta$ chain anomalies (Table 7-1 and Figure 7-3), and many are in the heme pocket. Others, such as Hb Gun Hill, also involve $\alpha_1\beta_2$ contact amino acids resulting in instability, heme loss, and increased $O_2$ affinity.

(6) In a number of instances, different substitutions at the same site have been identified (Table 7-3). The substituted amino acid rather than the site itself may determine the clinical severity. For example, a

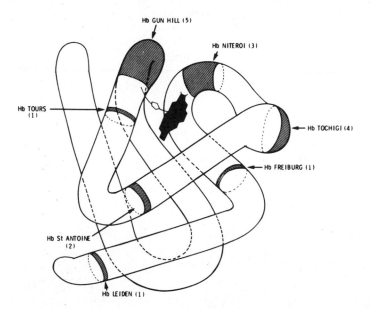

**Figure 7-3.** $\beta$ chain amino acid deletions in unstable hemoglobin disease. The shaded areas are the approximate sites where deletions have occurred. Multiple deletions have been found only on or near interhelical corners. [From J.M. White.[32]]

157

Table 7-3
Multiple Substituted Sites Resulting in UHD

| Unstable hemoglobin | Residue (helical number) | Substitution | mRNA codon |
|---|---|---|---|
| Riverdale-Bronx | $\beta^{24}$(B6) | Gly→Arg | GGU→CGU |
| Savannah | | Gly→Val | GGA→GUA |
| St. Louis | $\beta^{28}$(B10) | Leu→Gln | CUA→CAA |
| Genova | | Leu→Pro | CUU→CCU |
| Hammersmith | $\beta^{42}$(CD1) | Phe→Ser | UUU→UCU |
| Louisville | | Phe→Leu | UUU→UUA |
| Sidney | $\beta^{67}$(E11) | Val→Ala | GUU→GCU |
| Bristol | | Val→Asp | GUU→GAU |
| Tours | $\beta^{88}$(F4) | Leu→O | CCU→O |
| Borås | | Leu→Arg | CUU→CGU |
| Santa Ana | | Leu→Pro | CUU→CCU |
| Ferrara | $\alpha^{47}$(CD5) | Asp→Gly | GAC→GGC |
| Hasharon | | Asp→His | GAC→CAC |

substitution for valine at B⁶⁷(E11) results in either Hb Sidney (Val→Ala) or Hb Bristol (Val→Asp). The former is associated with mild hemolysis, whereas Hb Bristol is extremely unstable and the hemolysis is severe. The presence of charged aspartic acid in the heme pocket is obviously more hazardous to the stability and function of hemoglobin than uncharged alanine.

## Clinical Features

**Demography**    Unstable hemoglobin disease is a rare disorder when compared to sickle cell and thalassemia syndromes. Hb Köln disease is the most common of the 70 different unstable hemoglobinopathies and yet fewer than 50 cases have been reported. Single or at most two or three cases per family have been described in most of the other entities. Although the distribution of UHD is worldwide, the true incidence in any population has not been ascertained. Many isolated abnormalities have been detected by serendipity in large-scale population surveys. The fact that most patients are from the Western Hemisphere and Europe or are of European background is more likely a testament to technologic development and medical-diagnostic sophistication rather than to a geographic concentration in any racial or ethnic groups. Hb Köln disease has been reported in black[15] and Hispanic Americans[16] and in Malaysians.[17]

**Genetics**    An autosomal dominant mode of inheritance predominates in UHD (Figure 7-4). Well-documented cases of spontaneous mutations have been reported in disorders generally

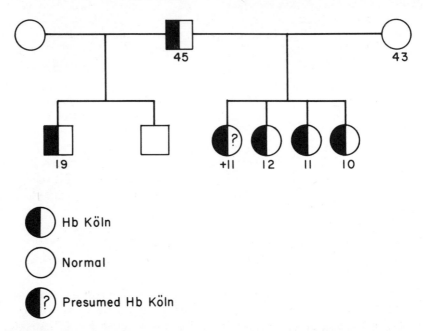

**Figure 7-4.** Autosomal dominant mode of inheritance in a family with Hb Köln disease. The presumed heterozygote had clinical symptoms identical to those of her siblings, but was not available for investigation, having died at age 11 of infection.

associated with more severe clinical manifestations—Hb Hammersmith,[18] Hb Bristol,[19] Hb Olmsted,[20] Hb Sabine,[21] and Hb Köln.[22] On the basis of data with Hb Hammersmith, a mutation rate of $1 \times 10^{-7}$ per nucleotide or $1 \times 10^{-4}$ per gene has been proposed.[23] Affected patients are heterozygotes; it is unlikely that homozygosity is compatible with life. Double heterozygosity has been reported in two cases: Hb Peterborough ($\beta$111 Val→Phe [G13])-Hb Lepore,[24] and Hb Duarte ($\beta$62 Ala→Pro [E6])-$\beta$-thalassemia.[25]

Generally, the amount of abnormal hemoglobin varies from 10% to 30% of the total hemoglobin complement, considerably less than that seen in heterozygotes with structural defects, suggesting an associated defect in biosynthesis of the abnormal hemoglobin or reflecting exaggerated denaturation and removal of the unstable molecules. An exception is Hb Duarte-$\beta$ thalassemia, in which the majority of the hemoglobin was the unstable variant because of deficient synthesis of normal $\beta$ chains.

As stated above, the genetic lesion lies in either single point mutation in the DNA codon or in deletion of single (Hb St. Etienne) or multiple (Hb Gun Hill) codon triplets.

Associated congenital malformations, chromosomal abnormalities, other diseases, or exposure to mutagens have not been documented. Although there appears to be a consistency in the clinical severity of a particular UHD within families, there is great variability between unrelated families.[26,27]

**Signs, Symptoms, and Physical Findings**   Patients with UHD often present at any age with the triad of hemolysis—pallor, jaundice, and splenomegaly. Hyperbilirubinemia and compensated hemolysis may be present in the newborn period, particularly if the amino acid substitution occurs in the $\alpha$ chain (Hb Hasharon $\alpha$47 Asp→His [CD5])[28] or in the $\gamma$ chain (Hb F-Poole $\gamma$130 Tyr→Gly [136 $\gamma$136 Gly] [H8]).[29] It is now presumed that some cases of congenital Heinz body hemolytic anemia in the newborn period represent unstable hemoglobinopathies. In older children intermittent episodes of jaundice accompanied by dark brown urine may be misdiagnosed as hepatitis. The discoloration is caused by the presence of dipyrrolic urinary pigments derived from degraded heme.[30] The presence of these compounds is not specific for UHD, as they are also found in patients with thalassemia (which in a broad sense can be considered a Heinz body or unstable hemoglobin hemolytic anemia because of the instability and precipitation of excess $\alpha$ or $\beta$ chains). Patients may have perioral cyanosis caused by methemoglobinemia or decreased oxygen affinity. In other patients with more severe chronic hemolysis, frontal bossing and, rarely, malleolar ulcers are seen. As with other chronic congenital hemolytic anemias, reticulocytopenic crises due to erythroid hypoplasia in association with infection may occur. Increased hemolysis, with fatigue, fever, and dark urine, often accompanies these infections. Drug-induced hemolysis has been observed with Hb Hasharon,[31] Hb Zürich,[5] Hb Torino,[32] Hb Shepherds Bush,[32] Hb Leiden,[32] and in some,[33] but not other,[22] cases of Hb Köln.

Although cholelithiasis may occur, the frequency is much less than in the sickle cell and thalassemia syndromes, reflecting the milder degree of hemolysis in many types of UHD. Death from overwhelming pneumococcal infection has been reported in a splenectomized child with Hb Hammersmith.[32]

## Laboratory Findings

**Standard Hematologic Studies**   The levels of hemoglobin may vary from normal to low, and indices reveal a normocytic, hypochromic anemia with decreased MCH and MCHC. Presplenectomy, erythrocyte morphology is abnormal, with polychromatophilia, moderate anisocytosis, occasional poikilocytosis and microspherocytosis,

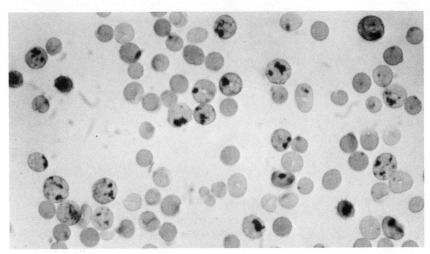

**Figure 7-5.** Heinz bodies in erythrocytes of a 12-year-old boy with Hb Köln disease, postsplenectomy.

and rare punctate basophilia. Heniz bodies, which require supravital staining, are not seen in fresh blood presplenectomy but can be induced by incubation with brilliant cresyl blue for 24 hours at 37°C. Postsplenectomy, in some types of UHD one or more large inclusions may be seen in many red cells after brief staining with methyl violet (Figure 7-5).

Although reticulocytosis is moderate to mild in most patients, expression of reticulocytes as absolute concentration rather than as percentage of total red cells indicates that some patients have a six- to eight-fold increase in erythropoiesis. These latter patients have marked erythroid hyperplasia. Thrombocytopenia, perhaps related to hypersplenism, has been reported in some patients, but granulocyte and platelet counts are usually normal.

**Nonspecific Tests of Hemolysis**   Haptoglobin and hemopexin are decreased or absent, and a mild elevation of unconjugated bilirubin is present. Other markers of intravascular hemolysis, such as increased methemalbumin and hemosiderinuria, are present in some patients. The Coombs' and Ham's (acid hemolysis) tests and tests for urinary coproporphyrins and porphobilinogens are negative. The results of the autohemolysis test are variable. When abnormal, a "type I" pattern with partial correction by glucose is seen. More useful information is provided by the presence of Heinz bodies and the generation of significant amounts of methemoglobin after 24 to 48 hours incubation at 37°C under the sterile conditions of the autohemolysis test (Figure 7-6).[22]

The osmotic fragility of fresh Hb Köln cells is slightly decreased, but after 24 hours incubation it decreases markedly and reflects a

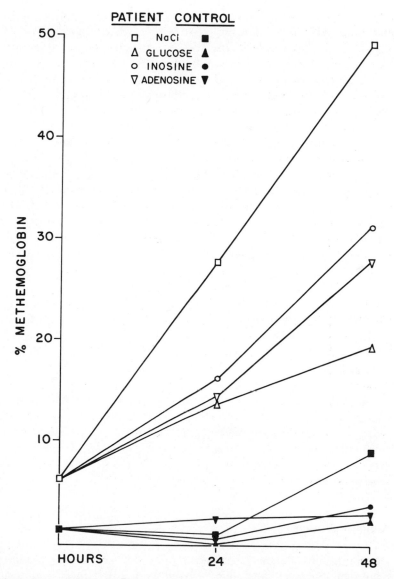

**Figure 7-6.** Methemoglobin formation after 24 and 48 hours of sterile incubation at 37°C in a patient with Hb Köln disease and in a normal individual. Methemoglobin levels were lower in the presence of nutrient additives. [From D.R. Miller et al,[22] with permission of Grune and Stratton.]

marked reduction in intracellular $K^+$ and a disproportionately smaller increment in $Na^+$, the hallmarks of the "dessicyte" or "xerocyte" or dehydrated erythrocyte.[22]

**Red Cell Survival**   Erythrocyte survival as measured by the half-life (T½) of $^{51}Cr$-labeled autologous cells is decreased and correlates with the absolute reticulocyte count but not with the level of hemoglobin.[34] Although the use of $^{51}$Cr, which is bound preferentially to $\beta$ chains, and particularly to unstable $\beta$ chains, has been criticized[35] because falsely low survival might be measured in unstable $\beta$-chain variants, simultaneous studies with DF$^{32}$P and $^{51}$Cr have revealed identical erythrocyte survival in patients with unstable hemoglobins.[34]

Surface scanning over the liver, spleen, and heart has revealed marked splenic sequestration in Hb Köln disease and combined hepatic and splenic uptake in Hbs Genoa, Philly, Zürich, and Seattle.

**Ferrokinetics**  Representative studies in a family with Hb Köln disease are shown in Table 7-4.[36] Increased serum iron, normal total iron binding capacity, and near total saturation of transferrin have been observed in severely affected patients. Plasma clearance time of $^{59}$Fe is reduced and plasma iron turnover is markedly increased. Red cell utilization of radioiron is normal, demonstrating that erythropoiesis is effective. Brisk erythropoiesis is verified by a marked increase in red cell iron turnover and rapid marrow transit time.

**Table 7-4**
**Ferrokinetics in Hb Köln Disease**

|  | Hb Koln | Normal |
|---|---|---|
| Serum Fe, $\mu$g/dl | 259 | 100 |
| TIBC, $\mu$g/dl | 280 | 300 |
| Saturation, % | 93 | 33 |
| $^{59}$Fe plasma clearance, t½, min. | 27 | 60–120 |
| Plasma iron turnover, mg/dl blood/24hr | 5.4 | 0.4–0.8 |
| RBC utilization, % | 95 | 80–100 |
| RBC Fe turnover, mg/dl blood/24hr | 5.1 | 0.4–0.7 |
| Marrow transit time, days | 2.5 | 5.7 |

## Hemoglobin Studies

**Hemoglobin Stability**  The heating of hemolysates from patients with unstable hemoglobins in a phosphate or TRIS buffer for ten minutes at 50°C results in the precipitation of hemoglobin. Heat disrupts weakened heme-globin or interchain binding sites or permits the unfolding of the $\alpha$-helical formation, exaggerating the pre-existing structural instability. The isopropanol test[37] is a simple and specific test for unstable hemoglobins and is based upon the principle that the solvent isopropanol is relatively nonpolar, weakening the internal hydrophobic bonding forces of the protein molecule and decreasing its stability. The test has a further advantage in that the precipitated unstable hemoglobin can be recovered for further characterization.

False-positive reactions have been reported with aging of the sample and with elevated fetal hemoglobin levels (>4%).[38] These problems can be obviated with storage of whole blood at 4°C and by the addition of a small amount of 2% KCN to the hemolysate before testing.[39] The sulfhydryl reagent, parachloromercuribenzoate (PCMB), also causes the precipitation of unstable hemoglobins and can be used for screening purposes.[40] Mechanical shaking may also be used to detect and to quantify unstable hemoglobins.[41]

**Hemoglobin Electrophoresis**  The electrophoretic pattern on starch gel or cellulose acetate in UHD depends in most instances on any charge differences conferred by the mutation; it may show unexpected abnormalities due to charges in the tertiary structure of the molecule. Hb J Guantanamo ($\beta$128 Ala→Asp [H6]), an unstable hemoglobin with two additional negative charges, migrates predictably faster than Hb A on starch gel at pH 8.6,[42] and occupies the same position on starch gel as do other Hb J mutants. A change in net charge is not necessarily associated with an abnormal pattern of migration as the charge may be buried in the hydrophobic region of the molecule and be silent on routine hemoglobin electrophoresis (e.g., Hb Volga $\beta$27 Ala→Asp, $\beta$9).[43] Few of the unstable hemoglobins have charge alterations, as most involve substitutions of neutral amino acids. Some variants with neutral substitutions demonstrate alterations in charge and abnormal bands because of the effect of the mutant, substituted amino acid on its neighbors or because of loss of heme and alteration of structure of the heme pocket. In Hb Köln disease, methionine at $\beta$98 increases the tendency to lose hemin, and a smeared band migrating near the position of Hb F is noted (Figure 7-7). The trailing smeared band disappears when hemin is added to a hemolysate containing Hb Köln; free $\alpha$ chains may be found at the origin. Generally, the abnormal band(s) constitutes less than 10% to 15% of the total hemoglobin. The amount of true Hb $A_2$ and Hb F are usually normal although slight elevations of both have been observed.[35] If no abnormality is observed on starch gel or cellulose acetate electrophoresis, PCMB or isopropanol precipitation can be used to isolate the unstable fraction.[44] The identification of certain mutants poses severe technical difficulties and is dependent upon slight changes in peptide chromatographic mobility. Hb Christchurch ($\beta$77 Phe→Ser [E15]) was characterized with the use of $^{14}$C-labeled Hb A as a control.[45]

**Hemoglobin Synthesis**  The relative quantities of normal and unstable hemoglobin in the red cells of patients with UHD may be the result of two factors: (1) different rates of synthesis of the two components and (2) preferential destruction and loss of the unstable molecule.

The $\beta$ chains of the unstable variants and of Hb A may be synthesized at different rates (Table 7-5). In $\beta^{Gun\ Hill}$ the biosynthetic rate is

164

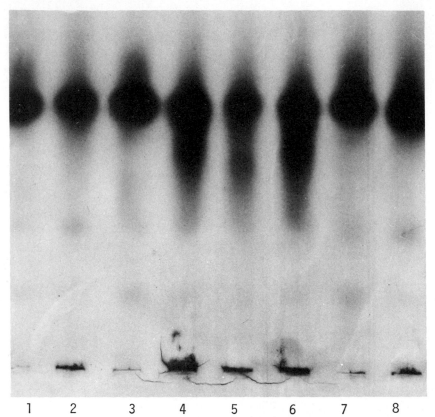

**Figure 7-7.** Starch gel electrophoresis, TRIS-EDTA-borate buffer, pH 8.6, of Hb A and Hb Köln. (1) Hb A, (2) Hb Köln + hemin, (3) Hb A + CO, (4) Hb Köln, (5) Hb Köln + CN⁻, (6) Hb Köln + hemin, (7) Hb A + hemin, (8) Hb Köln + hemin. Note disappearance of training smeared band when hemin was added to Hb Köln. Nonmigrating hemoglobin at origin (probable free alpha chains) is noted with Hb Köln (slots 2,4-6, and 8). Amido black stain. [From F.B. de Furia and D.R. Miller. *Blood* 39:398, 1972.]

increased relative to $\beta^A$.[46] In Hbs Köln,[47,48] Hammersmith,[49] Bristol,[50] and Shepherds Bush,[47] the rates of synthesis of the variant and normal $\beta$ chains are equal, and in Hbs Riverdale-Bronx,[51] Borås,[47] and Abraham Lincoln,[52] a decreased rate of production of the abnormal $\beta$ chain was observed.

In Hb Ann Arbor,[53] an $\alpha$-chain variant ($\alpha$80 Leu→Arg), the synthetic rate of the abnormal chain was much greater than that of normal $\alpha$ chains. Furthermore, decreased synthesis of normal $\beta$ chains was observed, suggesting that the $\beta$ chains released by degradation of preferentially destroyed $\alpha^{Ann\ Arbor}$ chains suppress the synthesis of new $\beta$ chains. Interestingly, Heinz bodies are not seen in Hb Ann Arbor, further suggesting that the abnormal hemoglobin is removed by proteolysis.

**Table 7-5**
**Synthesis of Globin Chains of Unstable Hemoglobins**

| Hemoglobin | % Abnormal Hb | Synthetic rate ($\beta^{variant}/\beta^a$) |
|---|---|---|
| β-Chain Variants | | |
| Gun Hill | 32 | 1.20 |
| Köln | 12 | 1.0 |
| Hammersmith | 40 | 1.0 |
| Bristol | 36 | 0.98 |
| Shepherds Bush | 25 | 1.0 |
| Genova | 20 | 1.0 |
| Riverdale-Bronx | 28 | 0.57 |
| Borås | 10 | 0.33 |
| Abraham Lincoln | 18 | 0.50 |
| β-Chain Variants | | |
| Ann Arbor | 14 | 2.60 |

The rate limiting step in the synthesis of heme involves the formation of δ-aminolevulinic acid (ALA) from succinylcoenzyme A and glycine and is catalyzed by the enzyme ALA synthetase. The activity of ALA synthetase, which is related directly to the number of immature red cells (reticulocytes and nucleated precursors), is significantly decreased in the erythrocytes of patients with Hb Köln disease.[16] Feedback repression of synthesis of the enzyme by excess heme or heme-induced inhibition of the membrane transport of iron and glycine[54] may cause the low levels of ALA synthetase, but the exact mechanism is still unclear.

**Hemoglobin Function**   Alterations in oxygen affinity of the unstable hemoglobins are attributed to heme depletion or displacement and weakened $\alpha_1\beta_2$ and heme-globin contacts. As noted in Table 7-1, some (50%) variant hemoglobins have increased affinity (low $P_{50}$) and others (30%) have decreased affinity (high $P_{50}$). Hemoglobin Köln,[55] the most extensively studied variant, has a high oxygen affinity and decreased heme-heme interaction. The residue FG5 is involved in heme-globin and $\alpha_1\beta_2$ binding and its substitution causes heme depletion, instability, and increased oxygen affinity.

The addition of hemin to solutions of purified Hb Köln in vitro decreases the oxygen affinity and increases heme-heme interaction, presumably by causing conformation changes which favor the deoxy conformation of the molecule.

The glycolytic intermediate, 2,3-diphosphoglycerate (2,3-DPG), reacts normally with purified Hb Köln and decreases the oxygen affinity of Hb Köln "stripped" of 2,3-DPG.[12]

The clinical implications of altered oxygen affinity are predictable.

Patients with disorders associated with high affinity hemoglobins (e.g., Hb Köln) usually have a well-compensated anemia with normal values of hemoglobin and red cell mass because of the leftward shift of the oxygen dissociation curve, which results in decreased delivery of oxygen to the tissues, increased erythropoietin formation, and increased erythrocyte production.[56] In the absence of compensating erythrocytosis, mixed venous oxygen tension is reduced, and evidence of latent hypoxia and decreased reserve are suggested by increased erythropoietin (two to six times normal), decreased mean end capillary pressure, and evidence of redistribution of blood flow. Renal blood flow is reduced by one-third to one-half, but cardiac output and oxygen consumption are normal.[57] These findings suggest that whereas patients with high affinity unstable hemoglobins are essentially asymptomatic at rest and with ordinary activity, they are more vulnerable to conditions that would further impair oxygen delivery. Postsplenectomy, erythrocytosis is observed in Hb Köln disease.

In Hb Seattle, associated with a rightward-shift of the oxygen dissociation curve and decreased oxygen affinity, patients have a relatively low hematocrit, considering the mild degree of hemolysis,[58] supporting Huehns and Bellingham, who have reported that the hemoglobin (and hematocrit) level in patients with unstable hemoglobins relates more closely to the position of the oxygen dissociation curve than to red cell life span.[59]

## Erythrocyte Metabolism

Glycolysis in the red cells of patients with UHD is brisk,[22,60,61,62] reflecting the activity of youth. Glucose utilization, lactate production, and selected enzymes of the pentose phosphate shunt and the Embden-Meyerhof pathway are increased. Glutathione (GSH) levels are normal[22,35] or slightly decreased.[20,44,63] Both normal[22] and increased GSH utilization[64,65,66] have been reported. Jacob and coworkers[65] found excessive GSH binding in mixed disulfide linkage to the $\beta^{93}$ cysteine of Hb Köln and suggested that Heinz bodies were attached to the inner erythrocyte membrane by disulfide linkages. More recently, however, Winterbourn and Carrell[13,66] were unable to detect blocked cysteine residues or covalent disulfide bonds between hemoglobin and the membrane.

A positive screening test for G6PD deficiency is obtained when nitrite-induced methemoglobin reduction is used as the indicator. Methemoglobin reduction progresses normally after nitrite is removed and the activities of NADH and NADPH dependent methemoglobin reductases are normal. The ascorbate-cyanide test of Jacob and

Jandl,[67] another screening test for G6PD deficiency, may also be positive in unstable hemoglobinopathies.[18]

The intracellular concentration of ATP is decreased in the erythrocytes of patients with unstable hemoglobins,[22,60] but remains stable after incubation. The ADP:ATP ratio and the rate of catabolism of adenine nucleotides to hypoxanthine are increased, suggesting that the low levels of ATP are the consequence of markedly increased utilization rather than decreased production. Increased expenditure of ATP in active cation transport occurs in Hb Köln cells. Active, ouabain-sensitive, ATP-dependent potassium influx is increased and potassium efflux ("leak") is 2.5-fold normal.[22,65] Nearly one-quarter of glucose utilization in Hb Köln cells can be inhibited by ouabain, whereas in normal erythrocytes about 10% of glycolysis is ouabain-inhibitable and presumably geared to active cation transport. These abnormalities are not specific and have been reported in patients with pyruvate kinase deficiency, hereditary stomatocytosis, $\beta$ thalassemia, sickle cell anemia, and other hereditary hemolytic anemias.[68,69,70]

During incubation in the absence of glucose, a marked reduction of intracellular potassium, a small sodium gain, and a large net total cation loss occurs. The deformability of the resulting dehydrated cells is decreased presplenectomy and decreases even further postsplenectomy because of the presence of Heinz bodies.[22]

## Pathogenesis of Hemolysis

We know a great deal about structure-function relationships in UHD but less about the exact mechanisms of hemolysis. Although subject to modification and embellishment, current concepts, based upon the studies of Jacob, Winterhalter, Rachmilewitz, Carrell, and Winterbourn, support the following model, which incorporates increased sulfhydryl reactivity, methemoglobin generation, hemichrome formation, heme-depletion, hemoglobin precipitation, and membrane damage (Figure 7-8). Because of structural defects either in the heme pocket or elsewhere in the globin chain, water gains entry to the hydrophobic heme pocket and binds to and oxidizes $Fe^{++}$ to $Fe^{+++}$ (methemoglobin). This process of auto-oxidation can occur under physiologic conditions and does not require additional oxidative stress. Superoxide radicals ($O_2^-$) are generated and in the presence of superoxide dismutase are converted to $H_2O_2$. The highly reactive species $O_2^-$ and $H_2O_2$ can attack sulfhydryl groups in hemoglobin ($\beta^{93}$ cysteine) and the red cell membrane and can be removed by catalase and glutathione peroxidase. Methemoglobin can be converted stepwise, first to reversible hemichromes (hemichrome 1) in which heme iron is bound to

168

both the imidazole groups of the proximal (F8) and distal (E7) histidines and then to irreversible hemichromes (hemichrome 2), which lose SH groups, are denatured, and precipitate as Heinz bodies. This pathway does not require heme depletion. Several unstable hemoglobins (Table 7-3, group II) are heme-depleted and as such are partially unfolded, deficient in helical content, and easily denatured. Heme-depleted hemoglobin can be converted into hemichromes and become denatured as outlined above or as isolated chains precipitated as Heinz bodies. Studies by Carrell and Winterbourn[13] have shown that

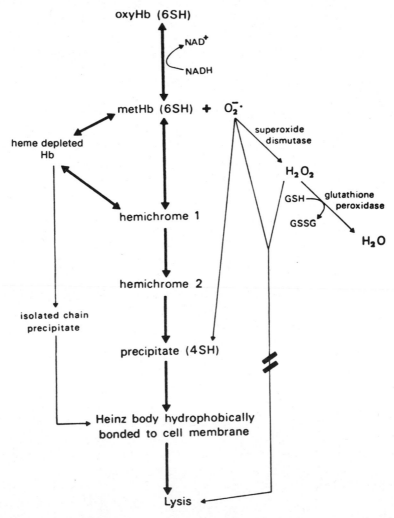

**Figure 7-8.** Proposed mechanism for intracellular denaturation of unstable hemoglobin resulting in Heinz body formation and hemolysis either through formation of hemichromes or through action of superoxide radicals ($O_2^-$) and $H_2O_2$. [From C. Winterbourn and R.W. Carrell.[13]]

Heinz bodies are bound hydrophobically to the cell membrane and not covalently, as proposed by Jacob and Winterhalter.[71] This attachment may alter membrane function, permitting the excess loss of $K^+$ and water from the cell and increasing membrane rigidity, which results in entrapment of nondeformable cells in the microcirculation of the spleen and liver where they are engulfed by reticuloendothelial cells (Figure 7-9). Carrell, Winterbourn, and Rachmilewitz[14] have proposed

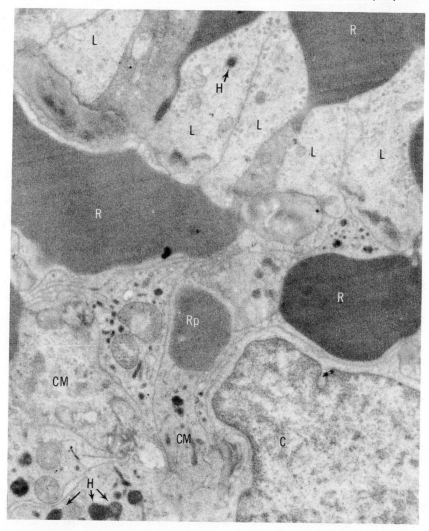

**Figure 7-9.** Electron micrograph of spleen from patient with Hb Köln disease. Erythrocytes (R) are in passage through splenic cord (C) and between sinus littoral cells (L) into splenic sinuses (S). Cordal macrophages (CM) are loaded with Heinz bodies (H) and one contains a phagocytosed erythrocyte (Rp). Single inclusion body is seen in sinus littoral cell (Pb citrate and uranyl acetate stain). × 10,000. [From D.R. Miller, et al. *Blood* 38:715, 1971.]

further that $H_2O_2$ can denature membrane SH groups, disrupting structural proteins and cation gradients and leading to lysis. These final steps are still unsettled.

Not all unstable hemoglobins follow the same pathway of denaturation. In Hb Köln there is increased thiol reactivity at $\beta^{93}$ with $O_2^-$ and $H_2O_2$ whereas in Hb Belfast and Hb Christchurch this reaction does not occur. In the latter variants, hemichrome formation and denaturation depend only upon the amount of methemoglobin produced and do not involve $O_2^-$ and $H_2O_2$ in the process.[72] Thus, the relative importance of auto-oxidation and superoxide production compared with hemichrome formation varies as the hemolytic process varies from one unstable hemoglobin to another.

## Treatment and Prognosis

The mainstays of therapy in hereditary hemolytic anemias are transfusions and splenectomy, but in UHD the former are rarely necessary and the latter may not always be salutary. Although patients with UHD who have undergone splenectomy may have an increase in packed cell volume and hemoglobin levels, this rise is not necessarily equated with clinical improvement or prolonged erythrocyte survival. A priori clinical benefit should be derived from the procedure because of the spleen's role in red cell removal. In some reported cases, [51]Cr and DF[32]P red cell survival improved,[15,22,35,73] and in patients with hypersplenism, thrombocytopenia resolved after surgery. The increase in hemoglobin concentration is more likely a function of the effect of a high affinity hemoglobin on erythropoiesis. The procedure should be reserved for patients with severe or moderate hemolytic anemia who have demonstrable splenic sequestration or hypersplenism. Documenting the specific molecular lesion may be useful to permit a comparison with past clinical experience, but good clinical judgment in an individual case rather than rigid guidelines is more appropriate.

Splenectomy is not without hazards. Deaths related to overwhelming pneumococcal infection and thromboembolism have been reported.[32,35] The common use of prophylactic penicillin and the recent availability of polyvalent pneumococcal vaccine should lessen the bacterial complications. The pediatrician should be aware that microbes other than the pneumococcus (e.g., *E. coli, H. influenzae*) may cause serious life-threatening infections that cannot be prevented by available prophylactic measures. Splenectomized patients should be seen promptly at the first signs of fever, appropriate cultures should be obtained, and the patients treated appropriately with antibiotics, according to the clinical situation.

Transfusions with packed red cells are indicated if patients develop hypoplastic crises and severe anemia or pulmonary infections which cause respiratory embarrassment. Chronic transfusion therapy is rarely required except in severe UHD (Hb Hammersmith, Hb Bristol) during the first year or two of life or in variants with low oxygen affinity when compensating mechanisms are inadequate.

Additional supportive measures include the administration of folic acid, 1 mg daily. Riboflavin, given with the aim of increasing the activity of GSH reductase and protecting hemoglobin sulfhydryl groups from oxidation, failed to have a beneficial effect on red cell survival.[35,74] Antioxidants and free radical scavengers such as tocopherol and 2,3-dihydroxybenzoic acid (2,3-DHB) have not received a clinical trial; 2,3-DHB significantly decreases in vitro the formation of malonyldialdehyde, considered to be a byproduct of membrane lipid peroxidation.[75]

**Future Perspectives**

Despite the exciting information provided by these fascinating disorders of hemoglobin structure and function, a number of unresolved issues remain. These include (1) the exact mechanism of oxidative denaturation, hemichrome formation, and hemolysis; (2) the technical difficulties in purifying, studying, and identifying certain variants; (3) the membrane abnormality; and (4) the control mechanisms in globin and heme synthesis. The continued study of the unstable hemoglobins should provide useful new information relating to the genetics, biochemistry, and molecular biology of hemoglobin.

**HEMOGLOBIN M DISEASE**

Methemoglobin is formed when heme iron is stabilized in the oxidized or $Fe^{3+}$ form. Methemoglobin cannot serve as a respiratory pigment because in its ferric state iron is unable to combine with molecular oxygen. Methemoglobinemia is caused by (1) excessive formation of methemoglobin due to the action of drugs and chemicals, (2) diminished conversion of endogenously formed methemoglobin secondary to a deficiency of the enzyme, NADH-dependent methemoglobin reductase, and (3) a structural abnormality in the globin chain of the hemoglobin molecule, resulting in what are collectively designated M hemoglobins.

**Historical Perspective**

The designation hemoglobin M was proposed[76] for a spectroscopically abnormal methemoglobin first described in 1948 by Horlein and Weber[77] in a family with congenital cyanosis. The spectral abnormality was present when patients' globin was combined with normal heme but not when patients' heme was hybridized with normal globin, thus proving that the abnormality resided in the globin moiety of hemoglobin. Subsequently, the abnormality was identified as Hb M Saskatoon. Gerald and Efron[78] characterized three hemoglobin M disorders—M Boston, M Saskatoon, and M Milwaukee; the first involving an abnormality of the $\alpha$ chain, the latter two, of the $\beta$ chains. Tyrosine replaced the E7 histidine (distal histidine) in Hb M Boston and the F8 histidine (proximal histidine) in Hb M Saskatoon. In Hb M Milwaukee, the substitution was identified as $\beta$67 (E11) Val→Glu. Shibata and coworkers[79] identified Hb M Iwate in Japanese patients with congenital cyanosis. In 1966, Heller et al[80] described the fifth Hb M variant, Hb M Hyde Park. In Hb M Hyde Park and Hb M Saskatoon, a mild hemolytic anemia and hemoglobin instability accompanies the methemoglobinemia. The properties of these five Hb M mutants are summarized in Table 7-6.

**Pathogenesis**

Normally, the fifth coordination position of heme iron is linked to the imidazole group of the proximal (F8) histidine of the $\alpha$ and $\beta$ chains. Oxygen binds to the sixth coordination position of iron on the opposite side of heme in proximity to the distal (E7) histidine of $\alpha$ and $\beta$ chains. Oxygen normally resides between the heme and distal histidine. This does not occur in hemoglobin M disorders because the substituting amino acids form ionic links with the iron atom, thereby stabilizing it in the ferric state. The substitution in four of the five M hemoglobins involves tyrosine for histidine—proximal $\alpha$ His (F8) in Hb M Iwate, proximal $\beta$ His in Hb M Hyde Park, distal $\alpha$ His (E7) in Hb M Boston, and distal $\beta$ His in Hb M Saskatoon. In methemoglobins associated with His→Tyr substitutions, the phenolic residues of tyrosine form covalent bonds with heme iron, stabilize the ferric form of iron, and produce methemoglobinemia.[78] It is not surprising that all four potential substitutions are associated with a distinctive M hemoglobinopathy. The His→Tyr substitutions reflect a single pyrimidine base-substitution in the DNA triplet codon for histidine (GTA or GTG) giving ATA or ATG which is transcribed to UAU or UAC, the mRNA codon for tyrosine. In Hb M Milwaukee, valine at $\beta$67 is replaced by glutamic acid which has a longer side chain forming a bond with iron.

**Table 7-6**
**Properties of M Hemoglobins**

| Hemoglobin | Substitution | Helical residue | Oxygen affinity | Bohr effect | Hill's $\eta$ (heme-heme interaction) | Quaternary deoxy Hb | Structure oxy Hb | Stability to heat |
|---|---|---|---|---|---|---|---|---|
| A | $\alpha_2\beta_2$ | — | | Present | 2.7 | T* | R† | Normal |
| M Boston[78,81] | $\alpha^{58}$ His→Tyr | E7 | 26 | | 1.2 | T | T | Increased |
| M Iwate[79,82,83] | $\alpha^{87}$ His→Tyr | F8 | | | 1.1 | T | T | — |
| M Milwaukee[78,84] | $\beta^{67}$ Val→Glu | E11 | | Present | 1.2 | T | R | Normal |
| M Saskatoon[78,85] | $\beta^{63}$ His→Tyr | E7 | Normal | Present | 1.2 | — | — | Unstable |
| M Hyde Park[80,83,86] | $\beta^{92}$ His→Tyr | F8 | Normal | Present | 1.3 | T | R | Unstable |

*T Tense or deoxygenated conformation.
† Relaxed or oxygenated conformation.

## Structure-Function Relationships

Hemoglobin function in the M hemoglobins is determined by the affected subunit rather than the specific histidine (distal or proximal) which is substituted. Oxygen affinity is decreased in Hb M Boston, Hb M Iwate, and Hb M Milwaukee, and is normal in Hb M Saskatoon and Hb M Hyde Park. The Bohr effect ($\Delta \log P50/\Delta pH$) is decreased in Hb M Boston and Hb M Iwate, and the heme-heme interaction (Hill's n value) is decreased in all since only two of the subunits can carry oxygen.

X-ray crystallography has established the quaternary structure of deoxygenated and oxygenated hemoglobin, the T (tense) and R (relaxed) conformations, respectively.[87,88,89] The change or transition from T to R conformation and altered equilibrium in the transition from T to R will increase oxygen affinity. Oxygen affinity will be decreased if the oxygenated hemoglobin is fixed in the T conformation or if the stability of the T conformation is increased; this occurs in Hb M Boston and Hb M Iwate.

## Clinical Features

M hemoglobin is transmitted as a Mendelian dominant characteristic although spontaneous mutations have been documented. The distribution of cases is worldwide. Patients are cyanotic but are entirely asymptomatic. Alpha chain defects (M Boston and M Iwate) are associated with cyanosis from birth, since the $\alpha$ chains of Hb F are also affected. Methemoglobinemia and cyanosis do not appear until after the first few months of life in a child with Hb M due to a $\beta$ chain defect. Methemoglobin constitutes 15% to 30% of the total hemoglobin in affected individuals with $\alpha$ chain Hb M disease and 40% to 50% in $\beta$ chain Hb M defects.

The diagnosis can be established by comparing the spectral characteristics of the suspected abnormal cyanmethemoglobin with normal cyanmethemoglobin (Figure 7-10). More sophisticated spectroscopic techniques employ electron paramagnetic resonance and offer the advantage of permitting specific identification of the variant hemoglobins. Agar gel electrophoresis at pH 7.1 or gel electrofocusing of ferricyanide-treated hemolysates generally permit a clear separation of Hb A and Hb M.[90]

Congenital methemoglobinemia caused by NADH-dependent methemoglobin reductase deficiency can be differentiated easily from Hb M disease. Infants with the enzyme deficiency have an autosomal recessive disorder and normal spectral analysis and hemoglobin electrophoretic patterns. Careful history should exclude drug-induced disease. An accurate and prompt diagnosis is essential to avoid unnecessary, expensive, and invasive procedures, such as cardiac catheterization, and useless therapy. In contrast to the therapeutic effect of methylene blue and ascorbic acid in patients with the established forms of congenital and drug-induced types of methemoglobinemia, Hb M disorders are totally unaffected by this therapy. Reassurance is the treatment of choice.

## HEMOGLOBINOPATHIES WITH ALTERED OXYGEN AFFINITY

A number of stable hemoglobin variants have been reported exhibiting either increased or decreased oxygen affinity.[84] Mutants with increased oxygen affinity (Hbs Chesapeake, J Capetown, Yakima, Kempsey, Hiroshima, Ranier, Philly) release a smaller proportion of oxygen to the tissues when compared with normal hemoglobin and are

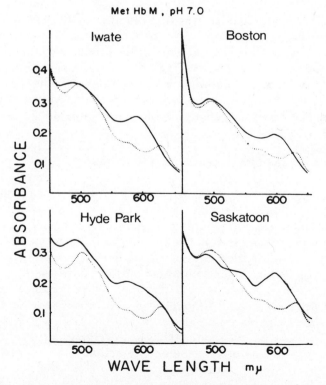

**Figure 7-10.** Absorption spectra of purified M hemoglobins after they are fully oxidized with ferricyanide. The absorption spectrum of normal methemoglobin A is shown by the dotted line. [From S. Shibata, et al. *Bull. Yamaguchi Med. Sch.* 14:141, 1967.]

frequently associated with erythrocytosis. Variants with lowered oxygen affinity (Hbs Kansas, Beth Israel) are associated with cyanosis caused by increased dissociation of oxygen from hemoglobin and an increased concentration of deoxyhemoglobin. A number of excellent reviews on hemoglobins with altered oxygen affinity have appeared recently.[91-94] The identification of these disorders has added considerably to our understanding of normal hemoglobin physiology.

The observed abnormalities of hemoglobin function are related to the site of the amino acid substitution. Perutz and associates[88,89] demonstrated that oxygen affinity is altered when the amino acid substitution affects oxygen binding by (1) changing the conformation of the heme surroundings, (2) altering the binding of hydrogen atoms (Bohr effect) or 2,3-DPG, or (3) shifting the allosteric equilibrium between the tertiary and quaternary oxy- and deoxyhemoglobin structures.

### Historical Perspective

Familial erythrocytosis was first reported by Nichamin in 1908.[95] Charache and coworkers[96] described the first hemoglobinopathy associated with increased oxygen affinity and erythrocytosis—Hb Chesapeake, $\alpha 92$, Arg→Leu. Hemoglobin Kansas was the first reported low affinity variant.[97] Subsequently, 26 other variants with altered oxygen affinity have been reported. The 23 variants with increased and five with decreased oxygen affinity are listed in Tables 7-7 and 7-8.

### Pathogenesis and Structure-Function Relationships

Amino acid substitutions affecting the $\alpha_1\beta_2$ interface binding sites for 2,3-DPG and the C terminus of the $\beta$ chain have a marked effect on hemoglobin function. Increased oxygen affinity occurs if substitutions at the $\alpha_1\beta_2$ interface result in the inability to stabilize the deoxyhemoglobin (T) conformation of the molecule (Figure 7-11); decreased oxygen affinity results if an amino acid substitution prevents a stabilized bond between $\alpha_1$ and $\beta_2$ in the oxyhemoglobin or R conformation (Hb Kansas, $\beta 102$ Asn→Ser). Although it is not the case for all abnormal hemoglobins with an amino acid substitution at the $\alpha_1\beta_1$ contact, Hb Philly ($\beta 35$ Tyr→Phe, $\alpha_1\beta_1$ contact) has an extremely high oxygen affinity and a complete lack of heme-heme interaction.[101]

Altered 2,3-DPG binding increases oxygen affinity. Decreased 2,3-DPG binding and increased oxygen affinity have been reported in Hb Helsinki,[102] Hb Rahere,[103] and Hb Providence,[104] all associated with a substitution at $\beta 82$ (EF6), a DPG binding site. Beta 143 histidine also binds 2,3-DPG, and both Hb Syracuse ($\beta$143 His→Pro)[105] and Hb Little Rock ($\beta$143 His→Gln)[106] have decreased 2,3-DPG binding.

**Table 7-7**
**Hemoglobin Variants with Increased Oxygen Affinity and Erythrocytosis***

| Variant | Substitution | Inferface | Bohr effect | Electrophoretic identification† |
|---|---|---|---|---|
| Chapel Hill[99] | $\alpha^{74}$ Asp→Gly | ? | N | S |
| Chesapeake | $\alpha^{92}$ Arg→Leu | $\alpha_1\beta_2$ | N | S,A,G, |
| J. Capetown | $\alpha^{92}$ Arg→Gln | $\alpha_1\beta_2$ | N | S |
| Tarrant[100] | $\alpha^{126}$ Asp→Asn | $\alpha_1\beta_1$ | ↓ | A |
| Olympia | $\beta^{20}$ Val→Met | $\alpha_1\beta_2$ | — | — |
| Philly[101] | $\beta^{35}$ Tyr→Phe | $\alpha_1\beta_1$ | — | A |
| Helsinki[102] | $\beta^{82}$ Lys→Met | 2,3-DPG | ↓ | |
| Rahere | $\beta^{82}$ Lys→Thr | 2,3-DPG | N | |
| Providence | $\beta^{82}$ Lys→Asn,Asp | 2,3-DPG | | |
| Creteil | $\beta^{89}$ Ser→Asn | | | G |
| Malmo | $\beta^{97}$ His→Gln | $\alpha_1\beta_2$ | N | G |
| Wood | $\beta^{97}$ His→Leu | $\alpha_1\beta_2$ | | G |
| Yakima | $\beta^{99}$ Asp→His | $\alpha_1\beta_2$ | N | S |
| Kempsey | $\beta^{99}$ Asp→Asn | $\alpha_1\beta_2$ | ↓ | S,G |
| Ypsilanti | $\beta^{99}$ Asp→Tyr | $\alpha_1\beta_2$ | | S |
| Brigham | $\beta^{100}$ Pro→Leu | $\alpha_1\beta_2$ | N | — |
| Heathrow | $\beta^{103}$ Phe→Leu | Heme | N | — |
| San Diego | $\beta^{109}$ Val→Met | $\alpha_1\beta_2$ | | G |
| Little Rock | $\beta^{143}$ His→Gln | $\beta\beta$ | N | A,G |
| Syracuse | $\beta^{143}$ His→Pro | $\beta\beta$ | ↓ | G |
| Andrew-Minneapolis | $\beta^{144}$ Lys→Asn | $\beta\beta$ | | S,G |
| Ranier | $\beta^{145}$ Tyr→Lys | $\beta\beta$ | ↓ | A |
| Bethesda | $\beta^{145}$ Tyr→His | $\beta\beta$ | ↓ | A |
| Ft. Gordon | $\beta^{145}$ Tyr→Asp | $\beta\beta$ | ↓ | |
| Hiroshima | $\beta^{146}$ His→Asp | $\beta\beta$ | ↓ | S,A,G |

*Modified from Bunn, Forget, and Ranney.[98]
†Starch gel (S) pH 8.6, agar gel (A) 6.0, or gel electrofocusing (G).

**Table 7-8**
**Hemoglobin Variants with Decreased Oxygen Affinity**

| Variant | Substitution | Interface | Bohr effect | Cyanosis |
|---|---|---|---|---|
| Titusville | $\alpha^{90}$ Asp→Asn | $\alpha_1\beta_2$ | ↓ | 0 |
| Agenogi | $\beta^{90}$ Glu→Lys | external residue | | 0 |
| Kansas | $\beta^{102}$ Asn→Thr | $\alpha_1\beta_2$ | N | + |
| Beth Israel | $\beta^{102}$ Asn→Ser | $\alpha_1\beta_2$ | N | + |
| Yoshizuka | $\beta^{108}$ Asn→Asp | $\alpha_1\beta_2$ | | 0 |

Due to their unstable deoxy conformation, certain high affinity hemoglobins (Hb Kempsey, Hb Chesapeake) dissociate into dimers at the $\alpha_1\beta_1$ interface when they are fully deoxygenated.

Substitutions at the C terminus of the $\beta$ chain (particularly involving $\beta$146 histidine) may alter the Bohr effect ($\Delta$ logP50/$\Delta$pH) because of an inability to form a salt bond with $\beta$94 aspartic acid. Indeed, as noted in Table 7-7, five of the seven hemoglobinopathies with altered $\beta\beta$ contact are associated with a decreased Bohr effect.

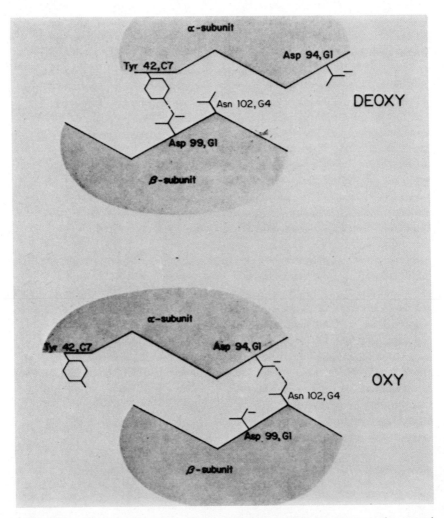

**Figure 7-11.** Changes at a portion of the $\alpha_1\beta_2$ interface upon oxygenation. The area of contact shifts in a dovetail fashion. Deoxyhemoglobin is stabilized by a hydrogen bond between $\alpha^{42}$ Tyr and $\beta^{99}$ Asp. In Hb Kempsey ($\beta$99 Asp→Asn) this bond cannot form and oxygen affinity is increased. Oxyhemoglobin is also stabilized by a bond between $\alpha$94 Asp and $\beta$102 Asn. This bond cannot form in Hb Kansas ($\beta$102 Asn→Thr), Hb Beth Israel ($\beta$102 Asn→Ser), and Hb Titusville ($\alpha$94 Asp→Asn), resulting in decreased oxygen affinity. [From M.F. Perutz. *New Scientist Sci. J.* June 1971.]

## Clinical Features

The inheritance pattern of structurally abnormal hemoglobins with altered oxygen affinity is autosomal dominant, although examples of apparent spontaneous mutations have been reported.[107] Polycythemia and increased red cell mass without leukocytosis and thrombocytosis are found in hemoglobinopathies with increased oxygen affinity; mild cyanosis in hemoglobinopathies is associated with decreased oxygen affinity. Most patients are asymptomatic, and often the diagnosis is not made until adulthood. Minor manifestations of headache, lethargy, occasional dizziness, and easy fatigability have been described in some children.[108] In the elderly, exercise intolerance, exertional dyspnea, and mild angina pectoris have been described. The patients have no splenomegaly or other physical signs except for a ruddy complexion and deeply injected conjunctivae. The cyanosis in Hb Kansas and Hb Beth Israel is of cosmetic importance only since oxygen unloading at the tissue level is normal. Minimal anemia in low affinity hemoglobinopathies is caused by the increased oxygen delivery and decreased erythropoietin-stimulated erythropoiesis.

Hemoglobin levels in patients with high affinity hemoglobins range between 16 and 24 g/dl. In children, the differential diagnosis of polycythemia includes disorders associated with (1) autonomous erythroid proliferation or polycythemia vera, exceedingly rare in children[109,110]; (2) inappropriate increase in erythropoietin occurring in certain neoplastic and nonneoplastic diseases of the kidneys, liver, and central nervous system; (3) increased production of erythropoietin in families with recessively-inherited erythrocytosis[111]; (4) hypoxemia with a secondary increase in erythropoietin as in cardiopulmonary disease, high altitude, alveolar hypoventilation, and left-to-right intra-cardiac shunts; and (5) abnormal hemoglobin function.

The laboratory evaluation of a patient with polycythemia should rule out hemoglobin dysfunction, although in children hypoxemia secondary to cardiopulmonary disease is more common. Assessment of oxygen affinity requires techniques often available only in research laboratories. Lichtman and coworkers[112] have described a simple technique using a single venous blood sample to calculate the $P_{50}$ at standard or at in vivo conditions by measurement of pH, $PO_2$, $PCO_2$ and $O_2$ saturation. The correlation between the calculated and measured $P_{50}$ is excellent.

Hemoglobin electrophoresis on starch gel, pH 8.6, or agar gel, pH 6.0, or gel electrofusing should detect most but not all variants with altered oxygen affinity. Some, with neutral amino acid substitutions, are silent (Hb Olympia, $\beta$20 Val→Met; Hb Brigham, $\beta$100 Pro→Leu; Hb Heathrow, $\beta$103 Phe→Leu; and Hb Philly, $\beta$35 Tyr→Phe). Other hemoglobins with neutral substitutions (Hb Kansas, $\beta$102 Asn→Thr)[113] have slightly altered electrophoretic mobility.

180

Additional hematologic studies should include measurement of red blood cell mass and blood volume. Erythropoietin is increased in high affinity hemoglobinopathies. When measured, levels of 2,3-DPG are normal. The $P_{50}$ of variant hemoglobins associated with substitutions at 2,3-DPG binding sites and hemoglobins "stripped" of 2,3-DPG increases minimally or not at all with exogenous 2,3-DPG. Ligand binding,[114] x-ray crystallography,[12] nuclear magnetic resonance, and electron paramagnetic resonance further characterize these variants.

## Treatment

Accurate diagnosis rather than treatment is the key to successful and appropriate management of these disorders. Therapeutic misadventures ([32]P for erroneously diagnosed polycythemia vera) must be avoided. Because blood viscosity increases exponentially when the packed red cell volume increases above 0.65 liter/liters, cautious phlebotomy has been recommended, particularly in symptomatic patients.

1. Cathie, I.A.B. Apparent idiopathic Heinz body anemia. *Great Ormond Street J.* 3:43, 1952.
2. Lange, R.D., and Ackeroyd, J.H. Congenital hemolytic anemia with abnormal pigment metabolism and red cell inclusion bodies, a new clinical syndrome. *Blood* 13:950, 1958.
3. Schmid, R., Brecher, G., and Clemens, T. Familial hemolytic anemia with erythrocyte inclusion bodies and a defect in pigment metabolism. *Blood* 14:991, 1959.
4. Scott, J.L., Haut, A., Cartwright, G.E., et al. Congenital hemolytic disease associated with red cell inclusion bodies, abnormal pigment metabolism and an electrophoretic hemoglobin abnormality. *Blood* 16:1239, 1960.
5. Frick, P.G., Hitzig, W.H., and Betke, K. Hemoglobin Zürich. I. A new hemoglobin anomaly associated with acute hemolytic episodes with Heinz bodies after sulfonamide therapy. *Blood* 20:261, 1962.
6. Grimes, A.J., and Meisler, A. Possible cause of Heinz bodies in congenital Heinz body anemia. *Nature* 194:190, 1962.
7. Grimes, A.J., Meisler, A., and Dacie, J.V. Congenital Heinz-body anaemia: Further evidence on the cause of Heinz-body production in red cells. *Br. J. Haematol.* 10:281, 1964.
8. Hutchison, H.E., Pinkerton, P.H., Waters, P., et al. Hereditary Heinz-body anemia, thrombocytopenia, and haemoglobinopathy (Hb Köln) in a Glasgow family. *Br. Med. J.* 2:1099, 1964.
9. Carrell, R.W., Lehmann, H., and Hutchison, H.E. Haemoglobin Köln ($\beta^{98}$ valine→methionine): An unstable protein causing inclusion body anaemia. *Nature* 210:915, 1966.
10. Perutz, M.F., and Lehmann, H. Molecular pathology of human haemoglobin. *Nature* 219:902, 1968.
11. Perutz, M.F. Structure and function of hemoglobin. *Harvey Lect.* 63:213, 1969.

12. de Furia, F.G., and Miller, D.R. Oxygen affinity in hemoglobin Köln disease. *Blood* 39:398, 1972.

13. Winterbourn, C.C., and Carrell, R.W. Studies of hemoglobin denaturation and Heinz body formation in the unstable hemoglobins. *J. Clin. Invest.* 54:678, 1974.

14. Carrell, R.W., Winterbourn, C.C., and Rachmilewitz, E.A. Activated oxygen and haemolysis. *Br. J. Haematol.* 30:259, 1975.

15. Pedersen, P.R., McCurdy, P.R., Wrightstone, R.N., et al. Hemoglobin Köln in a black: Pre- and post-splenectomy red cell survival (DF$^{32}$ and $^{51}$Cr) and the pathogenesis of hemoglobin instability. *Blood* 42:771, 1973.

16. Kolski, G.B., and Miller, D.R. Heme synthesis in hereditary hemolytic anemias: Decreased δ-aminolevulinic acid synthetase in hemoglobin Köln disease. *Pediatr. Res.* 10:702, 1976.

17. Lie-Injo, L.E., Lopez, C.G., Eapen, J.S., et al. Unstable haemoglobin Köln disease in members of a Malay family. *J. Med. Genet.* 9:340, 1972.

18. Dacie, J.V., Shinton, N.K., Gaffney, P.J., et al. Haemoglobin Hammersmith ($\beta^{42}$(CD1)Phe→Ser). *Nature* 216:663, 1967.

19. Steadman, J.H., Yates, A., and Huehns, E.R. Idiopathic Heinz body anaemia: Hb Bristol ($\beta^{67}$(E11)Val→Asp). *Br. J. Haematol.* 18:435, 1970.

20. Fairbanks, V.F., Opfell, R.W., and Burgert, E.O. Three families with unstable hemoglobinopathies (Köln, Olmstead and Santa Ana) causing hemolytic anemia with inclusion bodies and pigmenturia. *Am. J. Med.* 46:344, 1969.

21. Schneider, R.G., Ueda, S., Alperin, J.B., et al. Hemoglobin Sabine beta-91 (F7)Leu→Pro: An unstable variant causing severe anemia with inclusion bodies. *N. Engl. J. Med.* 280:739, 1969.

22. Miller, D.R., Weed, R.I., Stamatoyannopoulos, G., et al. Hemoglobin Köln disease occurring as a fresh mutation: Erythrocyte metabolism and survival. *Blood* 38:715, 1971.

23. Lehmann, A., and Carrell, W. Variations on the structure of human haemoglobin (with particular reference to the unstable haemoglobins). *Br. Med. Bull.* 25:14, 1969.

24. King, M.A.R., Wiltshire, B.G., Lehmann, H., et al. An unstable haemoglobin with reduced oxygen affinity. Haemoglobin Peterborough $\beta^{111}$(G13) valine→phenylalanine, its interaction with normal haemoglobin and haemoglobin Lepore. *Br. J. Haematol.* 22:125, 1972.

25. Beutler, E., Lang, A., and Lehmann, H. Hemoglobin Duarte ($\alpha_2\beta_2{}^{62}$[E6]Ala→Pro): A new unstable hemoglobin with increased oxygen affinity. *Blood* 43:527, 1974.

26. Sansone, G., and Pik, C. Familial haemolytic anaemia with erythrocyte inclusion bodies, bilifuscinuria and abnormal haemoglobin (haemoglobin Galliera Genova). *Br. J. Haematol.* 11:511, 1965.

27. Labie, D., Bernadou, A., Wajcman, H., et al. Familial case of Genova 28 (B10)Leu→Pro hemoglobin: Clinical, hematological, genetic and biochemical studies in a French family. *Nouv. Rev. Fr. Hematol.* 12:502, 1972.

28. Levine, R.L., Lincoln, D.R., Buchholz, W.M., et al. Hemogloblin Hasharon in a premature infant with hemolytic anemia. *Pediatr. Res.* 9:7, 1975.

29. Lee-Potter, J.P., Deacon-Smith, R.A., Simpkiss, M.J., et al. A new cause of haemolytic anaemia in the newborn. A description of an unstable fetal haemoglobin: F Poole, $\alpha_2^G\gamma_2{}^{130Trp\rightarrow Gly}$. *J. Clin. Pathol.* 28:317, 1975.

30. Kreimer-Birnbaum, M., Pinkerton, P.H., Bannerman, R.M., et al. Dipyrrolic urinary pigments in congenital Heinz-body anaemia due to Hb Köln and thalassemia. *Br. Med. J.* 2:396, 1966.

182

31. Adams, J.G., Heller, P., Abramson, R.K., et al. Sulfonamide-induced hemolytic anemia and hemoglobin Hasharon. *Arch. Int. Med.* 137:1449, 1977.

32. White, J.M. The unstable haemoglobin disorders. *Clin. Haematol.* 3:333, 1974.

33. Motulsky, A.G., and Stamatoyannopoulos, G. Drugs, anesthesia and abnormal hemoglobins. *Ann. NY Acad. Sci.* 151:807, 1968.

34. Bentley, S.A., Lewis, S.M., and White, J.M. Red cell survival studies in patients with unstable hemoglobin disorders. *Br. J. Haematol.* 26:85, 1974.

35. White, J.M., and Dacie, J.V. The unstable hemoglobins—molecular and clinical features. *Prog. Hematol.* 7:69, 1971.

36. Miller, D.R., and Kolski, G.B. Heme synthesis in hereditary hemolytic anemias. *Pediatr. Res.* 9:324, 1975.

37. Carrell, R.W., and Kay, R. A simple method for the detection of unstable haemoglobins. *Br. J. Haematol.* 23:615, 1972.

38. Carrell, R.W., Hemoglobin stability tests. Edited by R.M. Schmidt, T.H.J. Huisman, and H. Lehmann. In *The Detection of Hemoglobinopathies.* Cleveland: CRC Press, 1974.

39. Brosious, E.M., Morrison, B.Y., and Schmidt, R.M. Effects of hemoglobin F levels, KCN, and storage on the isopropanol precipitation test for unstable hemoglobins. *Am. J. Clin. Pathol.* 66:878, 1976.

40. Wrightstone, R.N., Wilson, J.B., Reynolds, C.A., et al. Methods for detection and analysis of unstable hemoglobins. *Clin. Chim. Acta* 44:217, 1973.

41. Asakura, T., Adachi, R., Shapiro, M., et al. Mechanical precipitation of hemoglobin Köln. *Biochim. Biophys. Acta* 412:197, 1975.

42. Martinez, G., Lema, F., and Colombo, B. Haemoglobin J Guantanamo (22 128 (H6) Ala-Asp). A new fast unstable haemoglobin found in a Cuban family. *Biochim. Biophys. Acta* 491:1, 1977.

43. Idelson, L.I., Didkovsky, N.A., Filippova, A.V., et al. Haemoglobin Volga, $\beta^{27}$(B9)Ala→Asp, a newly highly unstable haemoglobin with a suppressed charge. *FEBS Lett.* 58:122, 1976.

44. Honig, G.R., Green, D., Shamsuddin, M., et al. Hemoglobin Abraham Lincoln, B$^{32}$(B14)leucine→proline, an unstable hemoglobin variant producing severe hemolytic disease. *J. Clin. Invest.* 52:1746, 1973.

45. Carrell, R.W., and Owen, M.C. A new approach to haemoglobin variant identification. Haemoglobin Christchurch $\beta^{71}$(E15)phenylalanine→serine. *Biochim. Biophys. Acta* 236:507, 1971.

46. Rieder, R.F. Synthesis of hemoglobin Gun Hill: Increased synthesis of the heme-free $\beta^{GH}$ globin chain and subunit exchange with a free $\alpha$-chain pool. *J. Clin. Invest.* 50:388, 1971.

47. White, J.M. The synthesis of abnormal haemoglobins. *Ser. Haematol.* 4:116, 1971.

48. White, J.M., and Brain, M.C. Defective synthesis of an unstable haemoglobin: Haemoglobin Köln ($\beta^{98}$val→met). *Br. J. Haematol.* 18:195, 1970.

49. White, J.M., and Dacie, J.V. In vitro synthesis of Hb Hammersmith (CD1 Phe→Ser). *Nature* 225:860, 1970.

50. Steadman, J.H., Yates, A., and Huehns, E.R. Idiopathic Heinz body anaemia: Hb Bristol ($\beta^{67}$(E11)val→asp). *Br. J. Haematol.* 18:435, 1970.

51. Bank, A., O'Donnell, J.V., and Braverman, A.S. Globin chain synthesis in heterozygotes for beta chain mutations. *J. Lab. Clin. Med.* 76:616, 1970.

52. Honig, G.R., Mason, R.G., Vida, L.N., et al. Synthesis of hemoglobin Abraham Lincoln ($\beta^{32}$leu→pro). *Blood* 43:657, 1974.

53. Adams, J.G., Winter, W.P., Rucknagel, D.L., et al. Biosynthesis of hemoglobin Ann Arbor: Evidence of catabolic and feedback regulation. *Science*

176:1427, 1972.

54. Ponka, P., and Neuwirt, J. Use of reticulocytes with high non-haem iron pools for studies of regulation of haem synthesis. Br. J. Haematol. 19:593, 1970.

55. Sharma, V.S., Noble, R.W., and Ranney, H.M. Structure-function relation in Hemoglobin Köln ($\beta^{98}$val→met). J. Mol. Biol. 82:139, 1974.

56. Bellingham, A.J., and Huehns, E.R. Compensation in haemolytic anaemias caused by abnormal haemoglobins. Nature 218:924, 1968.

57. Woodson, R.D., Heywood, J.D., and Lenfant, C. Oxygen transport in hemoglobin Köln. Arch. Intern. Med. 134:711, 1974.

58. Stamatoyannopoulos, G., Parer, J.T., and Finch, C.A. Physiologic implications of a hemoglobin with decreased oxygen affinity (hemoglobin Seattle). N. Engl. J. Med. 281:915, 1969.

59. Huehns, E.R., and Bellingham, A.J. Diseases of function and stability of haemoglobin. Br. J. Haematol. 17:1, 1969.

60. Mills, C.G., Levin, W.C., and Alperin, J.B. Hemolytic anemia associated with low erythrocyte ATP. Blood 32:15, 1968.

61. Mills, G.C., Alperin, J.B., Hill, F.L., et al. Unstable hemoglobin hemolytic anemia: In vitro incubation studies on erythrocytes with hemoglobin Sabine. Biochem. Med. 5:212, 1971.

62. Mills, G.C., Alperin, J.B., Hill, F.L., et al. Additional biochemical studies on erythrocytes containing hemoglobin Sabine. Biochem. Med. 6:355, 1972.

63. Vaughan Jones, R., Grimes, A.J., Carrell, R.W., and Lehmann, H. Köln haemoglobinopathy. Further data and a comparison with other hereditary Heinz body anaemias. Br. J. Haematol. 13:394, 1967.

64. Carrell, R.W., and Lehmann, H. The unstable haemoglobin haemolytic anaemias. Semin. Hematol. 6:116, 1969.

65. Jacob, H.S., Brain, M.C., and Dacie, J.V. Altered sulfhydryl reactivity of hemoglobins and red blood cell membranes in congenital Heinz body hemolytic anemia. J. Clin. Invest. 47:2664, 1968.

66. Winterbourn, C.C., and Carrell, R.W. The attachment of Heinz bodies to the red cell membrane. Br. J. Haematol. 25:585, 1973.

67. Jacob, H., and Jandl, J.H. A simple visual screening test for G-6-PD deficiency employing ascorbate and cyanide. N. Engl. J. Med. 274:1162, 1966.

68. Orringer, E.P., and Parker, J.C. Ion and water movements in red blood cells. Prog. Hematol. 8:1, 1973.

69. Nathan, D.G., and Shoht, S.B. Erythrocyte ion transport defects and hemolytic anemia: "Hydrocytoses" and "desiccytosis." Semin. Hematol. 7:381, 1970.

70. Glader, B.E., Fortier, N., Albala, M.M., et al. Congenital hemolytic anemia associated with dehydrated erythrocytes and increased potassium loss. N. Engl. J. Med. 291:491, 1975.

71. Jacob, H.S., and Winterhalter, K.H. Unstable hemoglobins: The role of heme loss in Heinz body formation. Proc. Natl. Acad. Sci. USA 65:697, 1970.

72. Winterbourn, C.C., McGrath, B.M., and Carrell, R.W. Reactions involving superoxide and normal and unstable haemoglobins. Biochem. J. 155:493, 1976.

73. Bunn, H.F., Forget, B.G., and Ranney, H.M. Unstable hemoglobin variants — congenital Heinz body hemolytic anemia. In Human Hemoglobins. Philadelphia: W.B. Saunders Co., 1977.

74. Nomanbhoy, Y.T., and Fairbanks, V.F. Failure of riboflavin ingestion to modify the anemias and glutathione reductase activity of erythrocytes in three unstable hemoglobin disorders (Köln, H., Olmsted). Proc. XIII Congr. Int. Soc. Hematol. Munich, 1970.

75. Graziano, J.H., Miller, D.R., Grady, R.W., et al. Inhibition of membrane peroxidation in thalassemic erythrocytes by 2,3-dihydroxybenzoic acid. *Br. J. Haematol.* 32:351, 1976.

76. Singer, K. Hereditary hemolytic disorders associated with alterations of the hemoglobin molecule. *Am. J. Med.* 18:633, 1955.

77. Horlein, H., and Weber, G. Über chronische familiare Methanoglobinamie und eine neue Modifikation des Methamoglobins. *Dtsch. Med. Wochenschr.* 73:476, 1948.

78. Gerald, P.S., and Efron, M.L. Chemical studies of several varieties of Hb M. *Proc. Natl. Acad. Sci. USA* 47:1758, 1961.

79. Shibata, S., Miyaji, T., Iuchi, I., et al. Substitution of tryosine for histidine (87) in the $\alpha$ chain of hemoglobin M Iwate. *Acta Haematol. Jpn.* 27:13, 1964.

80. Heller, P., Coleman, R.O., and Yakulis, V. Structural studies of hemoglobin M-Hyde Park. *J. Clin. Invest.* 45:1021, 1966.

81. Suzuki, T., Akira, H., and Yamamura, Y. Functional abnormality of hemoglobin M Osaka. *Biochem. Biophys. Res. Commun.* 19:691, 1965.

82. Hayashi, N., Motokawa, Y., and Kikuchi, G. Studies on relationship between structure and function of hemoglobin M Iwate. *J. Biol. Chem.* 241:79, 1966.

83. Ranney, H.M., Nagel, R.L., Heller, P., et al. Oxygen equilibrium of hemoglobin M Hyde Park. *Biochim. Biophys. Acta* 127:280, 1966.

84. Ranney, H.M. Clinically important variants of human hemoglobin. *N. Engl. J. Med.* 282:144, 1970.

85. Suzuki, T., Hayashi, A., Shimizu, A., et al. The oxygen equilibrium of hemoglobin M Saskatoon. *Biochim. Biophys. Acta* 127:280, 1966.

86. Hayashi, A., Suzuki, T., Shimizu, A., et al. Some observations on the physicochemical properties of hemoglobin M Hyde Park. *Arch. Biochem.* 125:895, 1968.

87. Pulsinelli, P.D., Perutz, M.F., and Nagel, R.L. Structure of hemoglobin M Boston, a variant with a five coordinated ferric heme. *Proc. Natl. Acad. Sci. USA* 70:3870, 1973.

88. Perutz, M.F. Stereochemistry of cooperative effects of haemoglobin. *Nature* 228:726, 1970.

89. Morimoto, H., Lehmann, H., and Perutz, M.F. Molecular pathology of human haemoglobin: Stereochemical interpretation of abnormal oxygen affinities. *Nature* 232:408, 1971.

90. Gerald, P.S. The electrophoretic and spectroscopic characterization of Hgb M. *Blood* 13:936, 1958.

91. Charache, S. Haemoglobins with altered oxygen affinity. *Clin. Haematol.* 3:357, 1974.

92. Nagel, R.L., and Bookchin, R.M. Human hemoglobin mutants with abnormal oxygen binding. *Semin. Hematol.* 11:385, 1975.

93. Stamatoyannopoulos, G., Bellingham, A.J., Finch, C.A., et al. Abnormal hemoglobins with high and low affinity. *Annu. Rev. Med.* 22:221, 1971.

94. Bunn, H.F., Forget, B.G., and Ranney, H.M. *Hemoglobinopathies.* Philadelphia: W.B. Saunders Co., 1977, Chapter 6.

95. Nichamin, S.D. Ein Fall von Erythrämie. *Folia Hematol.* 6:301, 1908.

96. Charache, S., Weatherall, D.J., and Clegg, J.B. Polycythemia associated with a hemoglobinopathy. *J. Clin. Invest.* 45:813, 1966.

97. Reissmann, K.R., Ruth, W.E., and Nomura, T. A human hemoglobin with lowered oxygen affinity and impaired heme-heme interactions. *J. Clin. Invest.* 40:1826, 1961.

98. Bunn, H.F., Forget, B.G., and Ranney, H.M. Hemoglobinopathy due to abnormal oxygen binding. In *Human Hemoglobins*. Philadelphia: W.B. Saunders Co., 1977.

99. Orringer, E.P., Wilson, J.B., and Huisman, T.H.J. Hemoglobin Chapel Hill or $\alpha_2$ Asp→Gly $\beta_2$. *FEBS Lett.* 65:297, 1976.

100. Moo-Penn, W.F., Jue, D.L., Johnson, M.H., et al. Hemoglobin Tarrant $\alpha_{126}$ (H9) Asp→Asn: A new hemoglobin variant in the $\alpha_1\beta_1$ contact region showing high oxygen affinity and reduced cooperativity. *Biochim. Biophys. Acta* 490:443, 1977.

101. Asakura, T., Adachi, K., Wiley, J.S., et al. Structure and function of haemoglobin Philly (Tyr C1(35)$\beta$→Phe). *J. Mol. Biol.* 104:185–195, 1976.

102. Ikkala, E., Koskela, J., Pikkarainen, P., et al. Hb Helsinki: A binding site ($\beta_{82}$ (EF6) Lys→Met). *Acta Haematol.* 56:257, 1976.

103. Lorkin, P.A., Stephens, A.D., Beard, M.E.J., et al. Haemoglobin Rahere ($\beta_{82}$ Lys→Thr): A new high affinity haemoglobin associated with decreased 2,3-DPG binding and relative polycythemia. *Br. Med. J.* 4:200, 1975.

104. Charache, S., McCurdy, P., and Fox, J. Hemoglobin Providence (Hb Prov): A fetal-like hemoglobin. *Blood* 46:1030, 1975.

105. Jensen, M., Oski, F.A., Nathan, D.G., et al. Hemoglobin Syracuse ($\alpha_2\beta_2^{143(H21)His\rightarrow Pro}$): A new high affinity variant detected by special electrophoretic methods. *J. Clin. Invest.* 55:469, 1975.

106. Bare, G.H., Alben, J., Bromberg, P.A., et al. Hemoglobin Little Rock ($\beta_{143}$(H21) Hb→Gln). Effects of an amino acid substitution at the 2,3-DPG binding site. *J. Biol. Chem.* 249:773, 1974.

107. Bunn, H.F., Bradley, T.B., Davis, W.E., et al. Structural and functional studies on hemoglobin Bethesda ($\alpha_2\beta_2^{145His}$), a variant associated with compensatory erythrocytosis. *J. Clin. Invest.* 51:2299, 1972.

108. Abildgaard, C.F., Cornet, J.A., and Schulman, I. Primary erythrocytosis. *J. Pediatr.* 63:1072, 1963.

109. Dystra, O.H., and Halbertsma, T. Polycythemia vera in childhood; report of a case with changes in the skull. *Am. J. Dis. Child.* 60:907, 1940.

110. Kellman, L. Primary polycythemic manifestations. *Am. J. Dis. Child.* 58:146, 1939.

111. Adamson, J.W., Stamatoyannopoulos, G., Kontras, S., et al. Recessive familial erythrocytosis: Aspects of marrow regulation in two families. *Blood* 41:641, 1973.

112. Lichtman, M.A., Murphy, M., and Pogal, M. The use of a single venous blood sample to assess oxygen binding to haemoglobin. *Br. J. Haematol.* 32:85, 1976.

113. Bonaventura, J., and Riggs, A. Hemoglobin Kansas: A human hemoglobin with a neutral amino acid substitution and an abnormal oxygen equilibrium. *J. Biol. Chem.* 243:980, 1968.

114. Gibson, Q.H., and Nagel, R.L. Allosteric transition and ligand binding in hemoglobin Chesapeake. *J. Biol. Chem.* 249:7255, 1974.

# PART II

# Sickle Cell
# Disorders

# 8 Homozygous Sickle Cell Disease*

Marie O. Russell, M.D.
Kwaku Ohene-Frempong, M.D.

Homozygous sickle cell disease (Hb SS) occurs in one in 500 black infants born in the United States; it is characterized by significant morbidity, particularly in early childhood, and a shortened life span. Although there is presently no cure, improved management of complications has been achieved by early, precise diagnosis, a better understanding of the morbidity of this disease, the availability of antibiotics, and improved medical supervision. Natural history data available from Africa[1] and the United States[2,3] suggest that appropriate treatment of intercurrent infections, better nutrition, and consistent medical care improve the course of sickle cell disease.

At The Children's Hospital of Philadelphia all patients identified as having sickling disorders are offered the option of enrolling in a comprehensive care program supported by the Commonwealth of

*We are grateful to Rachel McClinton for her assistance in the preparation of this manuscript, to Janet Fithian for editorial assistance, and to hematology nurses Joanne Halus, Marie Martin, and Regina Butler for participation in the care of patients and in clinical studies.

Pennsylvania. All primary care and evaluation and management of acute illness are provided by a special staff which includes pediatric hematologists. A team of hematology nurse specialists, a social worker, and a counselor assist the physicians in assessment, patient education, and continuity of care. Prior to June 1978, 316 patients between one month and 18 years of age were enrolled. After age 18, patients are referred to a sickle cell center for adults. The hemoglobinopathy of each patient is defined as precisely as possible. The numbers and diagnoses of patients currently being cared for are listed in Table 8-1. Delineation of the course of these patients and similar groups receiving intensive specialized medical supervision in other centers should give important information about the prognosis for sickle cell patients obtaining this kind of care in the United States today.

**Table 8-1**
**Diagnosis, Age and Sex of 293 Sickle Cell Patients Currently Followed at The Children's Hospital of Philadelphia**

| | Diagnosis | | | | | | | | | |
|---|---|---|---|---|---|---|---|---|---|---|
| | SS | | SC | | $S\beta^0$ | | $S\beta^+$ | | Others* | |
| Age | M | F | M | F | M | F | M | F | M | F |
| <1 | 3 | 0 | 0 | 0 | 0 | 0 | 0 | 0 | 0 | 0 |
| 1–5 | 25 | 33 | 5 | 2 | 1 | 1 | 1 | 0 | 1 | 0 |
| 6–10 | 35 | 32 | 15 | 9 | 1 | 0 | 0 | 3 | 1 | 1 |
| 11–15 | 25† | 42† | 3 | 7 | 2 | 2 | 1 | 1 | 1 | 1 |
| 16–18 | 12† | 9 | 7 | 5 | 1 | 1 | 2 | 2 | 0 | 0 |
| 293 (Total) | 100 | 116 | 30 | 23 | 5 | 4 | 4 | 6 | 3 | 2 |

*Others (in order of increasing age)
    Males: S-O Arabia, S-δβThal, S-HPFH
    Females: S-β⁺Thal-αG, SC Harlem
†Four SS-α Thal patients are included in these groups.

## CLINICAL FEATURES

Clinical manifestations of homozygous sickle cell disease do not usually occur until five or six months of age.[1,4,5] Within the first months of life, reticulocytes are increased.[6] A low hemoglobin level or polychromasia in the peripheral blood smear may give early clues to the diagnosis, usually by the third or fourth month.[1,5,6] During the first year there is typically a hemolytic anemia with hemoglobin levels between 8 to 10 g/dl. The anemia worsens with illness. Polychromasia and normoblasts are seen on the blood smear. Although there is usually poikilocytosis, typical sickle forms may be infrequent or absent because in these patients Hb F levels decrease at a rate slower than normal and the high levels of Hb F may inhibit sickling.[6] Persistence of a mild elevation of unconjugated bilirubin may be noted. Although studies from Africa report early failure to thrive,[1] American series suggest that normal growth and development is the rule in early childhood.[5,7] Colic and irritability are reported to be common in young sickle cell patients. Splenomegaly and hepatomegaly are usually present by five or six months of age.

One of the most characteristic and often the earliest clinical manifestation of Hb SS is sickle cell dactylitis, or the hand-foot syndrome, first described by Watson in 1956.[8] Sickle cell disease should be the major consideration when painful swelling of the hands and feet of a black child is observed.

Functional asplenia usually develops between 6 and 13 months of age and is indicated by the appearance of Howell-Jolly bodies in the smear. Functional asplenia in conjunction with other defects causing increased susceptibility to infection increases the risk of septicemia and meningitis, particularly with pneumococcus. Such infection may result in sudden fever, shock, and death. In addition, severe anemia secondary to acute splenic sequestration[9,10] or aplastic episodes can lead to death from congestive heart failure. An evaluation of 64 infants with sickle cell disease in the first year of life revealed a 16% mortality.[5] Early diagnosis before such complications occur may reduce this mortality since it will allow parent education about serious complications, resulting in early medical intervention when fever, irritability, listlessness, or pallor develop.

After the first year of life, the hemoglobin gradually drops to 6 to 9 g/dl in most patients. Hemoglobin F falls below 20% and continues to decrease gradually until adolescence.[6] Sickle forms become more evident and normoblasts are commonly seen on the peripheral smear. The reticulocyte count increases. As the child gets older, other types of vaso-occlusive problems replace the hand-foot syndrome. The incidence of serious infection often decreases with age.

Care of children with sickle cell disease should include periodic assessment and health maintenance, as well as optimal management of complications. At our institution, newly diagnosed patients are seen at monthly intervals. Routine preventive pediatric care is provided along with parent education. Immunizations are given, with pneumococcal vaccine provided after the second birthday. Folic acid 0.5 to 1.0 mg is given daily to prevent megaloblastic anemia. Periodic dental, developmental, visual, and hearing screening is provided, and any problems are pursued. Routine clinic visits are extended to every three to six months when the parents are comfortable with the diagnosis and the child is doing well. After the age of ten, yearly retinal examinations with indirect ophthalmoscopy are performed. Adolescents are provided with an opportunity to learn the genetic implications of their disease. Female patients are referred for family planning services, and all adolescents are given information about sexuality and reproduction, with stress on the fact that oral contraceptives may be dangerous for patients with sickling disorders.

An important aspect of comprehensive care is to provide ongoing anticipatory guidance to the child with sickle cell disease and his parents about the psychological stresses of chronic disease in general and sickle cell disease in particular.[11] Despite the unpredictable course of the disease, patients can be expected to have many periods of well-being, and most will survive to adulthood, probably to middle age or older. These children should be encouraged to plan for the future and to develop skills, self-esteem, and independence. Parents need guidance in dealing with their feelings and fears and those of the child. Such guidance is best given as a continuum during many years by professionals who understand the disease and can suggest realistic goals to the family.

## SPECIFIC COMPLICATIONS AND THEIR MANAGEMENT

### Growth and Development

Children with sickle cell disease do not have physical features that readily distinguish them from other children. Growth and development in the first three years of life are usually normal,[2] but growth may be retarded in children with serious infections or other complications. Several studies have shown that as a group older children with sickle cell disease have lower heights and weights than their normal sibs or other controls,[12,13,14] but by the age of 20 the majority of patients are well-developed and normal in both height and weight. A small minority of patients develop an eunuchoid appearance, with long, slender arms, legs, hands and feet, and a short trunk.[2] Delayed bone age has been described, particularly after age 11.[14] Puberty may be delayed until 16 to 18 years in males and 15 to 17 years in females.[15]

The exact nature of the delayed growth and maturation is not known. Disturbances of pituitary and sex hormones have been reported, and they probably account for skeletal and pubertal delay in most cases. Zinc deficiency has been reported, as has improvement in growth after zinc supplementation.[16] Subjective evaluation by mothers often suggests that the underweight sickle cell child may be a poor eater. This may be a reflection of a poor sense of taste (hypogeusia), a condition in which saliva zinc is low.[17] Of course, poor nutrition will contribute to growth failure in these patients as it will in normal children.

## Fever and Infection

The physician and parents should always be alert to the possibility that febrile children with sickle cell disease may have bacterial infections. Appropriate cultures to rule out sepsis, to identify respiratory, urinary, or fecal pathogens, or to diagnose meningitis should be performed where indicated by the clinical situation. Observation in the hospital is often necessary. The decision to use appropriate parenteral antibiotic coverage while awaiting culture results should be based on clinical grounds, considering the height of fever, the degree of toxicity, and the age of the child.

## Vaso-Occlusive Problems

Vascular occlusion by sickle cells accounts for much of the morbidity associated with the disease by causing serious acute and chronic effects. Relatively rigid sickled erythrocytes can obstruct blood flow in capillaries and venules, leading to stagnation of blood flow. This causes hypoxia, resulting in additional sickling, vascular injury, vasospasm, leakage of fluid and cells into the perivascular spaces, hemoconcentration, and fibrin formation.[18] This chain of events seems to be the basis for the episodic painful vaso-occlusive crisis as well as the chronic organ damage seen in sickle cell disease. Prolonged ischemia from vaso-occlusion may lead to infarction and necrosis, causing pain or organ dysfunction. The contribution of platelets and coagulation to vaso-occlusive events needs to be determined by further investigation.[19]

Painful vaso-occlusive crisis is the most frequent complication of the disease, with certain areas of the body being particularly susceptible. The extremities, back, chest, and abdomen are the most frequent sites involved.

**The Hand-Foot Syndrome** Typically, the child presents with swollen, tender hands and/or feet, a moderate degree of fever, irritability, and an unwillingness to use the extremities involved. The edema is nonpitting, often symmetrical, and the skin may not be erythematous. Dactylitis is usually the earliest type of vaso-occlusive crisis and is most commonly seen between five months and four years. Initially, x-rays show soft tissue swelling, but no bone changes. After 7 to 14 days, extensive lytic lesions with distortion of the trabecular pattern and periosteal proliferation are seen on roentgenograms.[18] Histopathologic examination of one case[29] showed extensive infarction of marrow, medullary trabeculae, and inner layers of cortical bone, with periosteal elevation. It has been postulated that the predilection for vaso-occlusion in the hands and feet of the young child is due to marrow hyperplasia and poorly developed collateral circulation in these small bones.[21] This area is less susceptible to hypoxic injury later when the marrow is replaced by fat.

The major differential diagnosis is osteomyelitis due to bacteria, tuberculosis, or syphilis.[18] Recognition of the typical symmetry and location in the small bones of the hands and feet, negative blood cultures, and serologic tests help to distinguish the hand-foot syndrome from osteomyelitis. Symptoms from hand-foot syndrome usually last 10 to 14 days, but may last as long as 31 days.[22] The normal course is one of gradual resolution of the swelling and pain and complete and spontaneous healing of the bone defects without residual deformity. Hand-foot syndrome may recur at the same or different sites.

**Painful Crises in the Older Child**    Later in life, various locations are commonly involved in the painful crises which periodically interrupt the usual well-compensated steady state of the child with sickle cell disease. Pain lasting from a few hours to several days may occur in the extremities, the vertebrae, the chest, and the abdomen. Occasionally, vaso-occlusive phenomena such as cerebrovascular accidents, pulmonary infarcts, priapism, and massive organ infarcts occur.

Pain from vaso-occlusive crisis has been described as a gnawing, relentless type of pain. It may be so mild that no medical help is sought or so severe as to incapacitate the patient. The child is irritable, often crying, and may change positions constantly in a vain attempt to find a comfortable position, or may lie still, moaning but afraid to move because of pain. Fever is mild to moderate or absent, and there may be dehydration. Physical signs at the site of pain are sometimes present. Warmth or edema may be noted and pain may be exacerbated by touch or by motion of the affected part.

**Extremities**    Localized infarction of bone, bone marrow, periosteum, or periarticular tissues causes the severe pain in the extremities.[23] Symptoms may last hours or several days. Vaso-occlusive crisis must be distinguished from osteomyelitis when there is substantial local swelling, tenderness, fever, and leukocytosis. Blood cultures should be part of the initial evaluation of the child with significant fever, localized swelling, and bone pain. Findings of Döhle bodies, vacuoles, and toxic granules in neutrophils may suggest infection. Conventional radiographs are not useful, because symptomatology precedes bone changes by several days in bone disorders.

Where they are available, bone and bone marrow scans may be helpful in distinguishing bone and bone marrow infarcts from osteomyelitis.[24-27] Using $^{99m}$Tc-sulfur colloid for bone marrow imaging and $^{99m}$Tc-diphosphonate for bone scanning, Lutzker and Alavi[25,26] found a characteristic pattern in infarction of the bone marrow in vaso-occlusive crisis. Within five days of onset of symptoms, bone scans are

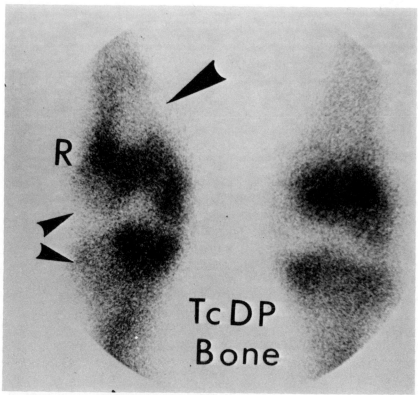

**Figure 8-1.** Bone scan with $^{99m}$Tc-diphosphonate performed within 5 days of onset of fever and pain in the right knee in a patient with bone and marrow infarction. Negative defects are present in the distal femur and knee area (arrows). [From L.G. Lutzker and B. Alavi.[25]]

normal or have small areas of decreased uptake in bone marrow infarction (Figure 8-1), but bone marrow scans show large areas of decreased uptake in the infarcted region (Figure 8-2).[25,27] In early osteomyelitis, intense localized increased uptake on bone scan may be seen as early as 24 hours after symptoms begin.[26] It is important to do such scans early, because after five days of infarction the bone scan can show increased uptake due to increased osteoblastic activity.[27] Culture of periosteal aspirates in equivocal cases may be useful.

Acute joint pain with swelling, warmth, and fever is common in sickle cell disease. It may be monoarticular or polyarticular, and may move from joint to joint. The association of joint symptoms with cardiomegaly, cardiac murmurs, ECG changes, leukocytosis, and fever in sickle cell disease has frequently been misdiagnosed as rheumatic fever or rheumatoid arthritis. Vascular occlusion occasionally causes joint effusion.[28] Joint aspiration is necessary if there are clinical indications of bacterial infection, since septic arthritis can also occur.[18]

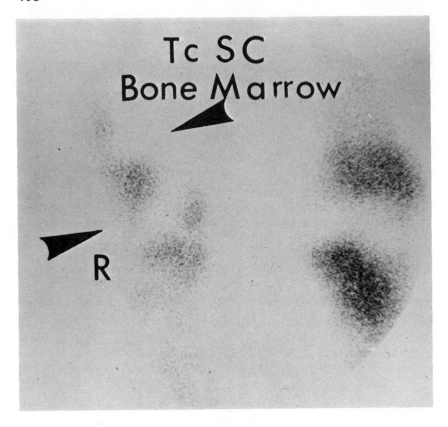

**Figure 8-2.** Bone marrow scan with $^{99m}$Tc-sulfur colloid in the same patient shows decreased activity over a larger area in the same location (arrows), indicating extensive marrow infarcts. [From L.G. Lutzker and B. Alavi.[25]]

**Abdomen** Abdominal crises are quite common in children, and are usually associated with low grade fever. In severe abdominal crises, high fever and prostration may be present. During severe episodes, the child may refuse all oral intake. The abdominal pain is usually diffuse, and vomiting may occur. On physical examination, guarding and rebound may be present, but bowel sounds are also present.

The causes of abdominal pain in sickle cell disease are not clearly understood. Pain may be due to vascular occlusion in the liver, spleen, mesentery, or abdominal wall. Sickle cell crisis may mimic several other conditions, such as hepatitis, cholecystitis, cholelithiasis, duodenal ulcer, appendicitis, intestinal obstruction, intussusception, perforated viscus, ureteral colic, pyelonephritis, and pelvic inflammatory disease.

**Back** Painful vaso-occlusive crisis involving the vertebral column may cause spasm of the back or neck muscles, simulating the symptoms of meningeal irritation. A lumbar puncture may be necessary to rule out meningitis.

**Chest**    Chest pain may be due to sternal, rib, or pulmonary infarction, or to pneumonitis. It may be difficult to distinguish pulmonary infarction from infection completely, and the two may coexist. Pulmonary infarcts are rare in younger children, and their chest complaints are more likely to be due to pneumonia than to vaso-occlusive problems. In older children or adults, sudden chest pain, especially when associated with tightness in the chest, pleural pain, tachycardia, dyspnea, cough, hemoptysis, or a friction rub, raises the possibility of pulmonary thrombosis or thromboembolism. Pneumonia may be preceded by upper respiratory infection, whereas painful crisis may precede acute pulmonary infarction or thromboembolism. Roent-genograms may be normal initially in pulmonary infarction, but later may show opacification similar to pneumonia. Radionuclide lung scans may be helpful in delineating infarction when x-rays are negative. It is unclear whether heparin therapy should be utilized in equivocal cases of pulmonary thrombosis, and the risk of anticoagulation may outweigh the possible benefit.[29] If pulmonary infarction is documented, heparin is indicated.

## Management of Vaso-Occlusive Crises

Even though the basic conditions for sickling exist constantly in sickle cell patients, painful vaso-occlusive crises occur only episodically and unpredictably. Diggs and Flowers[30] followed 177 children for two years and found an average of 3.9 painful crises per patient per year with great variation in different individuals and in the same individuals at different times. Factors other than the presence of red cells capable of sickling must influence the occurrence of painful crises.

Events reported to be associated with onset of crisis include infections, fever, exposure to wet or cold, dehydration, trauma, strenuous physical activity, bee stings, alcoholic intoxication, and emotional disturbance.[18] Except for cold exposure, direct cause and effect for these presumptive inducers of crises have never been clearly demonstrated. Patients do not develop painful crisis each time they are exposed to a given factor, and in many instances of painful crisis there are no clearly identifiable precipitating events. Children can go from a seemingly healthy state into severe pain within minutes.

The lack of understanding of the initiation of crisis has made it difficult to develop effective measures for preventing it. In addition, a safe, effective method to prevent or reverse sickling has not yet been found. Therefore, current management of vaso-occlusive crisis is supportive. Effective analgesia, hydration at one and one-half to twice the daily maintenance fluid requirement, and investigation for possible associated infections are standard measures. Maintaining warmth or application of heat to the affected part has been reported by some patients to provide additional relief from pain.

Appropriate analgesia ranges from aspirin or acetaminophen to narcotic analgesics, varying with the subjective needs of the patient. The aim of administration of analgesics should be to achieve good control of pain. Aspirin is quite effective in mild crisis. Its effectiveness may be enhanced by its anti-inflammatory and thrombopathic effects. Narcotic analgesics in effective doses are useful for severe pain until there is improvement. Intramuscular administration every three to four hours probably has a more sustained effect than intravenous use. Because crisis pain may vary in severity from episode to episode, medical personnel often question the need for narcotics and express concern about promoting addiction. Unfortunately, crisis pain is severe and may require intermittent use of narcotic analgesics. The rational use of these drugs in a hospital setting should permit the necessary relief without promoting misuse of drugs.

Parents can be educated to treat mild painful crisis at home. If the pain is severe or refractory to home treatment, an initial trial of intravenous fluids and more potent analgesics can be given for three or four hours in an emergency room or hospital holding area. Some crises will resolve, and hospital admission can be avoided. If pain is still severe after three or four hours, hospital admission is advisable until the crisis resolves. This usually occurs within four days, but occasionally patients have pain for a week or more.

There is controversy as to whether parenteral hydration is any more effective than oral hydration. Practically, many patients in pain may not feel well enough to maintain their increased fluid requirement by drinking, and we often use intravenous hydration in initial management. Studies in 1964[31] and more recently[32] have shown that the administration of alkali was no more effective than hydration alone. Oxygen administration is unnecessary except when pulmonary function is significantly impaired. Compounds, such as urea and cyanate, with antisickling properties which have been tested to date have proven to be ineffective, toxic, or too cumbersome to be adopted for general use. To date, no effective, safe, specific therapy has been found.

Although blood transfusion has been reported to shorten the duration of painful symptoms,[23,33,34] the evidence is inconclusive. The cost of transfusion to the patient—iron overload, infectious risks, and potential sensitization to red cell antigens—is unacceptable for most patients and unnecessary for painful crisis. Transfusion should be reserved for the very rare instance when vaso-occlusive events are damaging critical tissue.

## Special Vaso-Occlusive Problems

The following complications can result in serious functional disturbance and require special management.

**Stroke**    Stroke occurs in approximately 6% of children with sickle cell disease.[2] Signs of stroke can include intermittent loss of motor function or speech (transient ischemic episodes), cranial nerve palsies, monoparesis, hemiparesis, quadriparesis, or coma.[35,36] Most episodes appear to be secondary to thrombosis and arterial occlusion. Aneurysm and cerebral hemorrhage also occur with increased frequency in sickle cell disease and have a high mortality rate.[37] Recurrence of stroke has been reported to be as high as 70% in sickle cell disease, and each episode increases the risk of permanent and more extensive neurologic deficit.[38] To minimize damage during an acute episode of stroke, transfusion with blood from donors with the Hb A phenotype that contains adequate 2,3-DPG for normal oxygen transport should be given to dilute the sickle cells in the circulation and inhibit further sickling, which could increase cerebral ischemia or infarction. Exchange or repeated packed cell transfusion can be given depending on the patient's clinical status. We continue to transfuse the patients until the percentage of cells containing Hb S is reduced to 30% or less.[39] Densitometric scanning of cellulose acetate electrophoresis strips can be utilized to quantitate this percentage. Fluid and electrolyte balance should be carefully maintained. Appropriate electrolyte solutions should be provided to replace fluid loss and to avoid dehydration, but water intoxication must also be avoided.

Although radiographic dyes may induce sickling,[40] cerebral arteriography can be safely performed with proper safeguards after the patient is stabilized.[41,42,43] Transfusion with Hb A red cells until the Hb S level is less than 30% and careful hydration with one and one-half to twice the daily maintenance fluid requirement appear to reduce the hazards of arteriography. Cerebral arteriography is useful in defining the cause of stroke events in sickle cell disease[41,43] and in assessing the effect of prolonged transfusion therapy.[42,43] Another report defined its utility in detecting a cerebral aneurysm, allowing successful surgical intervention.[44]

Repeated transfusion for a prolonged period has been recommended after stroke because of the high rate of recurrence of stroke.[45] However, since all untransfused patients do not have recurrence, transfusion may not be necessary for every patient who has had stroke. Our experience with arteriography may help to establish a rational

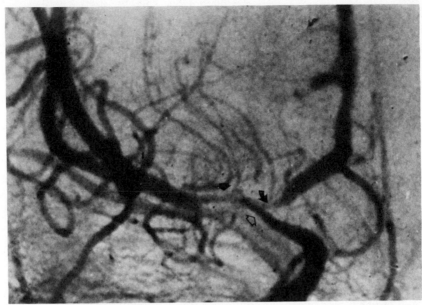

**Figure 8-3.** Anteroposterior view, right carotid arteriogram in a patient with stroke demonstrates the typical irregular narrowing of major arterial vessels seen in most sickle cell patients who have strokes. There is progressive stenosis of the right internal carotid artery (open arrow) and severe narrowing of the proximal portion of the anterior cerebral artery (curved black arrow) and the middle cerebral artery (straight black arrow).

basis for transfusion. Most patients with stroke have had arterial vascular disease that causes stenosis or occlusion of multiple major cerebral arteries (Figure 8-3).[43] The cause for this involvement of large vessels is not clear, but recent pathologic data have demonstrated intimal hyperplasia at these sites.[46] This abnormality could be expected to favor vascular occlusion. Prolonged transfusion therapy decreases the rate of recurrence of stroke in patients with stenosis of major arteries. The degree of vascular abnormality is variable. In mild cases, transfusion may favor reversal of the arterial changes, but the stenosis may recur when transfusion is stopped. Many patients have moderate to severe stenosis of major vessels at the time of stroke; this does not reverse with transfusion. In a smaller group of patients the major arteries are normal after stroke. These patients may not be at great risk for recurrence and may not require repeated transfusion. Further study of this problem is needed.

Recovery of neurologic function after stroke is variable. Although some residual motor or intellectual deficit may occur, many patients can resume ambulation, school attendance, and independence in daily living, particularly when recurrence of stroke is prevented. Prolonged physical therapy and special education may be necessary. If recurrence can be prevented and the problems of chronic transfusion managed, guarded optimism for patients with stroke may be permissible.

**Eye** Serious loss of vision can occur in Hb SS, Hb SC, and Hb S-$\beta$ thalassemia as a result of sickling in the retinal vessels.

**Priapism** Priapism is an infrequent form of vaso-occlusive crisis, but it is particularly difficult to manage.[47,48] Pain and edema of the penis are often severe, and there is concern that recurrent or prolonged priapism may result in impotence. Urinary retention may occur and require catheterization. Therapy should be instituted rapidly to attempt to relieve obstruction of blood flow and to provide relief from pain. Many therapeutic efforts have been suggested but remain untested, and some may be harmful. Intravenous hydration at two times the daily maintenance fluid requirements for a short period may help to relieve mild obstruction. If pain is severe or improvement is not noted within a few hours, packed red cell transfusion with Hb A blood having normal oxygen dissociation properties should be given until the hemoglobin level is raised to normal.[47] Transfusion should be accomplished as quickly as possible without compromising the patient's cardiovascular status.

Within 24 hours after blood administration, pain will usually resolve and the penis will gradually soften.[47] Exchange transfusion may be used in nonanemic patients (e.g., Hb SC disease) or to reduce Hb S to less than 30% in an attempt to relieve severe pain in a shorter time if symptoms cannot be controlled by narcotic analgesia. Local application of heat or cold to the penis or other local manipulation should be avoided. Aspiration of blood from the engorged penis is not recommended because this may lead to serious infection. Surgical evacuation by a caverno-spongiosal shunt may be effective. Its use should be limited to cases in which pain is severe and persistent despite good conservative management, since serious complications may result.[48] The possibility of impotence should be minimized by prompt attempts at therapy, since normal erections have been reported in boys managed as outlined above. For frequently recurring priapism, repeated transfusion for three to six months will prevent symptoms temporarily and may break the cycle of recurrence.

## Chronic Organ Damage

Chronic organ dysfunction is the result of recurrent sickling in various organs.

**Spleen** The spleen is destroyed early by sickling, usually becoming nonfunctional, small, and fibrotic during the first decade. Damage to this organ is the major cause of serious infectious complications in sickle cell disease.

**Liver**   Most Hb SS individuals have hepatomegaly and some degree of hepatic dysfunction.[49,50] These abnormalities may vary from minimal hepatomegaly with normal liver function test results to severe liver disease. Liver dysfunction tends to increase with age and is accompanied by a moderate elevation of liver enzymes. Icterus is common, and may be constant or intermittent. The total bilirubin level is usually less than 10 mg/dl and results from chronic hemolysis and posthepatocytic cholestasis. Children usually do not have symptoms of chronic liver disease.

Sickle cell patients may develop acute liver disease with markedly increased liver enzymes and bilirubin levels associated with abdominal and systemic complaints. Viral hepatitis, acute cholestatic disease, and sickle hepatopathy (intrahepatic sickling) have been the most frequent causes for severe hyperbilirubinemia in sickle cell patients. The course of viral hepatitis in sickle cell anemia may be similar to that in normal individuals except that extraordinary elevations of serum bilirubin levels may occur. However, hepatitis may be more serious in patients with pre-existing liver pathology.[51]

Cholestasis in sickling disorders results from intrahepatic sickling and increased bilirubin production, both of which predispose the patient to intrahepatic and extrahepatic biliary obstruction. Transient intrahepatic obstruction of bile occurs when liver sinusoids become blocked with sickled cells.[49,50,52] Severe hyperbilirubinemia without significant liver dysfunction is seen. Serum bilirubin may be as high as 50 to 100 mg/dl, divided evenly between direct and indirect fractions. SGOT and SGPT are only mildly elevated, and the alkaline phosphatase is usually normal. The patient is not acutely ill and may have only mild hepatomegaly with mild right upper quadrant discomfort. The clinical course is benign, and recovery occurs within three weeks without specific therapy. Some cases of hyperbilirubinemia greater than 25 mg/dl were associated with severe systemic illness, abdominal pain, and greatly elevated enzymes (SGOT > 1000).[53,54,55] Histopathology of the liver at autopsy revealed acute liver necrosis, which was greatest in the centrilobular area.[18] Engorgement of liver sinusoids and Kupffer cells with sickled cells was also noted. Treatment of severe hyperbilirubinemia consists of hydration and general supportive measures. Evaluation to rule out other acute liver diseases should be made. If there is any indication that continuing sickling may be causing liver failure, a trial of transfusion therapy to minimize further sickling may be indicated.

Extrahepatic biliary obstruction may occur because cholelithiasis is common in Hb SS. Gallstones occur in 6% to 37% of patients in various series,[56] and may be present as early as 5 years of age.[57] A review of literature revealed that 20% of patients with gallstones were less than 20 years of age.[56] Although the incidence of cholelithiasis diagnosed by radiologic methods is high, few patients ever demonstrate typical symptoms of cholecystitis or obstruction of common bile ducts by gallstones. Obstruction or inflammatory biliary disease may contribute to some of the abdominal pain seen in sickle cell patients, and appropriate evaluation should be made when indicated.

The management of cholelithiasis in sickle cell patients is controversial. It is argued that elective cholecystectomy would be safer than the complications of severe cholestatic disease,[56] but some patients have no symptomatology from their cholelithiasis and may not need surgery. Despite surgery, the process responsible for pigment stone formation will remain, and common bile duct obstruction may occur. Even though sickle cell patients can be managed with preoperative transfusion and careful anesthetic care through surgery, they are at greater risk for intra- and postoperative complications. A reasonable approach is to operate on patients when there is evidence of repeated or severe episodes of biliary colic or obstructive jaundice.

**Kidney** Renal pathology secondary to sickling is well described.[58,59,60] Clinical renal disease is not common in children, and it is more frequent in adults. The most common functional renal abnormality is a defect in the mechanism for concentrating urine. Transfusion can reverse this defect in children less than 15 years old but eventually the defect becomes fixed, leaving adults with maximum concentrating ability of about 400 mOsm/kg of water.[61] The hypertonic environment of the renal medulla causes Hb SS cells to sickle even at normal oxygen tension.[62] Constant vascular occlusion destroys the vasa recta which supply the long loops of Henle of juxtamedullary nephrons.[63] These loops are responsible for renal concentrating ability. Fourteen percent of the nephrons in the kidney have these long loops of Henle, and their loss of function apparently does not appreciably affect overall renal function.[63]

Massive hematuria may occur in any sickling disorder, including sickle cell trait.[64] Bleeding, which is four times more common in males than in females, more commonly comes from the left kidney and is probably related to its blood supply. Bleeding seems to result from papillary ulceration and hemorrhage secondary to papillary necrosis. Clinically, the hematuria is usually silent and painless. Mild trauma precedes some cases. Blood loss may continue for days or weeks and may lead to severe anemia. The management of hematuria depends on its duration. Nephrectomy has been performed in the past, but it should be considered only when there is potentially fatal exsanguination, since in one series hematuria recurred in half of the nephrectomized patients.[64] Initially, bed rest and parenteral hydration are recommended, and these measures should be continued as long as significant progress is seen. Therapy with iron or, rarely, transfusion of packed cells may be necessary to replace blood loss. Initial or prolonged episodes should be investigated radiologically and urologically. Causes of hematuria unassociated with sickling should not be overlooked. In severe cases lasting for more than three weeks, aminocaproic acid has been shown to be effective,[65] but it should be used cautiously since it may prevent dissolution of clots in the renal pelvis.

Urinary tract infection and pyelonephritis are more common in patients with sickle cell disease than in the general population.[66]

Glomerular changes, including glomerular enlargement with capillary engorgement, occur in sickle cell disease. Ultrastructural analysis reveals electron-dense deposits in mesangial cytoplasm, focal fusion of foot processes, and granular deposits in glomerular basement membrane. McCoy[59] postulated that the mesangial deposits are iron-protein complexes which may cause a glomerular protein leak. These changes have been seen in kidneys of sickle cell patients with or without evidence of renal disease.[60] Mild proteinuria is found frequently in sickle cell patients, but its significance is unclear. Alleyne[61] reports that in Jamaica a close association exists between proteinuria and streptococcal infection in leg ulcers. A few patients develop the nephrotic syndrome, and end-stage renal disease occurs only occasionally in sickle cell patients. The relation of the pathologic changes to sickling is unclear, and it is possible that the nephrotic syndrome and renal failure seen in patients are from causes unrelated to sickle cell disease. Hemodialysis and renal transplantation have been performed successfully in sickle cell patients with end-stage renal disease.

**Heart**   Children with sickle cell disease have cardiomegaly and cardiac murmurs common in chronic severe anemias.[67] A hyperactive precordium, systolic ejection murmurs along the left sternal border with wide radiation, and pansystolic murmurs loudest at the apex similar to mitral regurgitation may be present. A third heart sound is usually present. Many patients also have a mid-diastolic rumble. Radiologic examination usually shows moderate to severe cardiac enlargement involving all chambers. Left ventricular hypertrophy is common on the electrocardiogram, and biventricular hypertrophy is seen in 10% to 15% of patients. For most patients, the cardiac findings do not represent disease but, rather, efficient methods of coping with severe anemia. Congestive heart failure or clinical cardiac disease is rare in children, but it may occur in adulthood. When cardiac decompensation occurs in the absence of acute illness or with mild problems, the possibility that rheumatic heart disease, other valvular disease, or congenital heart disease may coexist should be considered. When necessary, cardiac catheterization can be safely performed for diagnosis if the patient is carefully hydrated and transfused to reduce Hb S to very low levels. Corrective cardiac surgery has been occasionally performed under the same conditions.[67]

Ischemic myocardial injury is unusual, despite the nearly complete oxygen extraction in the coronary circulation.[68] Perhaps this resistance to vaso-occlusive infarcts in the coronary vessels lies in the extensive collateral circulation and short transit time of the red cells from deoxygenation to oxygenation.[69]

Symptoms such as dyspnea or chest pain may result when pulmonary complications acutely stress the cardiovascular system. A child with severe pneumonia may show a markedly increased heart rate, an enlarged, tender liver, and neck vein distention. Cardiac findings present during the steady state may be exacerbated with this stress. Slow transfusion of relatively fresh packed red cells to increase the oxygen-carrying capacity may reduce cardiac stress. Some modification of fluid therapy may be necessary, but severe restriction is not warranted.

**Bones and Joints** Frequent infarctions in bone and bone marrow, profound marrow expansion, occasional joint effusions, and osteomyelitis predispose these patients to permanent changes in their bones and joints.[21,28]

Significant skull deformities are rare in sickle cell disease. Calvarial thickening, frontal bossing, "tower skull," and the radiologic "hair on end" appearance are seen only occasionally.[21] Facial bone abnormalities are also rare, at least in the United States, but Konotey-Ahulu[70] has described in African patients a peculiar maxillary bone hypertrophy, termed gnathopathy, which causes a "buck teeth" appearance. Of 595 Hb SS patients, 31% had gnathopathy, which was evident after age 5.

With increasing age, vertebral bodies become increasingly osteoporotic and flattened. They become H-shaped when they are deeply indented by the intervertebral discs, causing classical fish-mouth vertebrae. Vertebral collapse can cause pain from compression of nerve roots.

The long bones in young children usually show no obvious abnormalities on physical examination. Radiographs in older patients, however, often show the effects of recurrent bone and bone marrow infarcts. Localized areas of necrosis, new bone formation, or periosteal separation may be seen. Roentgenograms and radionuclide scans of the extremities at any time may reflect not only the present clinical situation, but the past effects of multiple infarcts in various stages of repair.

Aseptic necrosis of the femoral head is one of the most disabling complications of sickle cell disease.[21,27] Its clinical and radiographic features are similar to those of Legge-Calvé-Perthe disease. This complication occurs in older children and adults and has increased incidence in Hb SC patients. Avascular necrosis of the juxta-articular bone causes degeneration of cartilage and synovium, leading to occlusion of the joint space. The round head of the femur is flattened

206

by gravity, and the capital epiphysis can become fixed to the pelvis, causing complete ankylosis of the joint.[21] Surgical correction is necessary in severe cases, and occasionally total hip replacement may be required.[71]

**Leg Ulcers**  Leg ulcers are reported to be common complications of sickle cell disease, occurring in 75% of older children and adults.[72] They are rarely seen in children less than 10 years old. The ulcers occur on the lower third of the leg and begin either spontaneously or following minor trauma, such as an insect bite or abrasion. Without special care, the ulcers deepen into large craters. Large ulcers characteristically heal very slowly, may take years to resolve completely, and leave irregular pigmented scars. Secondary infection is common with organisms such as *Clostridium tetani* and hemolytic streptococci.[73] Acute glomerulonephritis secondary to infection of these skin lesions has been reported.[61,74] Conservative management of ulcers has included bed rest, elevation, cleaning with mild antiseptics, and debridement. Systemic or topical antibiotics may be useful. It has been reported that daily administration of oral zinc sulphate increased healing.[75] Elastic stockings or, in the severe cases, Unna boots may help protect the area.[76] Surgical management with skin grafts has been generally unsuccessful.[73] Blood transfusions for a period of time may help to heal refractory ulcers.[77]

**Anemic Crises**

Other crises in sickle cell disease cause acute exacerbations of anemia, which may be severe.

**Aplastic Crisis**  Infection with bacteria, mycoplasma, or viruses can lead to transient cessation of erythropoeisis in normal individuals.[78,79] In people with congenital and acquired hemolytic anemias, including sickle cell disease, significant anemia can develop because the red cell life span is short. The child typically becomes pale and increasingly lethargic a few days after infectious illness. The blood count may show a hemoglobin level as low as 2 g/dl with a very low reticulocyte count and an absence of nucleated red cells. Platelet and white cell counts are usually normal, but granulocyte counts may be low early in the course and platelet counts may be high later. Treatment includes close observation of the patient and transfusion when anemia is severe. The decision to transfuse should be based on the clinical state of the patient and an estimation of red cell maturation in the bone marrow. A well-compensated child whose marrow shows a predominance of late normoblasts probably does not need to be transfused because nucleated red cells and reticulocytes should be released into the circulation within a day or two. If there are few or only early red cell precursors in the marrow, several days will pass before red cells are released and transfusion is recommended if hemoglobin levels are 5 g/dl or less. If transfusion is given, small aliquots of 2 to 5 ml of packed red cells per kilogram body weight should be given slowly every 12 hours to prevent circulatory overload until the desired hemoglobin level is reached. In severe anemia, diuretics or partial exchange transfusion may be necessary. It is advisable to watch the children until adequate reticulocytosis is observed in the peripheral blood. Some of the hyperhemolytic crises described in sickle cell disease probably reflect the recovery phase of aplastic crisis.

**Splenic Sequestration**    Once the child with sickle cell disease develops splenomegaly, he is at risk for the sudden rapid pooling of blood in the spleen known as splenic sequestration crisis, which results in sudden hypovolemia, shock, or even death.[9,10] This life-threatening complication is usually seen in children between 9 months and 5 years of age. After fibrosis of the spleen, sequestration is no longer a problem. In patients whose splenomegaly persists, as in 10% of homozygotes and in patients with sickle cell variants, sequestration can occur in later years. The clinical picture is well described by Seeler and Shwiaki in a review of 20 cases.[9] Sequestration may occur *de novo* or may arise during an infection or after viral illness. There is usually a sudden change in the child, including profound weakness, sudden abdominal distention, respiratory distress, and thirst. On physical examination, the child may show signs of acute circulatory insufficiency. Tachypnea, tachycardia, cardiomegaly, and abdominal distention may be noted, and a large, tender spleen is palpated. Severe anemia with increased normoblasts and reticulocytes may be present. Leucocytosis in the range of 25–35 $\times$ 10$^9$/l and thrombocytopenia are common. As this complication is life-threatening,[9,10] treatment must be instituted immediately to restore blood volume and to correct anemia. Packed red cells should be administered as soon as possible. Because the patient is hypovolemic, 15 to 20 ml/kg of packed red cells can probably be given but the child should be monitored carefully for signs of congestive heart failure. When there is shock, volume expanders may be given until blood is available. Recovery is rapid; with restoration of circulation much of the blood is gradually released from the spleen, which decreases in size. The hemoglobin level increases more than would be expected by the amount of blood transfused. Occasionally, treatment and the release of pooled blood may result in acute circulatory overload which requires therapy with diuretics. Acute splenic sequestration may recur, often within a few months of the first episode. Splenectomy has been recommended after one or more recurrence.[9] However, because splenectomy adds an additional risk of overwhelming sepsis to patients already at great risk, it is desirable to avoid this procedure when possible. We have limited experience with repeated transfusion for periods of approximately six months after recurrent sequestration. In a few patients, there was no recurrence during or after the transfusion period. Further experience with this alternative to splenectomy is warranted.

**Hyperhemolytic Crisis**    The early literature on sickle cell disease described situations in which patients were more anemic than usual and had increased reticulocyte counts as hyperhemolytic crises. Actually, most of these episodes probably represented the recovery phase from aplastic crisis. A few patients seem to have occasional episodes of significant hemolysis during vaso-occlusive crises; concomitant G6PD deficiency is thought to be responsible for this.[80] Bacterial infection, malaria, or autoimmune hemolytic anemia[81] might be other causes for increased hemolysis. Hyperhemolytic crisis is probably not a true entity and another explanation for the laboratory findings should be sought.

## TRANSFUSION IN SICKLE CELL DISEASE

Occasionally, patients with sickle cell disease will require transfusion. Severe exacerbations of anemia may require treatment. Some patients may require a prolonged period of transfusion to suppress their Hb S production because of a serious complication, to prepare for a special study such as an arteriogram or cardiac catheterization, or to minimize the serious risks of surgery or pregnancy. A complete red cell antigen typing should be performed before transfusion to serve as a guide for further transfusion therapy if red cell sensitization should occur. Blood for transfusion in sickle cell patients should be from donors who do not have Hb S. It is also advisable to give blood which has a normal capability for oxygen delivery, that is, with a normal oxygen dissociation curve and normal 2,3-DPG levels. Blood collected in citrate-phosphate-dextrose solution (CPD) and stored fewer than five days has normal oxygen delivery. Blood stored more than five days in CPD or red cells frozen after this length of storage may provide poor oxygen delivery initially[82] and may possibly be responsible for the development of such problems as vaso-occlusive crisis after transfusion. To suppress Hb S production, we have found it useful to transfuse the patient until the hemoglobin level is greater than 10 g/dl and the percentage of Hb S is less than 30%. This may be accomplished rapidly in critical situations such as stroke, or in preparation for emergency surgery by whole blood exchange of one blood volume in anemic patients or by giving two or three packed cell transfusions sufficient to raise the hemoglobin level to 12 to 14 g/dl every two to three weeks until Hb S is less than 30%. Suppression of Hb S production can be maintained if necessary by periodic transfusion of packed red cells every three to five weeks. Chelation therapy should be considered for patients who develop significant iron overload.

## SURGERY AND SPECIAL PROCEDURES

Surgery and radiographic procedures which require intra-arterial injection of hypertonic radiographic dyes present special risks to the sickle cell patient and should be undertaken only in centers where adequate hematologic support is available, with hematologists sharing in the preparation and care of the patient. Transfusion of Hb A red cells to suppress Hb S to less than 30% and to increase the hemoglobin to normal; careful observation; and oxygenation and hydration of the patient before, during, and after the procedure can substantially reduce the risk so that procedures offering significant benefit to the patient can be attempted. Adequate hydration is crucial to a successful outcome. Since oral intake is usually restricted for several hours before such procedures, parenteral hydration at one and one-half to twice the daily fluid maintenance requirements should be begun at the time of restriction and continued until the patient can fully meet his needs by oral intake. For very short anesthesia, such as for myringotomy, transfusion may not be necessary if careful hydration and oxygenation is insured. With the above measures, numerous surgical and other procedures have been accomplished without complication at our institution. The goal of preoperative transfusion should be not only to correct anemia, but also to reduce Hb S substantially to approximately 30%, since significant complications were reported when transfusion was utilized only to raise the hemoglobin level to normal.[83,84,85]

With comprehensive care and optimal management of complications, the morbidity from sickle cell disease can be reduced. The life span for patients today has increased greatly, primarily because of better management of infection and improvements in supportive care. Although the disease has not been cured, our improving ability to control its complications offers increasing hope to the sickle cell patient for an increased life span and better quality of life.

## REFERENCES

1. Trowell, H.C., Raper, A.B., and Welbourn, H.F. The natural history of homozygous sickle cell anaemia in central Africa. *J. Med.* 26:401–422, 1957.
2. Powars, D.R. Natural history of sickle cell disease—the first ten years. *Semin. Hematol.* 12:267–285, 1975.

3. Karayalcin, G., Rosner, R., Kim, K.Y., et al. Sickle cell anemia—clinical manifestations in 100 patients and a review of the literature. *Am. J. Med. Sci.* 269:51–68, 1975.

4. Seeler, R.A., Deaths in children with sickle cell anemia. A clinical analysis of 19 fatal instances in Chicago. *Clin. Pediatr.* 11:634–637, 1972.

5. Porter, F.S., and Thurman, W.B. Studies of sickle cell disease. Diagnosis in infancy. *Am. J. Dis. Child.* 106:35–42, 1963.

6. Davis, L.R. Changing blood picture in sickle cell anemia from shortly after birth to adolescence. *J. Clin. Pathol.* 29:898–901, 1976.

7. Booker, C.R., Scott, R.B., and Ferguson, A.D. Studies in sickle cell anemia. XXII. Clinical manifestations of sickle cell anemia during the first two years of life. *Clin. Pediatr.* 3:111–115, 1964.

8. Watson, R.J., Hemoglobins and disease. Edited by W. Dock and I. Snapper. In *Advances in Internal Medicine*. Vol. 8. Chicago: Year Book Publishers, 1956.

9. Seeler, R.A., and Shwiaki, M.Z. Acute splenic sequestration crisis (ASSC) in young children with sickle cell anemia. Clinical observations of 20 episodes in 14 children. *Clin. Pediatr.* 11:701–704, 1972.

10. Jenkins, M.E., Scott, R.B., and Baird, R.L. Studies in sickle cell anemia. XVI. Sudden death during sickle cell anemia crises in young children. *J. Pediatr.* 56:30–38, 1960.

11. Whitten, C.F., and Fischoff, J. Psychological effects of sickle cell disease. *Arch. Intern. Med.* 133:681–689, 1974.

12. Winsor, T., and Burch, G.E. The habitus of patients with sickle cell anemia. *Human Biol.* 16:99–114, 1944.

13. Scott, R.B., Ferguson, A.D., Jenkins, M.E., et al. Studies in sickle cell anemia. VIII. Further observations on the clinical manifestations of sickle cell anemia in children. *Am. J. Dis. Child.* 90:682–691, 1955.

14. Whitten, C.F. Growth status of children with sickle cell anemia. *Am. J. Dis. Child.* 102:355–364, 1961.

15. Olambiwonnu, O., Penny, R., and Frasier, S.D. Sexual maturation in subjects with sickle cell anemia. *J. Pediatr.* 87:459–464, 1975.

16. Prasad, A.S., Schoomaker, E.B., Ortega, J., et al. Zinc deficiency in sickle cell disease. *Clin. Chem.* 21:582–587, 1975.

17. Henkin, R.I., Mueller, C.W., and Wolf, R.O. Estimation of zinc concentration of parotid saliva by flameless atomic absorption spectrophotometry in normal subjects and in patients with idiopathic hypogeusia. *J. Lab. Clin. Med.* 86:175–180, 1975.

18. Diggs, L.W. Sickle cell crisis. *Am. J. Clin. Pathol.* 44:1–19, 1965.

19. Rickles, F.R., and O'Leary, D.S. Role of coagulation system in pathophysiology of sickle cell disease. *Arch. Intern. Med.* 133:635–641, 1974.

20. Weinberg, A.G., and Currarino, G. Sickle cell dactylitis: Histopathologic observations. *Am. J. Clin. Pathol.* 58:518–523, 1972.

21. Diggs, L.W. Bones and joint lesions in sickle cell disease. *Clin. Orthop.* 52:119–143, 1967.

22. Worrall, V.T., and Butera, V. Sickle cell dactylitis. *J. Bone Joint Surg. (Am.)* 58:1161–1163, 1976.

23. Pearson, H.A., and Diamond, L.K. The critically ill child: Sickle cell disease crises and their management. *Pediatrics* 48:629–635, 1971.

24. Alavi, A., Bond, J.P., Kuhl, D., et al. Scan detection of bone marrow infarcts in sickle cell disorders. *J. Nucl. Med.* 15:1003–1007, 1974.

25. Lutzker, L.G., and Alavi, A. Bone and marrow imaging in sickle cell disease, diagnosis of infarction. *Semin. Nucl. Med.* 6:83–93, 1976.

26. Alavi, A., Schumacher, R., and Dorwart, B. Bone marrow scan evaluation of arthropathy in sickle cell disorders. *Arch. Intern. Med.* 136:436–440, 1976.

27. Alavi, A., and Kim, H. Detection of bone and marrow infarction in sickle cell disorders. Manuscript in preparation.

28. Schumacher, H.R., Andrews, R., and McLaughlin, G. Arthropathy in sickle cell disease. *Ann. Intern. Med.* 78:203–211, 1973.

29. Barrett-Connor, E. Pneumonia and pulmonary infarction in sickle cell anemia. *JAMA* 224:997–1000, 1973.

30. Diggs, L.W., and Flowers, E. Sickle cell anemia in the home environment. *Clin. Pediatr.* 10:697–700, 1971.

31. Schwartz, E., and McElfresh, A.E. Treatment of painful crisis of sickle cell disease: A double blind study. *J. Pediatr.* 64:132–133, 1964.

32. Co-operative Urea Trials Group. Clinical trials of therapy for sickle cell vaso-occlusive crises. *JAMA* 228:1120–1124, 1974.

33. Charache, S. The treatment of sickle cell anemia. *Arch. Intern. Med.* 133:698–705, 1974.

34. Brody, J.I., Goldsmith, M.H., Park, S.K., et al. Symptomatic crises of sickle cell anemia treated by limited exchange transfusion. *Ann. Intern. Med.* 72:327–330, 1970.

35. Greer, M., and Schotland, D. Abnormal hemoglobin as a cause of neurologic disease. *Neurology* 12:114–123, 1962.

36. Portnoy, B.A., and Herion, J.C. Neurological manifestations in sickle cell disease with a review of the literature and emphasis on the prevalence of hemiplegia. *Ann. Intern. Med.* 76:643–652, 1972.

37. Falter, M.L., Sutton, A.L., and Robinson, M.G. Massive intracranial hemorrhage in sickle cell anemia. *Am. J. Dis. Child.* 124:415–416, 1973.

38. Powars, D., Wilson, B., Imbus, C., et al. The natural history of stroke in sickle cell disease. *Am. J. Med.* 65:461–471, 1978.

39. Russell, M.O., and Schwartz, E. Management of stroke patients with sickle cell disease. *Urban Health* 4:17, 1975.

40. Richards, D., and Nulsen, F.E. Angiographic media and the sickling phenomenon. *Surg. Forum* 22:403–404, 1971.

41. Stockman, J.A., Nigro, M.A., Muskin, M.M., et al. Occlusion of large cerebral vessels in sickle cell anemia. *N. Engl. J. Med.* 287:846–849, 1972.

42. Russell, M.O., Goldberg, H.I., Reis, L., et al. Transfusion therapy for cerebrovascular abnormalities in sickle cell disease. *J. Pediatr.* 88:382–387, 1976.

43. Russell, M.O., and Goldberg, H.I. Unpublished data.

44. Cheatham, M.L., and Brackett, C.E. Problems in management of subarachnoid hemorrhage in sickle cell anemia. *J. Neurosurg.* 23:488–493, 1965.

45. Lusher, J.M., Haghighat, H., and Khalifa, A.S. A prophylactic transfusion program for children with sickle cell anemia complicated by CNS infarction. *Am. J. Hematol.* 1:265–273, 1976.

46. Merkel, K.H.H., Ginsberg, P.L., Parker, J.C., et al. Cerebrovascular disease in sickle cell anemia: A clinical, pathological and radiological correlation. *Stroke* 9:45–52, 1978.

47. Seeler, R.A. Intensive transfusion therapy for priapism in boys with sickle cell anemia. *J. Urol.* 110:360–363, 1973.

48. Kinney, T.R., Harris, M.B., Russell, M.O., et al. Priapism in association with sickle hemoglobinopathies in children. *J. Pediatr.* 68:241–242, 1975.

49. Green, T.W., Conley, C.L., and Berthrong, M. The liver in sickle cell anemia. *Bull. Johns Hopkins Hosp.* 92:99–127, 1953.

50. Rosenblate, H.J., Eisenstein, R., and Holmes, A.W. The liver in sickle cell anemia. A clinical pathologic study. *Arch. Pathol.* 90:235–245, 1970.

51. Sheehy, T.W. Sickle cell hepatopathy. *South Med. J.* 70:533–538, 1977.

52. Buchanan, G.R., and Glader, B.E. Benign course of extreme hyperbilirubinemia in sickle cell anemia. Analysis of six cases. *J. Pediatr.* 91:21–24, 1977.

53. Barrett-Connor, E. Sickle cell disease and viral hepatitis. *Ann. Intern. Med.* 69:517–527, 1968.

54. Owen, D.M., Aldridge, J.E., and Thompson, R.B. An unusual hepatic sequelae of sickle cell anemia: A report of five cases. *Am. J. Med. Sci.* 249:175–185, 1965.

55. Bogoch, A., Casselmen, W.G.B., and Margolies, M.P. Liver disease in sickle cell anemia. A correlation of clinical, biochemical, histologic, and histochemical observations. *Am. J. Med.* 19:583–609, 1955.

56. Ariyan, S., Shessel, F.S., and Pickett, L.K. Cholecystitis and cholelithiasis masking as abdominal crises in sickle cell disease. *Pediatrics* 58:252–258, 1976.

57. Flye, M.W., and Silver, D. Biliary tract disorders and sickle cell disease. *Surgery* 72:361–367, 1972.

58. Mostofi, F.K., Vorder Bruegge, C.F., and Diggs, L.W. Lesions in kidneys removed for unilateral hematuria. *Arch. Pathol.* 62:336–351, 1957.

59. McCoy, R.C. Ultrastructural alterations in the kidney of patients with sickle cell disease and the nephrotic syndrome. *Lab. Invest.* 21:85–95, 1969.

60. Buckalew, V.M., and Someren, A. Renal manifestations of sickle cell disease. *Arch. Intern. Med.* 133:660–669, 1974.

61. Alleyne, G.A.O., Statius Van Eps, L.W., Addae, S.K., et al. The kidney in sickle cell anemia. *Kidney Int.* 7:371–378, 1945.

62. Perillie, P.E., and Epstein, F.H. Sickling phenomenon produced by hypertonic solutions: A possible explanation for the hyposthenuria of sicklemia. *J. Clin. Invest.* 42:570–580, 1963.

63. Statius Van Eps, L.W., Pineda-Veels, C., de Vries, G.H., et al. Nature of the concentration defect in sickle cell nephropathy: Microradioangiographic studies. *Lancet* 1:450–452, 1970.

64. Lucas, W.M., and Bullock, W.H. Hematuria in sickle cell disease. *J. Urol.* 83:733–741, 1960.

65. Black, W.D., Hatch, F.F., and Acchiardo, S. Amino caproic acid in prolonged hematuria of patients with sicklemia. *Arch. Intern. Med.* 136:678–681, 1976.

66. Barrett-Connor, E. Bacterial infection and sickle cell anemia. *Medicine* 50:97–112, 1971.

67. Lindsay, J., Jr., Meshel, J.C., and Patterson, R.H. The cardiovascular manifestations of sickle cell disease. *Arch. Intern. Med.* 133:643–651, 1974.

68. Craenen, J., Kilman, J., Hosier, D.M., et al. Mitral valve replacement in a child with sickle cell disease. *J. Thorac. Cardiovasc. Surg.* 63:797–799, 1972.

69. Baroldi, G. High resistance of the human myocardium to shock and red blood cell aggregation (sludge). *Cardiologia* 54:271–277, 1969.

70. Konotey-Ahulu, F.D. Effect of environment on sickle cell disease in West Africa: Epidemiologic and clinical considerations. Edited by H. Abramson, J.F. Bertles, and D.L. Wethers. In *Sickle Cell Disease: Diagnosis, Management, Education and Research.* St. Louis: C.V. Mosby, 1973.

71. Chung, S.M., Alavi, A., and Russell, M.O. Management of osteonecrosis in sickle cell anemia and its genetic variants. *Clin. Orthop.* 130:158–174, 1978.

72. Diggs, L.W. Anatomic lesions in sickle cell disease. Edited by H. Abramson, J.F. Bertles, and D.L. Wethers. In *Sickle Cell Disease: Diagnosis Management, Education and Research.* St. Louis: C.V. Mosby, 1973.

73. Serjeant, G.R. Leg ulceration in sickle cell anemia. *Arch. Intern. Med.* 133:690–694, 1974.

74. Svartman, M., Finklea, J.F., Earle, D.P., et al. Epidemic scabies and acute glomerulonephritis in Trinidad. *Lancet* 1:249–251, 1972.

75. Serjeant, G.R., Galloway, R.E., and Gueri, M.C. Oral zinc sulphate in sickle cell ulcers. *Lancet* 2:891–892, 1970.

76. Ward, L.S., and Dugan, W.M., Jr. Sickle cell leg ulceration—A nonoperative outpatient method of management. *J. Indiana State Med. Assoc.* 67:985, 1974.

77. Chernoff, A.I., Shapleigh, J.B., and Moore, C.V. Therapy of chronic ulceration of legs associated with sickle cell anemia. *JAMA* 155:1487–1491, 1954.

78. MacIver, J.E., and Parker-Williams, E.J. The aplastic crisis in sickle cell anemia. *Lancet* 1:1086–1089, 1952.

79. Singer, K., and Fisher, B. Studies on abnormal hemoglobins; distribution of type S (sickle cell) hemoglobin and type F (alkali resistant) hemoglobin within red cell populations in sickle cell anemia. *Blood* 7:1216–1226, 1952.

80. Smits, H.L., Oski, F.A., and Brody, J.I. The hemolytic crisis of sickle cell disease. The role of glucose-6-phosphate dehydrogenase deficiency. *J. Pediatr.* 74:544–551, 1969.

81. Wilkinson, L., Yam, P., Petz, L., et al. Erythrocyte autoantibodies in sickle cell disease. *Transfusion* 15:512–513, 1975.

82. Asakura, T., and Festa, R.S., Unpublished data.

83. Gilbertson, A.A. Anaesthesia in West African patients with sickle-cell anemia, haemoglobin SC disease, and sickle-cell trait. *Br. J. Anaesth.* 37:614–622, 1965.

84. Spigelman, A., and Warden, M.J. Surgery in patients with sickle cell disease. *Arch. Surg.* 104:761–764, 1972.

85. Howells, T.H., and Huntsman, R. Anaesthesia in sickle cell states. *Anaesthesia* 28:339–341, 1978.

# 9 Variants of Sickle Cell Disease*

Haewon C. Kim, M.D.

Persons with variants of sickle cell disease are doubly heterozygous for either Hb S and another abnormal hemoglobin or Hb S and thalassemia. Affected individuals have varying degrees of hemolytic anemia and a clinical expression ranging from asymptomatic to a degree of severity indistinguishable from that of homozygous sickle cell disease (HB SS). In contrast with Hb SS, in which sickled red cells are usually seen on the peripheral blood smear, sickled red cells may not always be found on the blood smear of patients with variants of sickle cell disease, although sickling can be readily induced under reduced oxygen tension.

The reasons for the difference in the severity of various sickle hemoglobinopathies are not completely understood; however, previous studies have indicated that at least three factors are known to be responsible for modifying the expression of sickle cell disease.[1-4]

*The author is greatly appreciative to Janet Fithian for excellent editorial help and to Rachel McClinton and Sandra Termini for typing the manuscript. This work was supported in part by a contract from the Commonwealth of Pennsylvania, NIH grant AM 16691, and the Tommy Fund.

215

The first factor is the degree of interaction between Hb S and other hemoglobins. Studies on this interaction have demonstrated that the minimum concentration of Hb S required for gelation of hemoglobin solution varies greatly, depending on the type of hemoglobin present with Hb S in erythrocytes. Several residues, such as $\beta^{73 \ Asp}$, $\beta^{121 \ Glu}$, or $\alpha^{23 \ Glu}$, are known to affect the gelling tendency of sickle hemoglobin. The presence of Hb F or Hb Korle Bu increases the minimum gelling concentration and reduces the gelling and sickling tendency,[5] while the presence of Hb O Arab of Hb D Punjab increases the gelling tendency.[1,6,7] The other two factors are the intracellular hemoglobin concentration (MCHC) and the concentration and distribution of sickle hemoglobin and nonsickle hemoglobin(s), particularly fetal hemoglobin, in the red cells. These two factors may play a role in the modification of the severity of disease in sickle-thalassemia syndromes since reduced MCHC diminishes sickling and the presence of Hb A or increased levels of Hb F decreases or ameliorates sickling. These properties appear to correlate well with clinical severity in variants of sickle cell disease,[1,3] which are summarized in Table 9-1 (pp. 220–222).

## HEMOGLOBIN SC DISEASE
(Hb SC Disease: $\alpha_2 \beta^{6 \ Val} \beta^{6 \ Lys}$)

The high frequency of sickle cell trait (Hb AS) (8% to 10%) and the relatively high frequency of Hb C trait (Hb AC) (2% to 3%)[8,9] in American blacks make Hb SC disease the most common of the sickling disorders other than homozygous sickle cell disease and sickle cell trait. The incidence of Hb SC disease at birth is about one in 800 in American blacks[9]; the incidence is negligible in the nonblack population although several white persons have been reported to have Hb SC disease.[10,11] Geographically, Hb SC disease is found in black populations of West Africa as well as in West Indians and North and Central American blacks who originated from West Africa. Since the genes for Hb S and Hb C are alleles, a person with Hb SC disease should receive a gene for Hb S from one parent and a gene for Hb C from the other parent. There are approximately equal amounts of Hb S and Hb C in the red cells of Hb SC patients.

Hb C was first identified in 1950 by Itano and Neel using the paper electrophoresis method.[12] The following year, Kaplan et al first described the clinical features in three patients with electrophoretically-proven Hb SC disease.[13] There is a considerable variation in clinical expression of Hb SC disease, and it is generally characterized by a longer life expectancy, a milder degree of hemolytic anemia, and less frequent vaso-occlusive crises than is homozygous sickle cell disease.

## Hematologic Findings

Persons with Hb SC disease have a mild to moderate degree of anemia and reticulocytosis.[11,14,15,16] The anemia is primarily the result of increased destruction of erythrocytes[17,18] secondary to the abnormal properties of Hb SC red cells. These erythrocytes have reduced solubility and intraerythrocytic crystal formation upon dehydration due to Hb C,[19,20] in addition to the abnormal physical properties of Hb S that may cause membrane damage and shortened red cell survival. It is still controversial whether the anemia in this disorder is also due to inadequate bone marrow response to the degree of anemia,[17,18] although bone marrow usually shows erythroid hyperactivity.[11,21] The average hemoglobin value in pediatric patients is about 10 g/dl,[14,16,21] with a range of 8.0 to 13.0 g/dl, and reticulocyte counts are less than 5%. Red cell indices are generally normal, although decreased mean cell volume (MCV) and mean cell hemoglobin (MCH) frequently have been reported[11,14,16,21] in the absence of $\alpha$ thalassemia or iron deficiency.[16] Examination of the peripheral blood film reveals a mild degree of anisocytosis, polychromasia, and numerous target cells usually comprising less than 50% of total erythrocytes,[11,14] although more than 50% have been reported.[10,11,17,21] Poikilocytosis is not common and sickle cells are not usually seen.[11,14] When sickle cells do occur, they are atypical forms with an absence of filamentous processes and with a thick rather than elongated appearance (oat cells). All erythrocytes containing Hb SC are easily sickled by sodium metabisulfite. The solubility and shake tests[22] are positive. Upon incubation with 3% NaCl solution, hexagonal crystals within the red cells can be readily demonstrated.[23] Target cells and the intraerythrocytic crystals may be due to the properties of Hb C. Osmotic fragility of the erythrocytes is reported to be reduced,[14] which is probably due to the predominance of target cells. There is not a great deal of information regarding erythrokinetics, but mean erythrocyte life span has been reported to be shortened to 18 to 56 days.[17,18,24] The oxygen dissociation curve is shifted to the right.[25] Patients with Hb SC disease have normal (non-$\alpha$)/$\alpha$ globin synthesis ratios (Figure 9-1) and normal free radioactive $\alpha$ chain pools (Figures 9-1, 9-2).[16] The white blood cell counts are generally normal to slightly increased with a normal differential during asymptomatic periods; leukocytosis often occurs during a crisis.[15,18]

## Clinical Manifestations

Persons with Hb SC disease have a similar symptomatology to those with Hb SS, but there is a considerable variation in severity.

**Table 9-1**
**Variants of Sickle Cell Disease**

| Sickling disorder | Genotype | S | Non-S | A₂ | F | Ethnic group | Number of patients reported |
|---|---|---|---|---|---|---|---|
| | | | % Hb present | | | | |
| **I. Association of Hb S and other β-chain mutations** | | | | | | | |
| SS | $\alpha_2\beta_2^{6Glu \rightarrow Val}$ | 80-98 | | 1.8-4.3 | 1.9-10.6 | African and American blacks, Mediterraneans, Turks, Arabs, southern Indians | 1:625 in American blacks* |
| AS | $\alpha_2\beta^A\beta^S$ | 38.1-45.2 | | 1.9-3.4 | N | Same as in Hb SS | 1:12 in American blacks* |
| SC | $\alpha_2\beta^S\beta^{6Glu \rightarrow Lys}$ | 45-55 | 45-55 | 0.2-8.1 | | American and African blacks | 1:833* |
| SC Harlem** | $\alpha_2\beta^S\beta^{6Val,73Asn}$ | 49.9 | 43.6 | | 7.2 | American blacks | 3 |
| SD Los Angeles* or SD Punjab | $\alpha_2\beta^S\beta^{121Glu \rightarrow Gln}$ | 45 | | 3.2 | 2.3-20.0 | Whites of English, Spanish, Mexican, and Cuban extraction, American blacks | 8 |
| SD Ibadan* | $\alpha_2\beta^S\beta^{87Thr \rightarrow Lys}$ | 20 | 80 | | | African black | 1 |
| SE** | $\alpha_2\beta^S\beta^{26Glu \rightarrow Lys}$ | 60-64.2 | | | 1.3 | Eti-Turks, American blacks | 5 1:100,000 in American blacks* |
| SO Arab** | $\alpha_2\beta^S\beta^{121Glu \rightarrow Lys}$ | 48.0-56.3 | 41.3-45.6 | | 2-28 | African and American blacks, Arabs | 12 |
| SG Galveston* (or SG Texas) | $\alpha_2\beta^S\beta^{43Glu \rightarrow Ala}$ | | | | 3.6 | American black | 1 |
| SG San Jose* | $\alpha_2\beta^S\beta^{7Glu \rightarrow Gly}$ | | < 2.5 | | | American blacks | 2 |
| S Korle Bu* | $\alpha_2\beta^S\beta^{73Asp \rightarrow Asn}$ | 40 | 60 | N | | African blacks | 2 |
| S Ocho-Rios* | $\alpha_2\beta^S\beta^{52Asp \rightarrow Ala}$ | | | 3.3 | N | Jamaican black | 1 |
| S Osu-Christiansborg* | $\alpha_2\beta^S\beta^{52Asp \rightarrow Asn}$ | 42 | 56 | N | 1.0 | African and American blacks | 3 |
| S Richmond* | $\alpha_2\beta^S\beta^{102Asn \rightarrow Lys}$ | | | 3.5 | | American blacks | 2 |
| S Camden*** | $\alpha_2\beta^S\beta^{131Gln \rightarrow Glu}$ | 34 | 66 | | | American black | 1 |
| S Deer Lodge | $\alpha_2\beta^S\beta^{2His \rightarrow Arg}$ | 36 | 54 | 4.1 | 6 | American black | 1 |
| S Hope*** | $\alpha_2\beta^S\beta^{136Gly \rightarrow Asp}$ | 45.6 | 51.3 | 2.7 | 1.3 | American blacks | 2 |
| SJ Baltimore*** | $\alpha_2\beta^S\beta^{16Gly \rightarrow Asp}$ | 29-44 | 56-67.8 | 3.0-3.2 | < 2.7 | African and American blacks | 5 |
| SJ Bangkok*** | $\alpha_2\beta^S\beta^{56Gly \rightarrow Asp}$ | 38.7, 38.9 | 58.5, 59.1 | 2.8, 2.0 | 0.1, 1.1 | American blacks | 2 |
| SK Cameroon*** | $\alpha_2\beta^S\beta^X$ | 25 | 75 | | | African black | 1 |
| SK Woolwich*** | $\alpha_2\beta^S\beta^{132Lys \rightarrow Gln}$ | 60 | 40 | | | African blacks | 7 |

| Clinical severity | Hb (g/dl) | Retic (%) | MCV (fl) | MCH (pg) | MCHC (g/dl) | Red cell morphology | PB globin synthesis ratio (non-$\alpha$)/$\alpha$ | PB free $\alpha$-chain radioactivity (%) | References |
|---|---|---|---|---|---|---|---|---|---|
| Marked | 6.5-9.6 | 2.2-26.1 | 80-98 | 26.1-32.1 | 31.0-36.6 | ISC (0%-40%), targets, moderate anisopoikilocytosis | 0.98-1.12 | 14.0-17.5 | -3,9,16 |
| ...nptomatic | 12.1-16.5 | N | 82.1-91.8 | 27-31 | | N | 0.96-1.04‡ | | 9,148,149 |
| Mild to moderate | 8.8-11.8 | 0.4-6.2 | 65-95 | 24.0-30.7 | 32.1-36.2 | Targets (30%-50%), rare ISC | 0.91-1.03 | 9.9-18.6 | 9,14-16 |
| Mild to moderate | 8.4-10.6 | 6.2-11.0 | 85-98 | 29.8-31.1 | 31.8-35.1 | Targets, ISC | 1.06,1.15 | 18.4, 18.5 | 150,151 |
| ...derate to marked | 6.9-9.9 | 4.0-14.4 | 81-120 | 26.0-34.5 | 28.7-33.0 | Numerous ISC, targets, mild anisocytosis | | | 1,7,53-59 |
| ...ptomatic | 14.8 | 1.0 | | | | N | | | 61 |
| ...ptomatic to mild | 8.4-14.6 | 1.5-4.0 | 71-97 | 24,26 | 25,27 | Rare ISC, targets, mild anisocytosis | | | 152-155 |
| ...derate to marked | 6.8-9.1 | 0.8-32 | 74-110 | 23.0-34.5 | 30-36 | Frequent ISC, targets, anisopoikilocytosis | | | 18,63,71-74 |
| ...otomatic | 16.3 | 1.4 | | | | N | | | 62 |
| ...otomatic | N | | | | | | | | 156 |
| ...tomatic | N | | | | | | | | 5,76 |
| ...tomatic | 15.4 | 2.0 | | | | Occasional targets | | | 157 |
| ...tomatic | 13.8 | 1.5 | | | | | | | 62,158 |
| ...tomatic | 13.4-14.2 | | | | | | | | 159 |
| ...tomatic | N | | | | | N | | | 160 |
| ...tomatic | 12.8 | 3.0 | | | | Mild anisopoikilocytosis | | | 161 |
| ...omatic | Hct 34.5 | < 2.0 | | | | | | | 162 |
| ...omatic | 12.1-14.4 | 0.9-1.0 | 71-84 | 21.0-24.5 | 28.0-30.5 | N or mild microcytosis and hypochromia | | | 1,163,164 |
| ...omatic | 11.6, 9.8 | 2.5, 2.1 | 84, 79 | 27.2, 26.5 | 33, 34 | N | | | 165 |
| ...omatic | | | | | | | | | 166 |
| ...omatic mild | 15.1 | 1.2 | 85.2 | 24.7 | 29.0 | N | | | 167,168 |

**Table 9-1** *(continued)*
**Variants of Sickle Cell Disease**

| Sickling disorder | Genotype | % Hb present | | | | Ethnic group | Number of patients reported | M(e) (g/ |
|---|---|---|---|---|---|---|---|---|
| | | S | Non-S | A₂ | F | | | |
| SN Baltimore*** | $\alpha_2\beta^s\beta$95Lys→Glu | | | | | | 3 families | 38 |
| S Pyrgos*** | $\alpha_2\beta^s\beta$83Gly→Asp | 35.2 | 62.2 | 2.6 | 0.7 | Greek | 1 | |
| S Saki or S Dakar-Saki | $\alpha_2\beta^s\beta$141Leu→Pro | 57 | 41 | 2 | | African black | 1 | |
| S Leslie | $\alpha_2\beta^s\beta$131Del | 60.9 | 34.1 | 4.8 | 0.8 | American black | 1 | |
| **II. Association of Hb S and α-chain mutations** | | | | | | | | |
| AS-G Philadelphia | $\alpha^A\alpha$68Asn→Lys$\beta^A\beta^s$ | 38-43.1 | | | 0.9-2.3 | American blacks | Several families | |
| SS-G Philadelphia | $\alpha^A\alpha$68Asn→Lys$\beta_2{}^s$ | 62-63.1 | | | 0.8-3.4 | American blacks | 4 | |
| | | (excluding 1-year-old child) | | | | | | |
| SC-G Philadelphia | $\alpha^A\alpha$68Asn→Lys$\beta^s\beta^c$ | 22,35 | | | 2.7,3.7 | American blacks | 2 | |
| AS-G Georgia | $\alpha^A\alpha$95Pro→Leu$\beta^A\beta^s$ | 28.6 | | 2.0 | | American black | 1 | |
| SS Memphis | $\alpha^A\alpha$23Glu→Gln$\beta_2{}^s$ | | | | 6-10 | American blacks | 3 | |
| AS-Stanleyville-II | $\alpha^A\alpha$78Asn→Lys$\beta^A\beta^s$ | | | | | African blacks | 11 | |
| SS-Stanleyville-II | $\alpha^A\alpha$78Asp→Lys$\beta_2{}^s$ | | | | 4.7-10 | African blacks | 2 | |
| AS-Hopkins-2*** | $\alpha^A\alpha$112His→Asp$\beta^A\beta^s$ | 45 | | | | | 6 | |
| **III. Association of Hb S with Thalassemia** | | | | | | | | |
| AS-α thal. | $\alpha^A\alpha$Thal$\beta^A\beta^s$ | 24.7-34.8 | 62.8-75.9 | 1.1-3.8 | 0.3-1.3 | American blacks, Arabs | | |
| SS-α thal.* | $\alpha^A\alpha$Thal$\beta_2{}^s$ | | | 2.3-4.2 | 2.3-33.3 | American and African blacks, Turks | 12 (1:20,000 in American blacks*) | |
| SS-Hb H*** | $\alpha$Thal¹$\alpha$Thal²$\beta_2{}^s$ | 40.7 | 14.0 | | 43.7 | Arab | I | |
| SC-α thal.** | $\alpha^A\alpha$Thal$\beta^s\beta^c$ | 50.5 | 47.7 | | 1.8 | American black | 1 | |
| SO Arab-α thal.** | $\alpha^A\alpha$Thal$\beta^s\beta$oArab | 54 | 46 | | < 2 | American black | 1 | |

| Clinical severity | Hb (g/dl) | Retic (%) | MCV (fl) | MCH (pg) | MCHC (g/dl) | Red cell morphology | PB globin synthesis ratio (non-α)/α | PB free α-chain radioactivity (%) | References |
|---|---|---|---|---|---|---|---|---|---|
| symptomatic | N | | | | | | | | 169 |
| symptomatic | 12.6 | 1.3 | 69.6 | 21.9 | 31.5 | Mild anisocytosis, microcytosis, hypochromia | | | 170 |
| symptomatic | 12.2 | | 93 | 29.7 | 32.1 | | | | 171 |
| symptomatic | 10.1 | | 75 | 24.5 | 33.0 | | | | 172 |
| symptomatic | 13.2-15.8 | | 77-87 | 25.1-27.9 | | N or slight anisopoikilocytosis, slight hypochromia | 0.42-0.75‡ | | 77,173 |
| Marked | 6.0-8.8 | 9.4-17.4 | 80-94 | 26.9-33.4 | 33.4-35.2 | Numerous ISC, targets, anisopoikilocytosis | | | 74,78,80 |
| Moderate to marked | 8.3,9.6 | 4.5 | 64.9,81 | 20.7,27 | 31.9 | Anisopoikilocytosis, targets, microcytosis, hypochromia | | | 77,81 |
| symptomatic | 10.9 | 3.2 | | | | | | | 174 |
| Mild | 7-10 | 5-24 | 88 | | 35.2 | ISC, poikilocytosis | | | 82-84 |
| symptomatic | N | | | | | N | | | 175,176 |
| Moderate to marked | 4-10 | 3-40 | | | | ISC, targets, anisopoikilocytosis | | | 175,176 |
| symptomatic | N | N | N | N | N | N | | | 177 |
| symptomatic | 12.2-16.3 | | 68-79 | 23-28 | | Mild microcytosis | 0.67-0.82‡ | | 149 |
| Mild to marked | 7.8-9.7 | 2.0-18.4 | 59-79 | 19.9-28.1 | 31.0-34.4 | ISC, microcytosis, hypochromia, targets, anisopoikilocytosis | 1.04-2.32 | 3.2-6.4 | 16,89,126 128,129 |
| symptomatic | 8.9 | | 70 | 20 | 28 | Hypochromia, anisopoikilocytosis | | | 127 |
| symptomatic | 7.9 | 7.2 | 53 | 16.2 | 30.6 | Numerous targets, marked hypochromia, microcytosis, anisopoikilocytosis | 1.47 | | 178 |
| Moderate | 11.8 | 6.3 | 73 | 24 | 33 | ISC(8%-11%), targets, anisopoikilocytosis | 1.41 | | 75 |

**Table 9-1** *(continued)*
**Variants of Sickle Cell Disease**

| Sickling disorder | Genotype | % Hb present | | | | Ethnic group | Number of patients reported | N ( |
|---|---|---|---|---|---|---|---|---|
| | | S | Non-S | A₂ | F | | | |
| S-$\beta^0$ thal.* | $\alpha_2\beta^s\beta$Thal$^0$ | 70-95 | | 2.2-6.9 | 1.6-20 | American blacks, Mediterraneans | 1:23,000 in blacks⁺ | |
| S-$\beta^+$ thal. | $\alpha_2\beta^s\beta$Thal$^+$ | 52.2-90.5 | 8.7-33 | 3.1-6.7 | 0.8-20.3 | American blacks, Mediterraneans | 1:5000 in blacks⁺ | |
| SS-ð thal.* | | | | 1.4 | | American black | 1 | |
| S-$\alpha\beta^+$ thal.* | $\alpha^A\alpha$Thal$\beta^s\beta$Thal$^+$ | 60.2 | 27.4 | 3.3 | 9.1 | American black | 1 | |
| S-ð$\beta$ thal.* | $\alpha_2\beta^s(\delta\beta)$Thal | 59.8-79.1 | | 1.4-3.4 | 15-37.1 | American blacks, Greeks, Italians | 9 | |
| S-Lepore (or S-Pylos)* | $\alpha_2\beta^s\beta^{\delta \times \beta}$ | 62.7-90 | 10-11 | 0.9-2.6 | 9.3-25.0 | Greeks, Italian, Jamaican black | 5 | |
| S-HPFH* | | 60-80 | | 1.1-2.2 | 15-34 | blacks | 27 | |
| S-$\beta^+$ thal-G Philadeliphia | $\alpha^A\alpha^G\beta^s\beta$Thal$^+$ | 57.7 | | | 4.1 | American black | 1 | |

*Similar to Hb SS by Hb electrophoresis at alkaline pH
**Similar to Hb SC by Hb electrophoresis at alkaline pH
***Hb S and fast Hb by Hb electrophoresis at alkaline pH
+Incidence
MGC Minimum gelling concentration

Crises are generally less frequent and less severe than in Hb SS disease.[11,14,15] In contrast to patients with Hb SS disease, in which the onset of symptoms almost always occurs during the first one or two years of life, approximately half of the individuals with Hb SC disease may not have their onset of symptoms under the age of ten years,[11] and some individuals may not have any symptoms until late adulthood.[11,15] These persons generally have normal physical appearance and sexual maturation,[11,14] but extensive radiologic changes of skeleton have been reported, with these changes being more obvious with age.[14,26] The most common symptom at the time of presentation is pain, particularly in the extremities, abdomen, or chest.

Although painful crises are generally less common in Hb SC disease than in Hb SS disease, there is a relatively high incidence of some vaso-occlusive–thrombotic episodes,[11,14,15,27] such as aseptic necrosis of the femoral head, serious ocular lesions and hematuria, and multiple complications, including pulmonary infarction, during

| Clinical severity | Hb (g/dl) | Retic (%) | MCV (fl) | MCH (pg) | MCHC (g/dl) | Red cell morphology | PB globin synthesis ratio (non-α)/α | PB free α-chain radioactivity (%) | References |
|---|---|---|---|---|---|---|---|---|---|
| Moderate to marked | 6.3-12.4 | 2.7-18.7 | 63-88 | 20.8-28.9 | 29.8-35.4 | ISC (rare to frequent), hypochromia, microcytosis, targets, anisopoikilocytosis | 0.35-0.81 | 36.1-53.0 | 95,102,105, 107,108,121 |
| Mild to moderate | 6.8-13.8 | 1.4-5.6 | 62-84 | 20.4-27.3 | 32.2-34.9 | Rare ISC, microcytosis, hypochromia, anisopoikilocytosis | 0.2-0.91 | 14.0-31.4 (bone marrow) | 95,101, 102-109 |
| Mild to moderate | 6.9-8.1 | 9.2 | 91 | 30 | 31 | Frequent ISC, targets, anisopoikilocytosis | | | 179 |
| Mild | 10.8 | 2.6 | 73 | 20.7 | 27.8 | Rare ISC, targets, anisopoikilocytosis, microcytosis, hypochromia | 0.66 | 18.9 | 121 |
| Asymptomatic to mild | 8.8-15.9 | 1.2-3.1 | 76-96 | 25.6-31.0 | 32.4 | Rare ISC, mild microcytosis | 0.66-1.00 | | 95,133-138 |
| Mild to severe | 8.0-12.5 | 3.3-8.0 | 77.7-83.0 | 24.3-27.6 | 33.1-35.3 | Few ISC, targets, slight poikilocytosis | | | 145-147 |
| Asymptomatic | 7.4-18 | 0.5-3.2 | 75-88.4 | 24.2-29.3 | | No ISC, occasional targets, slight hypochromia | 0.71-1.04 | | 106,139-141 |
| Mild | 11.6 | 4.6 | 67 | 25 | 36.9 | Rare ISC, microcytosis, hypochromia, anisopoikilocytosis | 0.70 | 13.4 | 180,181 |

N Normal
‡α/(non-α) ratio
PB Peripheral blood
ISC Irreversibly sickled cells

pregnancy. These complications seem to occur more frequently with advancing age. Despite the milder nature of hemolytic disease,[15] serious thrombotic complications do occur which may be due to a higher viscosity of venous blood since hematocrit values are higher in Hb SC than in Hb SS disease. There is a higher incidence of aseptic necrosis of the femoral head in Hb SC than in Hb SS disease.[28,29]

The effects of increased viscosity of blood containing Hb SC on ocular tissues are notable. The ocular manifestations are similar to those in Hb SS, although proliferative retinopathy with resultant vitreous hemorrhage and retinal detachment is much more common in Hb SC patients than in Hb SS patients.[30,31] The retina undergoes a series of progressive changes, beginning with diminished blood flow, progressive occlusion of arterioles and capillary beds with resultant ischemia and infarction, compensatory arteriovenous anastomoses, neovascularization, and proliferation of these new vessels (sea fans).[30-33] If these lesions are not treated prophylactically, vitreous

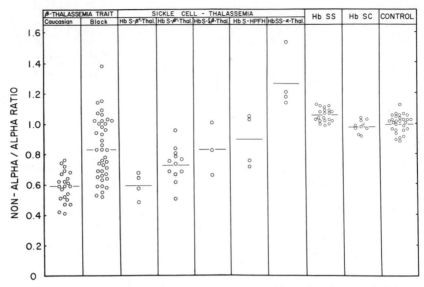

**Figure 9-1.** (Non-α)/α globin synthesis ratios in sickling disorders studied in our laboratory. The mean of each group is indicated by a horizontal line.

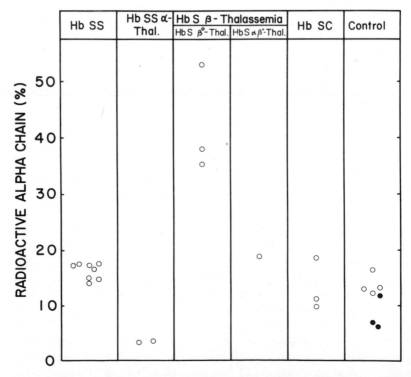

**Figure 9-2.** Percent of free radioactive α chain in the peripheral blood. Filled circles ( ● ) refer to percent of free radioactive α chain in iron-deficient controls.

hemorrhage and retinal detachment with blindness can occur. Clinically significant retinopathy is usually present in adults over the age of 20.[32] The proliferative lesions appear to be slowly progressive and somewhat age-dependent. Because of the common and serious nature of eye manifestations, periodic examination of eyes by indirect ophthalmoscopy and/or fluorescein angiography is recommended for patients older than ten years.

Since Hb SC disease may not be diagnosed in childhood and persons with this disorder may enter adulthood unaware of their disease, accurate diagnosis of sickle hemoglobinopathies is important in teenage girls as there are serious fetal and maternal complications with pregnancy.[34-37] Severe anemia, infections, and thromboembolic episodes in the third trimester of pregnancy and during intrapartum and puerperium occur rather frequently. Placental infarction with fetal wastage and pulmonary infarction or stroke, often with maternal death, can occur. High mortality rates in both the fetus and the mother have been reported in the literature.[34,35]

In contrast to patients with Hb SS disease, in which the spleen usually becomes nonpalpable and nonfunctional before the age of 5 years, about 60% of patients with Hb SC disease have persistent mild splenomegaly into adulthood.[11] There have been reports of increased risk of splenic sequestration or infarction upon exposure to reduced oxygen tension, such as in aircraft or during mountain travel,[38,39] but these episodes can also occur at low altitudes[40] without the precipitating cause being demonstrated.[11] In this disorder, splenic sequestration crises usually occur in late childhood or even in adulthood. Therefore, when a splenic sequestration crisis occurs after late childhood, a variant of sickle cell disease, especially Hb SC disease or Hb S-$\beta$ thalassemia, should be considered. Although functional asplenia in this disorder is not well recognized in the literature, it probably occurs more frequently than is generally thought. Only one case has been described, transient functional asplenia in a 22-year-old woman during a painful crisis.[41] We have observed functional asplenia in eight out of 57 patients with Hb SC disease, ranging in age from 14 months to 18 years. The 14-month-old child developed functional asplenia following a splenic sequestration crisis.

There is a relatively high frequency of hematuria, probably due to renal papillary necrosis.[42,43] A mild defect in urine concentrating ability has also been demonstrated.[44,45]

Patients with Hb SC often present with acute pulmonary syndromes due either to respiratory infections, with pneumonia reported to be common in children,[14] or to pulmonary infarction. Sudden death from pulmonary embolization following marrow infarction has been reported.[46,47] Serious bacterial infections are not common, with no deaths from infections reported in the literature.[48] This may be explained by the fact that the onset of functional asplenia is delayed until late childhood. However, there seems to be an increased incidence of gram-negative bacterial infections, particularly salmonella osteo-myelitis.[49,50] Some patients have cardiac murmurs which may be associated with slight cardiac enlargement, but usually there are no electrocardiographic abnormalities.[11,14] The impairment of hepatocellular function is not evident; however, jaundice, mild hepatomegaly, and elevation of alkaline phosphatase have been reported. Gallstones often occur in adulthood.[1,1] Leg ulcers usually do not occur. Cerebral vascular thrombosis and intracranial hemorrhages have been reported,[34,51] although these are rare compared to their incidence in patients with Hb SS.

## Diagnosis

Although Hb SC disease can be strongly suspected on the basis of clinical and hematologic findings and family studies, diagnosis should be confirmed by both acid and alkaline hemoglobin electrophoresis. Hemoglobins that migrate identically with Hb C, such as Hb E, Hb O Arab, or Hb C Harlem, should be differentiated from Hb C by agar gel electrophoresis and by incubation with 3% NaCl. Red cells containing Hb SC usually show intraerythrocytic crystals, but red cells with Hb S in combination with other hemoglobins do not have crystals. When red cell indices are decreased without iron deficiency, the combination of $\alpha$ thalassemia with Hb SC disease can be confirmed either by family studies or by globin synthesis and free radioactive $\alpha$ chain pool studies.[16] However, decreased red cell indices do not necessarily indicate the presence of $\alpha$ thalassemia in this disorder.[16]

## SICKLE CELL Hb D DISEASE
(Hb SD Los Angeles: $\alpha_2\beta^{6 \ Val}\beta^{121 \ Gln}$)

Shortly after the discovery of Hb S and Hb C, a third abnormal hemoglobin, Hb D, was identified by Itano in 1951.[52] Hb D is found mainly in India among Sikhs and Punjab Hindus and has a frequency of about 3% in Punjab (Hb D Punjab). Hb D Punjab is the most common type of Hb D and is now called Hb D Los Angeles, as Hb D was first described in Los Angeles before being discovered in Punjab and their amino acid substitutions are identical ($\alpha_2\beta_2^{121 \ Gln}$). Hemoglobin D is also found in populations of English, French, Austrian, Portuguese, Mexican, Cuban, and Turkish extraction, as well as in blacks. There is an incidence of 0.1% to 0.4% in American blacks.[53] More than 20 cases of Hb SD disease have been reported in the literature, most commonly in persons from England; however, structural analysis of Hb D was not done in most cases. Only five whites and three blacks have been proven to have Hb SD Los Angeles.[54-58] These patients had a moderate to severe degree of hemolytic anemia with hemoglobin levels ranging from about 6 to 10 g/dl and reticulocyte counts from 4.3% to 14%. Red cell morphology was characterized by numerous sickle cells, target cells, mild anisocytosis, and polychromasia. Hemoglobin $A_2$ levels were normal[56] and Hb F levels were elevated to 5% except for young infants.[54,56] Red cell survival with $^{51}Cr$ in two patients revealed half-lives of 9.5 and 12 days.[56,58] Most patients had frequent episodes of severe bone and joint pains, and one had recurrent pulmonary infarctions, aseptic necrosis of hip, and an episode of hemiparesis.[1,53] The spleen was not palpable except in two infants less than one year of age in whom marked splenomegaly was present.[57,59] In most cases of Hb SD disease reported in which Hb D was not structurally identified, there were hematologic and clinical findings similar to those in Hb SD Los Angeles. Two blacks with Hb SD were reported to be asymptomatic and nonanemic.[60,61] In one of these, Hb D was identified as Hb D Ibadan ($\alpha_2\beta_2^{87\ Lys\to Thr}$).[61] The mechanism of the interaction of Hb D and Hb S is not well understood. Hb SD has the same electrophoretic pattern as Hb SS at alkaline pH; thus, it might be overlooked as Hb SS in blacks. About 25 nonsickle hemoglobins are known to migrate similarly to Hb S at alkaline pH and are usually called either Hb D or Hb G. Of these abnormal hemoglobins, at least 21 have a single amino acid substitution in the $\beta$-polypeptide chain,[62] and nine of these hemoglobins have occurred with Hb S; only two resulting conditions, Hb SD Los Angeles and Hb S Lepore, have the manifestations of sickle cell disease.

### Diagnosis

When subjects have an electrophoretic pattern similar to that of Hb SS at alkaline pH, agar gel electrophoresis using a citrate buffer should be performed, as Hb D or Hb G can be separated from Hb S because they migrate to a position similar to that of Hb A. The parents should be studied since one parent's red cells should not sickle despite an electrophoretic pattern similar to that in sickle cell trait. For identification of the specific type of Hb G or Hb D, further studies, including structural analysis, are usually needed.

### SICKLE CELL Hb O Arab
(Hb SO Arab: $\alpha_2\beta^{6\ Val}\beta^{121\ Lys}$)

Hb O Arab was first described in 1960 by Ramot et al in an Arab family in Israel in whom Hb S occurred with Hb O.[63] Two years prior to this, a similar electrophoretic variant of slow mobility was discovered in Indonesia (Hb O Indonesia).[64] Later, Baglioni and Lehmann analyzed these two hemoglobins and found that Hb O Arab has a lysine at the position 121 of normal $\beta^A$-polypeptide chain instead of glutamic acid ($\beta$ 121 [GH4] Glu→Lys), and that Hb O Indonesia has a substitution in the $\alpha$ chain ($\alpha_2^{116\ Glu→Lys}\beta_2$).[65] Hemoglobin O Arab is a relatively uncommon variant of human adult hemoglobin and has been found sporadically in different races from different parts of the world, with the highest incidence probably in Bulgaria and Yugoslavia.[66,67,68] The exact incidence and origin of Hb O Arab is not well known; however, this hemoglobin was not found in Saudi Arabia,[69] although about one in 1000 persons in northern Sudan was found to have Hb O Arab trait, suggesting that this hemoglobin probably originated in non-Arab peoples of pre-semitic Egypt.[70]

Heterozygotes for Hb O Arab are asymptomatic and not anemic, with Hb O comprising about 35% to 45% of the total hemoglobin. Levels of Hb $A_2$ and Hb F are normal, and an abnormal red cell morphology characterized by slight anisopoikilocytosis, hypochromia, and some target cells has been reported.[68] Only 12 patients with Hb SO Arab—Arabs in Israel,[63] Sudanese,[71] and blacks from Jamaica[6] and America[18,72,73,74]—and one American black with Hb SO Arab-$\alpha$ thalassemia[75] have been reported. Hb SO Arab is characterized by a moderately severe form of sickle cell disease and is often indistinguishable from Hb SS. The clinical severity is reflected in the interaction of Hb O Arab with Hb S to enhance the gelling tendency.[6]

## Hematologic Findings

Most patients have a moderate to severe degree of anemia with hemoglobin levels of 6 to 9 g/dl and reticulocyte counts in the 5% to 15% range. Red cell indices are usually normal. The peripheral blood smear is similar to that in Hb SS, with numerous sickle forms, Howell-Jolly bodies, and normoblasts, but target cells and anisopoikilocytosis are more pronounced than in Hb SS. Hemoglobin F levels are increased, with higher levels in Arabs (10%, 28%) than in blacks (2% to 7%). Red cell survival with $^{51}Cr$ revealed a great variation in results, with a half-life of 6 days in one study[6] and 23.7 days in another study.[18] The oxygen dissociation curve was shifted to the right, similar to values in Hb SS.[6]

## Clinical Manifestations

The spectrum in this disorder is similar to that in sickle cell disease. These patients experience frequent, severe vaso-occlusive crises, with hand-foot syndromes, joint pains, and serious bacterial infections occurring early in life, probably due to the development of functional asplenia. Sickle retinopathy, leg ulcers, and gallstones are also described. In most patients, the spleen is not palpable except during childhood.

The one patient with Hb SO Arab-$\alpha$ thalassemia has mild anemia (10.8 to 12.5 g/dl), reticulocytosis (2.2% to 6.4%), and a mild clinical course, perhaps due to the effect of the $\alpha$-thalassemia gene.[75] Hemoglobin F was slightly elevated and the amounts of Hb S and Hb O were similar, with 54% Hb S and 46% Hb O Arab. A striking feature was the decreased red cell indices. Despite the mild nature of the disease compared to that in the usual patient with Hb SO Arab, red cell survival with $^{51}$Cr showed a short half-life of 14 days. The $\alpha$/(non-$\alpha$) globin synthesis ratios in peripheral blood and bone marrow were 0.71 and 0.75, respectively, similar to those in $\alpha$-thalassemia trait.

### Diagnosis

Since Hb O Arab migrates identically to Hbs C, E or C Harlem on alkaline electrophoresis, Hb SO Arab can be mistaken for Hb SC. However, hematologically and clinically Hb SO Arab may be differentiated from Hb SC, which is a relatively mild disorder without severe anemia and reticulocytosis or numerous sickle forms on peripheral smear. The differentiation of Hb O Arab from Hbs C, E, and C Harlem should be confirmed by citrate agar electrophoresis in which Hb O Arab migrates between Hb A and Hb S but nearer to Hb A, differing from Hbs C, E, and C Harlem. The differentiation from Hb SC can also be made by incubation with 3% NaCl solution, as Hb SO Arab red cells do not form intraerythrocytic crystals.

### SICKLE CELL Hb KORLE BU
(Hb S Korle Bu: $\alpha_2\beta^{6Val}\beta^{73\ Asn}$)

Hemoglobin Korle Bu was found to inhibit gelling of hemolysate containing Hb S.[5] Consequently, double heterozygotes for Hb S and Hb Korle Bu would be expected to have even milder sickling manifestations than persons with Hb AS. A father and a daughter with Hb S Korle Bu were reported to be nonanemic and asymptomatic.[76] Hemoglobin Korle Bu migrates as Hb S on alkaline electrophoresis, but migrates as Hb A on agar gel electrophoresis with the presence of approximately 60% of Hb Korle Bu and normal concentrations of Hb $A_2$.

## SICKLE CELL Hb G PHILADELPHIA
(Hb SS-G Philadelphia: $\alpha^A\alpha^{68\ Lys}\beta_2^{6\ Val}$)

Hemoglobin G Philadelphia, the most common $\alpha$ chain mutant ($\alpha_2^{68\ Asn \rightarrow Lys}\beta_2$), is relatively common in American blacks[77]; however, only a few families have been reported to have the combination of Hb G Philadelphia and sickle cell trait[74,77-80] or homozygous sickle cell disease.[74,78,80] The hematologic and clinical manifestations of persons heterozygous for Hb G Philadelphia and homozygous for Hb S are indistinguishable from those with Hb SS. Double heterozygotes for Hb S and Hb G Philadelphia are similar to persons with sickle cell trait, suggesting that Hb G Philadelphia does not interact with Hb S.[74] Four patients with Hb SS-G Philadelphia have been reported and have a severe degree of anemia with hemoglobin values of 6.0 to 8.8 g/dl and reticulocyte counts of 9.4% to 17.4%. Red cell indices were normal and sickle forms were present on the peripheral blood smear. Hemoglobin F levels were 0.8% to 3.4%. These persons experience severe, frequent painful crises, and stroke has occurred.[74] Two children with Hb SC in conjunction with Hb G Philadelphia have been reported, one having a course similar to that of Hb SS[77] and the other having a mild course with a nonpalpable spleen.[81]

### Diagnosis

In patients with Hb G Philadelphia in combination with Hb SS, there are two major components on electrophoresis, with the larger fraction having the mobility of Hb S and the smaller fraction having the mobility of Hb C due to two types of molecules ($\alpha_2^G\beta_2^S$ and $\alpha_2^A\delta_2$), and a minor component (less than 2%) that is slower than Hb $A_2$ due to the presence of Hb $G_2$ ($\alpha_2^G\delta_2$). This pattern could be confused with that of Hb SC disease. Differentiation between the two disorders can be made easily, since persons with Hb SC disease have about equal amounts of Hb S and Hb C, while here the Hb S band is about twice as dense as the Hb C-like band ($\alpha_2^G\beta_2^S + \alpha_2^A\delta_2$). However, the presence of Hb C should be ruled out by agar gel electrophoresis, as Hb G Philadelphia, differing from Hb C, migrates to the position of Hb A.

When Hb G Philadelphia occurs with Hb AS, there will be three major components: one with the mobility of Hb A ($\alpha_2^A\beta_2$, 35% to 40%), another with that of Hb S (about 50%) due to a mixture of Hb S ($\alpha_2^A\beta_2^S$) and Hb G Philadelphia ($\alpha_2^G\beta_2^A$), and a third with that of Hb C (10% to 18%) due to a mixture of the hybrid hemoglobin ($\alpha_2^G\beta_2^S$) and Hb $A_2$. Hemoglobin $G_2$, migrating even more slowly, is less than 2% of the total hemoglobin. There is more than 10% of hemoglobin at the position of Hb $A_2$ (usually 10% to 15%) in this disorder, clearly differentiating it from Hb S-$\beta^+$ thalassemia, in which Hb A$_2$ is less than 7%. Presumptive diagnosis for the $\alpha$ chain mutant in conjunction with the $\beta$ chain mutant can be made by electrophoretic methods; however, structural analysis is helpful for accurate diagnosis.

## SICKLE CELL Hb MEMPHIS
(Hb SS-Memphis: $\alpha^A\alpha^{23\ Gln}\beta_2^{6\ Val}$)

When the $\alpha$ chain mutant, Hb Memphis ($\alpha^{23Glu \rightarrow Gln}$), occurs with homozygous sickle cell disease, the result is a mild variant of sickle cell disease. The molecular defect of the $\alpha$ chain changes the deoxy quaternary structure of hemoglobin, interfering with sickling and thus protecting the person from the severe manifestations of a sickling disorder.

Three black patients from 40 to 72 years of age with Hb SS-Memphis were reported to have a very mild clinical course, with a moderate degree of anemia and marked reticulocytosis.[82,83,84] Hemoglobin F levels were elevated (6.0% to 10.1%).

## SICKLE CELL-THALASSEMIA

The sickle cell-thalassemia syndromes include sickle cell-$\beta$ thalassemia (Hb S-$\beta$ thalassemia), sickle cell-$\alpha$ thalassemia (Hb SS-$\alpha$ thalassemia), sickle cell-$\delta$ thalassemia (Hb SS-$\delta$ thalassemia), sickle cell-$\alpha\beta$ thalassemia (Hb S-$\alpha\beta$ thalassemia), sickle cell-$\delta\beta$ thalassemia (Hb S-$\delta\beta$ thalassemia), sickle cell-Lepore syndrome (Hb S-Lepore), and sickle cell-hereditary persistance of fetal hemoglobin (Hb S-HPFH). There is a biochemical and clinical heterogeneity of the expression of the thalassemia genes in these disorders; most are milder than homozygous sickle cell disease. There is hypochromia, microcytosis, and variation in red cell size and shape with relatively higher Hb F levels than in Hb SS. Each disorder will be discussed separately.

## SICKLE CELL-$\beta$ THALASSEMIA
(Hb S-$\beta$ thalassemia)

Sickle cell-$\beta$ thalassemia, the combination of sickle cell trait and $\beta$-thalassemia trait, is the second most common variant of sickle cell disease in American blacks. In this population, the gene frequency for high Hb A$_2$ $\beta$ thalassemia is approximately 0.8% to 1.4%[85,86,87] and the incidence of Hb S-$\beta$ thalassemia is about one in 5000.[9,85] Hemoglobin S-$\beta$ thalassemia is the most common variant of sickle cell disease in persons of Mediterranean ancestry, since $\beta$ thalassemia is prevalent in

Mediterranean areas and the incidence of the sickle cell gene is increased in certain parts of Italy and Greece. This disorder has also been found in other racial groups, including Indians,[88] Turks,[89] and Rumanians.[90] The syndrome has been well characterized since the first description of patients with sickle cell-thalassemia by Silvestroni and Bianco in 1944[91] and the widespread use of various hemoglobin electrophoresis methods. There are two types of $\beta$ thalassemia: $\beta0$,[92] which may be further subdivided into the Ferrara[93] and another type, in which there is complete suppression of the synthesis of the normal $\beta$-globin chain ($\beta^A$) and which is found mostly in nonblack populations of Mediterranean or Asian ancestry; and $\beta^+$,[92] in which there is partial suppression of the synthesis of $\beta^A$ chain and which is the common type found in blacks of African ancestry. The presence or absence of Hb A in an individual is genetically determined. The clinical expression of disease is variable in both major forms of Hb S-$\beta$ thalassemia, ranging from asymptomatic to severe, but it is generally milder than that in sickle cell disease.[94,95,96] These patients usually have elevated Hb $A_2$ values (4% to 7%). Both types of sickle cell-$\beta$ thalassemia are characterized by a variable degree of chronic hemolytic anemia, ranging from absence of anemia to a severe anemia with microcytosis and hypochromia, often in association with anisocytosis, poikilocytosis, target cells, and sometimes basophilic stippling of red cells. The mean cell volume and mean cell hemoglobin are usually decreased. Sickle forms may or may not be present, but sickling can easily be induced by sodium metabisulfite. The osmotic fragility of the erythrocytes is decreased.[89,94] The oxygen dissociation curve is shifted to the right,[95] similar to that in Hb SS. Mean cell life span is shortened to about one-half to two-thirds that of normal.[97,98] Persistent splenomegaly is common. Generally, the degree of anemia and clinical expression is more severe in Hb S-$\beta0$ thalassemia than in Hb S-$\beta^+$ thalassemia,[96,99] perhaps because of the presence of Hb A in the $\beta^+$ variety, which lowers the gelling tendency with the result of less sickling and less hemolysis.[3] However, there are exceptions, with some patients with Hb S-$\beta^+$ thalassemia having a severe clinical course,[95,97] suggesting that other factors may be responsible for modifying the clinical picture. It is known that homozygous $\beta$ thalassemia in blacks is milder than in whites[100]; similarly, the clinical picture of Hb S-$\beta$ thalassemia in blacks is also milder than in whites.[99]

## Hb S-$\beta^+$ Thalassemia

In this most common form of sickle-$\beta$ thalassemia, Hb S occurs with high $A_2$ $\beta^+$ thalassemia. Due to a thalassemia gene, Hb A is present in lesser amounts than Hb S, comprising less than 40% of the total hemoglobin. Hemoglobin F is usually less than 10% of total hemoglobin, but some patients have more than 20% Hb F.[89] There seem to be two different types of Hb S-$\beta^+$ thalassemia[96]: the milder, usual form, in which more than 20% of Hb A is present; and the moderate form, in which less than 15% of Hb A is present. However, some patients with more than 20% Hb A have a severe clinical course[95,97] while some others with less than 10% Hb A have a mild clinical course.[101]

**Hematologic Findings**   Persons with the milder form have no anemia or reticulocytosis or mild anemia with reticulocytosis less than 5%. Hemoglobin values range from 9 to 13 g/dl.[94,95,96,101] In comparison with the peripheral smear of the $\beta^0$ type, anisopoikilocytosis is usually less obvious, and sickle forms, nucleated red cells, and Howell-Jolly bodies are not usually seen. However, differentiation between the two types cannot be made on the basis of the smear alone. The bone marrow shows erythroid hyperplasia.[97] The (non-$\alpha$)/$\alpha$ globin synthesis ratios in the 12 black patients with Hb S-$\beta^+$ thalassemia studied in our laboratory, including five patients previously reported,[101,102,103] were 0.50 to 0.95 (Fig. 9-1), similar to those in 15 blacks reported by others (0.42 to 0.90),[104-108] but values in five whites were decreased to 0.44 to 0.75,[101,109] similar to those with $\beta$-thalassemia trait.[110] Interestingly, there is a discrepancy in the (non-$\alpha$)/$\alpha$ globin synthesis ratios between blacks and nonblacks, with a wide range of globin synthesis ratios in blacks. The findings of normal and decreased (non-$\alpha$)/$\alpha$ ratios in blacks with Hb S-$\beta^+$ thalassemia are similar to those in a group of blacks with $\beta$-thalassemia trait,[102,111] of whom approximately half have peripheral blood (non-$\alpha$)/$\alpha$ ratios in the range of normal control groups, while the remainder have ratios in the range of white heterozygotes for $\beta$ thalassemia (Figure 9-1). The percentage of newly synthesized radioactive free $\alpha$ chains in bone marrow was increased to 14% to 31.4%,[112] indicating a large nonradioactive $\alpha$ chain pool. These excess free $\alpha$ chains may be precipitated, resulting in ineffective erythropoiesis. The values in the bone marrow were close to unity, which may be due to the precipitation of excess free $\alpha$ chains,[113] to proteolysis,[114] or to modifications of synthesis of specific globin chains.

**Clinical Manifestations**   Persons with this disorder are usually asymptomatic[115] or have a mild clinical course[96,99] with normal body habitus and life span. Adults with this disease are often identified during screening programs or during studies for unrelated symptoms. They may have an occasional painful crisis, with joint pain being a most common presenting symptom.[96] Aplastic crises[97,116] or splenic sequestration crises[95,96,116] may occur. In one series of 57 children with Hb S-$\beta$ thalassemia, 14% developed splenic sequestration crisis,[116] indicating that this is a rather common complication. Splenic infarction is known to occur during air travel. There is an increased incidence of pneumonia reported in children.[116] In comparison to complications in Hb SS, Hb SC, or Hb S-$\beta$0 thalassemia, hematuria,[107] avascular necrosis of the femoral head,[29,117,118] ocular changes,[119] and leg ulcers occur less frequently. Although most women with this disorder tolerate pregnancy well, maternal morbidity is common, with some patients developing serious complications during pregnancy, such as severe vaso-occlusive crisis, aggravation of anemia due to either folate deficiency or hemolytic crisis, or cerebrovascular accident.[35,120] One report shows a high perinatal mortality rate.[35]

### Hb S-$\beta$0 Thalassemia

**Hematologic Findings**    When Hb S occurs in conjunction with $\beta$0 thalassemia, the electrophoretic pattern shows Hbs S, F, and A$_2$, a pattern indistinguishable from that of Hb SS. Hemoglobin F is usually elevated to 5% to 30% of hemoglobin.[89,94,95] Hematologic findings are generally similar to those in Hb SS and in the severe form of Hb S-$\beta^+$ thalassemia, with marked anemia and reticulocytosis.[108] The hemoglobin value ranges from 6 to 10 g/dl and the reticulocyte count from 10% to 20%. Globin synthesis studies in nine blacks[102,107,121] and in six patients of Mediterranean ancestry with Hb S-$\beta$0 thalassemia[105,108,122] showed $\beta^S/\alpha$ ratios ranging from 0.35 to 0.81, values similar to those found in $\beta$-thalassemia trait in whites. There is no significant difference in mean (non-$\alpha$)/$\alpha$ ratios between Hb S-$\beta$0 thalassemia and Hb S-$\beta^+$ thalassemia.[108] However, in contrast to the $\beta^+$ type, where normal $\beta/\alpha$ ratios have been found in some patients, none with Hb S-$\beta$0 thalassemia has been reported to have normal $\beta/\alpha$ ratios. The radioactive free $\alpha$ chain pool in the peripheral blood has been reported to be much higher (35.1% to 53%) than in persons with Hb SS or controls (Figure 9-2).[121] Thus, Hb S-$\beta$0 thalassemia can be differentiated from Hb SS by globin synthesis studies.

**Clinical Manifestations**    Clinical expression is markedly variable, from mild[108] to a degree of severity similar to that of Hb SS, with frequent, severe vaso-occlusive crises, including hand-foot syndrome in early childhood,[95] and an increased mortality rate in childhood.[116] Some patients develop functional asplenia early in life, resulting in an increased incidence of serious bacterial infections. However, many of these patients have persistent splenomegaly into adulthood,[96] in contrast to patients with Hb SS; thus, functional asplenia may not occur until later in life.

### Diagnosis of S-$\beta$ Thalassemia

When Hb S and Hb A are present, with amounts of Hb S being greater than Hb A in the absence of transfusion, Hb S-$\beta^+$ thalassemia is indicated. Increased Hb A$_2$, decreased MCV and MCH, and abnormal red cell morphology in persons with Hb SS are strongly suggestive of a Hb S-$\beta$o thalassemia. When Hb A is absent, it is difficult to differentiate between Hb S-$\beta$o thalassemia and Hb SS in the absence of family studies or globin synthesis studies. Although elevated Hb A$_2$ may indicate Hb S-$\beta$o thalassemia, accurate measurement of Hb A$_2$ is difficult in the presence of Hb S, and elevated levels of Hb A$_2$ have been reported in Hb SS.[123] Therefore, family studies should be done to make a precise differentiation between Hb S-$\beta$o thalassemia and Hb SS; a person with Hb S-$\beta$o thalassemia receives a gene for Hb S from one parent and a gene for $\beta$ thalassemia from the other parent. When family members are not available for study, diagnosis can be confirmed by globin biosynthesis studies, as there is no overlapping between (non-$\alpha$)/$\alpha$ ratios in Hb SS and Hb S-$\beta$o thalassemia.

### SICKLE CELL-$\alpha$ THALASSEMIA
(Hb SS-$\alpha$ Thalassemia)

The combination of a sickle cell gene and one or more genes for $\alpha$ thalassemia has only recently become widely recognized because it is difficult to differentiate this disorder from Hb SS by routine electrophoretic and hematologic studies. It is not surprising to find this disorder primarily in the black population, since the incidence of $\alpha$-thalassemia trait in black newborns is estimated to be about 2.0% to 7.0%,[124,125] with Hb SS-$\alpha$ thalassemia occurring in about one in 20 thousand blacks.[126] It may also be quite common in peoples from Saudi Arabia, since there is a relatively high frequency of genes for both Hb S and $\alpha$ thalassemia in this population.[127] However, only 13 patients, including 11 blacks,[121,128,129] one Arab,[127] and one Turk,[89] have been reported to have Hb SS in combination with $\alpha$ thalassemia. This disorder has not been well characterized, but it has been suggested that the presence of $\alpha$ thalassemia may modify the clinical picture of Hb SS,[127] resulting in a mild sickle cell disease which may be due to the reduced intracellular hemoglobin concentration.[128,129] The clinical course in the patients reported varies from asymptomatic to severe.

Two Ghanian women with sickle cell disease and a benign clinical course have been reported with elevated Hb F levels, decreased red cell indices, and decreased bone marrow $\alpha/\beta^s$ specific activity globin synthesis ratios (0.43, 0.75).[128] The women were presumed to have $\alpha$ thalassemia, but they had severe iron deficiency, which may also account for low red cell indices and decreased $\alpha/\beta^S$ globin synthesis ratios.[130]

We have reported four black children with Hb SS-$\alpha$ thalassemia[121] in whom the mean hemoglobin and Hb F levels were higher and reticulocyte counts and MCV and MCH were lower than in patients with Hb SS. The mean levels for hemoglobin, reticulocytes, and Hb F were 9.1 g/dl, 4.2%, and 13.3%, respectively. Globin synthesis studies of peripheral blood revealed decreased $\alpha/\beta^S$ ratios (0.65 to 0.85) in three and a normal ratio (0.89) in one patient (Figure 9-1), ratios similar to those in blacks with $\alpha$-thalassemia trait previously reported,[131] indicating that the gene for $\alpha$ thalassemia in blacks may not be detected or confirmed by globin synthesis ratios in some patients. However, the radioactive free $\alpha$ chain pools were decreased (3.2% to 6.4%) and were clearly below those of patients with Hb SS or normal control subjects (Fig. 9-2).[121]

Five black children were also reported to have Hb SS-$\alpha$ thalassemia.[129] In all patients, one of the parents had sickle cell trait with $\alpha$ thalassemia. One patient had 3.9% of Hb Bart's. All had mild clinical disease and a moderate degree of anemia, with hemoglobin levels ranging from 7.8 to 9.7 g/dl and reticulocyte counts of 6.2% to 18.4%. Hemoglobin $A_2$ levels were normal (2.3% to 3.6%) and Hb F levels were elevated (2.3% to 33.3%). All had microcytosis, numerous target cells, and poikilocytosis, but sickle forms were rarely observed. The peripheral blood $\alpha$/(non-$\alpha$) globin synthesis ratios were decreased to normal (0.83% to 0.96%).

An asymptomatic 4-year-old Saudi Arabic child with Hb SS and Hb H disease has been described.[127] Mild anemia with decreased red cell indices was noted, and there were high levels of Hb F (43.7%) and Hb Bart's (14.0%). The persistence of Hb Bart's past the newborn period differentiates this syndrome from the combination of Hb SS and two functioning $\alpha$-globin genes, instead of the usual four.

In all patients with Hb SS-$\alpha$ thalassemia reported, Hb F levels were elevated, ranging from 2.3% to 33.3%, and Hb $A_2$ levels were either normal or elevated despite the presence of $\alpha$ thalassemia. Red cell indices were all decreased. It is interesting to note that the clinical features varied from mild to severe, regardless of Hb F levels, although a high Hb F level has been known to protect against sickling.[1]


## Diagnosis

When patients with Hb SS have decreased red cell indices without iron deficiency, one should consider the concomitant presence of one of the thalassemia types with Hb SS. Hemoglobin $A_2$ and F levels are not helpful in differentiating this syndrome from Hb SS. In diagnosing Hb SS-$\alpha$ thalassemia, quantitation of Hb A and Hb S in parents is important, since one parent should have a decreased percentage of Hb S from that normally found in sickle cell trait, with perhaps decreased red cell indices and abnormal red cell morphology. When family studies cannot be done or are not conclusive, the measurement of radioactive free $\alpha$ chain pools in combination with the determination of $\alpha/\beta^s$ ratios differentiates this disorder from Hb SS or from Hb S-$\beta^0$ thalassemia.[121]

## SICKLE CELL-$\alpha\beta^+$ THALASSEMIA
(Hb S-$\alpha\beta^+$ Thalassemia)

Only one black patient with Hb S in combination with $\alpha\beta^+$ thalassemia has been described.[121] This patient had mild anemia and a very benign clinical course, similar to patients with the mild form of Hb S-$\beta^+$ thalassemia. The Hb F value was increased and the Hb $A_2$ value was high normal, similar to three black children doubly heterozygous for $\alpha\beta$ thalassemia.[132] The globin synthesis study revealed a decreased (non-$\alpha$)/$\alpha$ ratio (0.66), similar to that in Hb S-$\beta^+$ thalassemia, and a free radioactive $\alpha$ chain pool of 18.9% in the peripheral blood, which is at the upper part of the normal range but much higher than in Hb SS-$\alpha$ thalassemia and below that in Hb S-$\beta^0$ thalassemia.

## SICKLE CELL-$\delta\beta$ THALASSEMIA
(Hb S-$\delta\beta$ Thalassemia)
## AND
## SICKLE CELL-HEREDITARY PERSISTENCE OF FETAL HEMOGLOBIN
(Hb S-HPFH)

Complete absence of $\beta$-polypeptide chain synthesis occurs in homozygous states for $\beta^0$ thalassemia, $\delta\beta$ thalassemia, Hb Lepore syndrome, and hereditary persistence of fetal hemoglobin (HPFH). Delta chain synthesis is also completely suppressed in all of these disorders with the exception of $\beta^0$ thalassemia. Homozygotes with $\delta\beta$ thalassemia, Hb Lepore, or HPFH have no Hb A or Hb $A_2$, but only Hb F. When Hb S occurs with $\delta\beta$ thalassemia or HPFH, the hematologic and clinical findings are very similar, although Hb S-HPFH appears to be milder than Hb S-$\delta\beta$ thalassemia. The major laboratory differences between Hb S-$\delta\beta$ thalassemia and Hb S-HPFH are in the amount of $\gamma$-chain synthesis and in the cellular distribution of fetal hemoglobin. In Hb S-HPFH, Hb F levels tend to be higher than in Hb S-$\delta\beta$ thalassemia; there is a more homogeneous distribution of fetal hemoglobin in red cells in Hb S-HPFH than in Hb S-$\delta\beta$ thalassemia. A total of nine patients with Hb S-$\delta\beta$ thalassemia, including five blacks[95,133,134] and four whites,[135-138] and more than 25 blacks with Hb S-HPFH[106,139-142] have been reported.

## Hematologic Findings

In both disorders, there is mild anemia to no anemia present with normal to slightly elevated reticulocyte counts. Red cell indices vary from decreased to normal. There are mild abnormalities in red cell morphology with anisopoikilocytosis, target cells, and microcytosis, but microcytosis is more common in Hb S-$\delta\beta$ thalassemia. Sickle cells are not present in Hb S-HPFH, and can rarely be seen in Hb S-$\delta\beta$ thalassemia. Hemoglobin F levels are elevated in both, in the 15% to 40% range, and Hb A$_2$ levels are decreased to normal, 1.3% to 3.4%. By the acid elution (Kleihauer-Betke) technique, the distribution of fetal hemoglobin in the red cells in Hb S-$\delta\beta$ thalassemia is heterogeneous (2% to 98% of cells with Hb F) in contrast to Hb S-HPFH, in which the distribution of Hb F is homozygous (99% to 100%).[143] The $\beta^S/\alpha$ globin synthesis ratios in three blacks with Hb S-$\delta\beta$ thalassemia were 0.66 to 1.00[134] and in seven blacks with Hb S-HPFH were 0.7 to 1.11 (Figure 9-1).[106,141,142] The values of decreased to normal ratios in either disorder are similar to those in blacks with Hb S-$\beta^+$ thalassemia.

## Clinical Manifestations

Persons with Hb S-$\delta\beta$ thalassemia or Hb S-HPFH are generally asymptomatic, but infrequent mild musculoskeletal pains may occur. Avascular necrosis of the femoral head also has been reported in two patients with Hb S-HPFH.[139]

## Diagnosis

When Hb S occurs with high levels of Hb F (15% to 40%), the following sickling disorders should be considered: Hb S in combination with $\beta^0$, $\alpha$ or $\delta\beta$ thalassemia, Hb Lepore, or HPFH. Family studies are important for diagnosis. Measurements of Hb A$_2$ and globin biosynthesis studies may be useful but not conclusive in differentiating these disorders. Hemoglobin A$_2$ levels are normal or elevated in Hb SS and Hb SS-$\alpha$ thalassemia, usually elevated in Hb S-$\beta^0$ thalassemia, and normal or decreased in Hb S-Lepore, Hb S-$\delta\beta$ thalassemia, and Hb S-HPFH. The globin synthesis ratios may be overlapping among these disorders, with $\beta^S/\alpha$ ratios being normal in Hb SS, decreased to normal in Hb S-$\delta\beta$ thalassemia and Hb S-HPFH, always decreased in Hb S-$\beta^0$ thalassemia, and normal to increased in Hb SS-$\alpha$ thalassemia (Figure 9-1). Although the acid elution technique is known to distinguish Hb S-$\delta\beta$ thalassemia from Hb S-HPFH, it is sometimes difficult to differentiate these disorders by this technique, due either to technical error or to misinterpretation of results because the percentage of F cells (red cells containing Hb F) are similar in both disorders, with over 90% F cells in Hb S-$\delta\beta$ thalassemia in contrast to 99% to 100% F cells in Hb S-HPFH. As there are several variants of HPFH, including heterocellular HPFH,[144] diagnosis should be confirmed by family studies since one parent of a patient with Hb S-HPFH should have a mild to moderate elevation of Hb F.

## SICKLE CELL-Hb LEPORE
(Hb S-Lepore)

In the individual who is doubly heterozygous for Hb S and for Hb Lepore, the hematologic and clinical pictures are similar to those of Hb S-$\beta^0$ thalassemia. Hemoglobin Lepore, characterized by a fusion between $\delta$- and $\beta$-polypeptide chains, migrates identically to Hb S on alkaline electrophoresis, but does not cause sickling. To date, five patients have been reported, including two Greeks with Hb S-Pylos (Lepore-like hemoglobin),[145] two Italians with Hb S-Lepore,[146] and one Italian with Hb S-Lepore Washington.[147] Although there is variation in the severity of disease, this disorder is characterized by a mild to moderate degree of anemia with hemoglobin levels ranging from 8.0 to 12.5 g/dl, reticulocyte counts of 3.5% to 33%, and thalassemic red cell morphology. Sickle cells were present on the peripheral smear. Red cell indices were slightly decreased to normal. Hemoglobin Lepore or Hb Pylos were about 10% of the total hemoglobin. The Hb F level was elevated, from 9.3% to 25%, and Hb A$_2$ was normal or reduced, from 0.9% to 2.6%. These patients had bone and joint symptoms that varied greatly. All but one patient[147] had hepatosplenomegaly.

## CONCLUSION

Variants of sickle cell disease should be considered in persons with sickle cell disease who have atypical or delayed onset of manifestations of the sickling phenomenon. Methods are available to detect the association of sickle hemoglobin with thalassemia or with other hemoglobins having abnormal $\alpha$- or $\beta$-polypeptide chains; therefore, every effort should be made to identify variants of sickle cell disease precisely. An accurate diagnosis is important for studies of clinical severity, in assessing prognosis, and for genetic counseling.

## REFERENCES

1. Charache, S., and Conley, C.L. Rate of sickling of red cells during deoxygenation of blood from persons with various sickling disorders. *Blood* 24:25–48, 1964.

2. Bertles, J.F., and Milner, P.F. Irreversibly sickled erythrocytes: A consequence of the heterogeneous distribution of haemoglobin types in sickle cell anemia. *J. Clin. Invest.* 47:1731–1741, 1968.

3. Bookchin, R.M., and Nagel, R.L. Interactions between human hemoglobins: Sickling and related phenomena. *Semin. Hematol.* 11:577–595, 1974.

4. Moffat, K. Gelation of sickle cell hemoglobin: Effects of hybrid tetramer formation in hemoglobin mixtures. *Science* 185:274–277, 1974.

5. Bookchin, R.M., Nagel, R.L., and Ranney, H.M. The effect of $\beta^{73Asn}$ on the interactions of sickling hemoglobins. *Biochim. Biophys. Acta* 221:373–375, 1970.

6. Milner, P.F., Miller, C., Grey, R., et al. Hemoglobin O Arab in four Negro families and its interaction with hemoglobin S and hemoglobin C. *N. Engl. J. Med.* 283:1417–1425, 1970.

7. McCurdy, P.R. Clinical and physiologic studies in a Negro with sickle-cell hemoglobin D disease. *N. Engl. J. Med.* 262:961–964, 1960.

8. Schneider, R.G. Incidence of electrophoretically distinct abnormalities of hemoglobin in 1550 Negro hospital patients. *Am. J. Clin. Pathol.* 26:1270–1276, 1956.

9. Motulsky, A.G. Frequency of sickling disorders in U.S. blacks. *N. Engl. J. Med.* 288:31–33, 1973.

10. Chernoff, A.I. The human hemoglobins in health and disease. *N. Engl. J. Med.* 253:416–423, 1955.

11. River, G.L., Robbins, A.B., and Schwartz, S.O. S-C hemoglobin: A clinical study. *Blood* 18:385–416, 1961.

12. Itano, H.A., and Neel, J.V. New inherited abnormality of human hemoglobin. *Proc. Natl. Acad. Sci. USA* 36:613–617, 1950.

13. Kaplan, E., Zuelzer, W.W., and Neel, J.V. A new inherited abnormality of hemoglobin and its interaction with sickle cell hemoglobin. *Blood* 6:1240–1259, 1951.

14. Tuttle, A.H., and Koch, B. Clinical and hematological manifestations of hemoglobin SC disease in children. *J. Pediatr.* 56:331–342, 1960.

15. Serjeant, G.R., Ashcroft, M.T., and Serjeant, B.E. The clinical features of haemoglobin SC disease in Jamaica. *Br. J. Haematol.* 24:491–501, 1973.

16. Kim, H.C., Weierbach, R.G., Friedman, Sh., et al. Globin biosynthesis in sickle cell, Hb SC, and Hb C disease. *J. Pediatr.* 91:13–18, 1977.

17. Prindle, K.H., Jr., and McCurdy, P.R. Red cell life span in hemoglobin C disorders (with special reference to hemoglobin C trait). *Blood* 36:14–19, 1970.

18. McCurdy, P.R., Mahmood, L., and Sherman, A.S. Red cell life span in sickle cell-hemoglobin C disease with a note about sickle cell-hemoglobin O Arab. *Blood* 45:273–279, 1975.

19. Charache, S., Conley, C.L., Waugh, D.F., et al. Pathogenesis of hemolytic anemia in homozygous hemoglobin C disease. *J. Clin. Invest.* 46:1795–1811, 1967.

20. Murphy, J.R. Hemoglobin CC disease: Rheological properties of erythrocytes and abnormalities in cell water. *J. Clin. Invest.* 47:1483–1495, 1968.

21. Kaplan, E., Zuelzer, W.W., and Neel, J.V. Further studies on hemoglobin C. II. The hematologic effects of hemoglobin C alone and in combination with sickle cell hemoglobin. *Blood* 8:735–746, 1953.

22. Asakura, T., Ohnishi, T., Friedman, Sh., et al. Abnormal precipitation of oxyhemoglobin S by mechanical shaking. *Proc. Natl. Acad. Sci. USA* 71:1594–1598, 1974.

23. Ringelhann, B., and Khorsandi, M. Hemoglobin crystallization test to differentiate cells with Hb SC and CC genotype from SS cells without electrophoresis. *Am. J. Clin. Pathol.* 57:467–470, 1972.

24. Movitt, E.R., Mangum, J.F., and Porter, W.R. Sickle cell-hemoglobin C disease quantitative determination of iron kinetics and hemoglobin synthesis. *Blood* 21:535–544, 1963.

25. Cawein, M.J., O'Neill, R.P., Danzer, L.A., et al. A study of the sickling phenomenon and oxygen dissociation curve in patients with hemoglobins SS, SD, SF and SC. *Blood* 34:682–690, 1969.

26. Serjeant, G.R., Ennis, J.T., and Middlemiss, H. Haemoglobin SC disease in Jamaica. *Br. J. Radiol.* 46:935–942, 1973.

27. Smith, E.W., and Conley, C.L. Clinical features of the genetic variants of sickle cell disease. *Bull. Johns Hopkins Hosp.* 94:289–318, 1954.

28. Barton, C.J., and Cockshott, W.P. Bone changes in hemoglobin SC disease. *Am. J. Roentgenol.* 88:525–532, 1962.

29. Chung, S.M.K., and Ralston, E.L. Necrosis of the femoral head associated with sickle cell anemia and its genetic variants. *J. Bone Joint Surg.* 51-A:33–58, 1969.

30. Condon, P.I., and Serjeant, G.R. Ocular findings in hemoglobin SC disease in Jamaica. *Am. J. Ophthalmol.* 74:921–931, 1972.

31. Armaly, M.F. Ocular manifestations in sickle cell disease. *Arch. Intern. Med.* 133:670–679, 1974.

32. Goldberg, M.F. Natural history of untreated proliferative sickle retinopathy. *Arch. Ophthalmol.* 85:428–437, 1971.

33. Goldberg, M.F. Classification and pathogenesis of proliferative sickle retinopathy. *Am. J. Ophthalmol.* 71:649–665, 1971.

34. Fort, A.T., Morrison, J.C., Berreras, L., et al. Counseling the patient with sickle cell disease about reproduction. Pregnancy outcome does not justify the maternal risk. *Am. J. Obstet. Gynecol.* 111:324–327, 1971.

35. Pritchard, J.A., Scott, D.E., Whalley, P.J., et al. The effects of maternal sickle cell hemoglobinopathies and sickle cell trait on reproductive performance. *Am. J. Obstet. Gynecol.* 117:662–670, 1973.

36. Necheles, T. Obstetric complications associated with haemoglobinopathies. *Clin. Haematol.* 2:497–514, 1973.

37. Morrison, J.C., and Wiser, W.L. The use of prophylactic partial exchange transfusion in pregnancy associated with sickle cell hemoglobinopathies. *Obstet. Gynecol.* 48:516–520, 1976.

38. Smith, E.W., and Conley, C.L. Sicklemia and infarction of the spleen during aerial flight: Electrophoresis of the hemoglobin in 15 cases. *Bull. Johns Hopkins Hosp.* 96:35–42, 1955.

39. Githens, J.H., Gross, G.P., Eife, R.F., et al. Splenic sequestration syndrome at mountain altitudes in sickle/hemoglobin C disease. *J. Pediatr.* 90:203–206, 1977.

40. Chu, J.Y., and Niederman, L.G. Splenic sequestration syndrome in sickle/hemoglobin C disease at low altitude. *J. Pediatr.* 91:350–351, 1977.

41. Josphe, G., Rothenberg, S.P., and Baum, S. Transient functional asplenism in sickle cell/C disease. *Am. J. Med.* 55:720–722, 1973.

42. Sharpe, A.R., Jr., Fox, P.G., Jr., and Dodson, A.I., Sr. Unilateral renal hematuria associated with sickle cell C disease and sickle cell trait. *J. Urol.* 81:780–783, 1959.

43. Mahurkar, S.D., Dunea, G., and Bush, I.M. Hematuria in sickle cell C disease: Precipitation by acidosis and correction by dialysis. *J. Urol.* 110:443–445, 1973.

44. Keitel, H.G., Thompson, D., and Itano, H.A. Hyposthenuria in sickle cell anemia. A reversible renal defect. *J. Clin. Invest.* 35:998–1007, 1956.

45. Statius Van Eps, L.W., Schouten, H., Romeny-Wachter, C.C.T.H., et al. The relation between age and renal concentrating capacity in sickle cell disease and hemoglobin C disease. *Clin. Chim. Acta.* 27:501–511, 1970.

46. Ober, W.B., Bruno, M.S., Simon, R.M., et al. Hemoglobin S-C disease with fat embolism. Report of a patient dying in crisis; autopsy findings. *Am. J. Med.* 27:647–658, 1959.

47. Shelly, W., and Curtis, E.M. Bone marrow and fat embolism in sickle cell anemia and sickle cell hemoglobin C disease. *Bull. Johns Hopkins Hosp.* 103:8–26, 1958.

48. Barrett-Connor, E. Infection and sickle cell-C disease. *Am. J. Med. Sci.* 262:162–169, 1971.

49. Widen, A.L., and Cardon, L. Salmonella Typhimurium osteomyelitis with sickle cell-hemoglobin C disease: A review and case report. *Ann. Intern. Med.* 54:510–521, 1961.

50. Waldvogel, F.A., Medoff, G., and Swartz, M.N. Osteomyelitis: A review of clinical features, therapeutic considerations and unusual aspects. *N. Engl. J. Med.* 282:316–322, 1970.

51. Abrams, J., and Schwartz, I.R. The sickle cell diseases in pregnancy. *Am. J. Obstet. Gynecol.* 77:1324–1327, 1959.

52. Itano, H.A. A third abnormal haemoglobin associated with hereditary hemolytic anemia. *Proc. Natl. Acad. Sci. USA* 37:775–779, 1951.

53. Smith, E.W., and Conley, C.L. Sickle cell-hemoglobin D disease. *Ann. Intern. Med.* 50:94–105, 1959.

54. Baglioni, C. Abnormal human hemoglobins. III. Chemical studies on hemoglobin D. *Biochim. Biophys. Acta* 59:437–449, 1962.

55. Babin, D.R., Jones, R.T., and Schroeder, W.A. Hemoglobin D Los Angeles: $\alpha_2\beta_2^{121}$ Glu NH$_2$. *Biochim. Biophys. Acta* 86:136–143, 1964.

56. Schneider, R.G., Ueda, S., Alperin, J.B., et al. Hemoglobin D Los Angeles in two Caucasian families: Hemoglobin SD disease and Hemoglobin D thalassemia. *Blood* 32:250–259, 1968.

57. Uriarte, A., Atencio, R.P., and Colombo, B. Haemoglobin D Punjab in a Cuban family and its interaction with haemoglobin S. *Acta Haematol.* 50:315–320, 1973.

58. Ringelhann, B., Lewis, R.A., Lorkin, P.A., et al. Sickle cell haemoglobin D Punjab disease: S from Ghana and D from England. *Acta Haematol.* 38:324–331, 1967.

59. Sturgeon, P., Itano, H.A., and Bergren, W.R. Clinical manifestations of inherited abnormal hemoglobins. I. The interaction of hemoglobin-S with hemoglobin-D. *Blood* 10:389–404, 1955.

60. Restrepo, A.M., and London, O.G. Sickle cell hemoglobin D disease in a Negro Columbian patient. *Ann. Intern. Med.* 62:1301–1306, 1965.

61. Watson-Williams, E.J., Beale, D., Irvine, D., et al. A new haemoglobin, D Ibadan ($\beta$-87 Threonine→Lysine) producing no sickle-cell haemoglobin D disease with haemoglobin S. *Nature* 205:1273-1276, 1965.

62. McCurdy, P.R., Lorkin, P.A., Casey, R., et al. Hemoglobin S-G(S-D) syndrome. *Am. J. Med.* 57(4):665-670, 1974.

63. Ramot, B., Fisher, S., Remez, D., et al. Haemoglobin O in an Arab family: Sickle-cell haemoglobin O trait. *Br. Med. J.* 2:1262-1264, 1960.

64. Eng, L.L., and Sadono. Haemoglobin O (Buginese X) in Sulawesi. *Br. Med. J.* 1:1461-1462, 1958.

65. Baglioni, C., and Lehmann, H. Chemical heterogeneity of haemoglobin O. *Nature* 196:229-232, 1962.

66. Kantchev, K.N., Tcholakov, B.N., Baglioni, C., et al. Haemoglobin O Arab in Bulgaria. *Nature* 205:187-189, 1965.

67. Kantchev, K.N., Tcholakov, B.N., Casey, R., et al. Twelve families with Hb O Arab in the Burgas District of Bulgaria. Observations on sixteen examples of Hb O Arab-$\beta^0$ thalassaemia. *Humangenetik* 26:93-97, 1975.

68. Efremov, G.D., Sadlkarlo, A., Stojancov, A., et al. Homozygous hemoglobin O Arab in a Gypsy family in Yugoslavia. *Hemoglobin* 1:389-394, 1977.

69. Lehmann, H., Maranjian, G., and Mourant, A.Z. Distribution of sickle cell haemoglobin in Saudi Arabia. *Nature* 198:492-493, 1963.

70. Vella, F., Beale, D., and Lehmann, H. Haemoglobin O Arab in Sudanese. *Nature* 209:308-309, 1966.

71. Ibrahim, S.A., and Mustafa, D. Sickle cell haemoglobin O disease in a Sudanese family. *Br. Med. J.* 3:715-717, 1967.

72. Javid, J. Hemoglobin SO Arabia disease in a black American. *Am. J. Med. Sci.* 265:266-274, 1973.

73. Klingensmith, W.C., III, Danish, E.H., Dover, G.J., et al. Delineation of peripheral bone infarcts in a child with a rare hemoglobinopathy (SO Arab) and purpura fulminans: Case report. *J. Nucl. Med.* 17:1062-1064, 1976.

74. Charache, S., Zinkham, W.H., Dickerman, J.D., et al. Hemoglobin SC, SS/G Philadelphia and SO Arab diseases. Diagnostic importance of an integrative analysis of clinical, hematologic and electrophoretic findings. *Am. J. Med.* 62:439-446, 1977.

75. Ballas, S.K., Atwater, J., and Burka, E.R. Hemoglobin S-O Arab $\alpha$-thalassemia-globin biosynthesis and clinical picture. *Hemoglobin* 1:651-662, 1977.

76. Konotey-Ahulu, F.I., Gallo, E., Lehmann, H., et al. Haemoglobin Korle-Bu ($\beta$ 73 aspartic acid→asparagine) showing one of the two amino acid substitutions of haemoglobin C Harlem. *J. Med. Genet.* 5:107-111, 1968.

77. Rucknagel, D.L., and Rising, J.A. A heterozygote for Hb $\beta^s$, Hb $\beta^c$ and Hb $\alpha^{G\ Philadelphia}$ in a family presenting evidence of heterogeneity of hemoglobin alpha chain loci. *Am. J. Med.* 59:53-60, 1975.

78. Pugh, R.P., Monical, T.V., and Minnich, V. Sickle cell anemia with two adult hemoglobins—Hb S and Hb G$^{Philadelphia}$/S. *Blood* 23:206-215, 1964.

79. Eng, L.L., Wang, A.C., and Burnett, R.C. Another family showing the interaction of the Hb AS/G slight anemia due to G/S hybrid. *Acta Haematol.* 40:286-298, 1968.

80. Rising, J.A., Sautter, R.L., and Spicer, S.J. Hemoglobin G-Philadelphia/S. A family study of an inherited hybrid hemoglobin. *Am. J. Clin. Pathol.* 61:92-102, 1974.

81. Atwater, J., Friedman, Sh., and Schwartz, E. Control of the production of hemoglobin in the presence of 1, 2 or 3 abnormal genes. *Abstracts of the XIV*

244

*International Congress of Hematology.* Abstract Sao Paula, Brazil, 1972, No. 395.

82. Kraus, L.M., Miyaji, T., Iuchi, I., et al. Characterization of $\alpha^{23Glu\ NH_2}$ in hemoglobin Memphis. Hemoglobin Memphis/S, a new variant of molecular disease. *Biochemistry* 5:3701–3708, 1966.

83. Kraus, A.P., Miyaji, T., Iuchi, I., et al. Hemoglobin Memphis/S. A new variant of sickle cell anemia. *Trans. Assoc. Am. Physicians* 80:297–304, 1967.

84. Cooper, M.R., Kraus, A.P., Felts, J.H., et al. A third case of hemoglobin Memphis/sickle cell disease. Whole blood viscosity used as a screening test. *Am. J. Med.* 55:535–541, 1973.

85. Goldstein, M.A., Patpongpanij, N., and Minnich, V. The incidence of elevated Hb $A_2$ levels in the American Negro. *Ann. Intern. Med.* 60:95–99, 1964.

86. Livingston, F.B. *Abnormal Hemoglobins in Human Populations: A Summary and an Interpretation.* Chicago: Aldine Publishing Company, 1967.

87. Pierce, H.I., Kurachi, S., Sofroniadou, K., et al. Frequencies of thalassemia in American blacks. *Blood* 49:981–986, 1977.

88. Chatterjea, J.B. Haemoglobinopathy in India. Edited by J.H.P. Jonxis and J.F. Delafresnaye. In *Abnormal Haemoglobins.* Oxford: Blackwell Scientific Publications, 1959.

89. Aksoy, M. The first observation of homozygous hemoglobin S-alpha thalassemia disease and two types of sickle cell thalassemia disease: (a) sickle cell-alpha thalassemia disease, (b) sickle cell-beta thalassemia disease. *Blood* 22:757–769, 1963.

90. Bratu, V., and Predeseu, C. Hemoglobin S, thalassemia and thalassemia associated with hemoglobin S in a family from Rumania. Fifth Congress of the Asian and Pacific Society of Haematology. Abstract p. 69. Kagit Basim Isleri, Turkey, 1969.

91. Silvestroni, E., and Bianco, I. Microdrepanocitoanemia in un soggeto di razza bianca. *Boll. Med. Roma* 70:347, 1944.

92. Fessas, P. The heterogeneity of thalassemia. In *Plenary Session Papers of the Twelfth Congress of the International Society of Hematology.* New York, 1968.

93. Pontremoli, S., Bargellesi, A., and Conconi, F. Globin chain synthesis in the Ferrara thalassemia population. *Ann. NY Acad. Sci.* 165:253–269, 1969.

94. Weatherall, D.J., and Clegg, J.B. *The Thalassemia Syndromes.* 2nd Ed. Oxford: Blackwell Scientific Publications, 1972.

95. Pearson, H.A. Hemoglobin S-thalassemia syndrome in Negro children. *Ann. NY Acad. Sci.* 165:83–92, 1969.

96. Serjeant, G.R., Ashcroft, M.T., Serjeant, B.E., et al. The clinical features of sickle-cell/$\beta$ thalassaemia in Jamaica. *Br. J. Haematol.* 24:19–30, 1973.

97. Monti, A., Feldhake, C., and Schwartz, S.O. The S-thalassaemia syndrome. *Ann. NY Acad. Sci.* 119:474–489, 1964.

98. Malamos, B., Belcher, E.H., Gyttaki, E., et al. Simultaneous radioactive tracer studies of erythropoiesis and red cell destruction in sickle-cell disease and sickle cell haemoglobin/thalassaemia. *Br. J. Haematol.* 9:487–498, 1963.

99. Weatherall, D.J. Biochemical phenotypes of thalassemia in the American Negro population. *Ann. NY Acad. Sci.* 119:450–462, 1964.

100. Braverman, A.S., McCurdy, P.R., Manons, O., et al. Homozygous beta thalassemia in American blacks: The problem of mild thalassemia. *J. Lab. Clin. Med.* 81:857–866, 1973.

101. Gill, F.M., and Schwartz, E. Synthesis of globin chains in sickle $\beta$-thalassemia. *J. Clin. Invest.* 52:709–714, 1973.

102. Friedman, Sh., Hamilton, R.W., and Schwartz, E. $\beta$-Thalassemia in the American Negro. *J. Clin. Invest.* 42:1453–1459, 1973.

103. Kim, H.C., and Friedman, Sh. Globin synthesis studies in patients with Hb S-$\beta^+$ thalassemia. Unpublished observation, 1977.

104. Wood, W.G., and Stamatoyannopoulos, G. Globin synthesis in fractionated normoblasts of $\beta$-thalassemia heterozygotes. *J. Clin. Invest.* 55:567–578, 1975.

105. Weatherall, D.J., Clegg, J.B., Na-Nakorn, S., et al. The pattern of disordered haemoglobin synthesis in homozygous and heterozygous $\beta$ thalassaemia. *Br. J. Haematol.* 16:251–267, 1969.

106. Natta, C.L., Niazi, G.A., Ford, S., et al. Balanced globin chain synthesis in hereditary persistence of fetal hemoglobin. *J. Clin. Invest.* 54:533–438, 1974.

107. Steinberg, M.H., and Dreiling, B.J. Clinical, hematologic and biosynthetic studies in sickle cell-$\beta^0$-thalassemia: A comparison with sickle cell anemia. *Am. J. Hematol.* 1:35–44, 1976.

108. Bank, A., Dow, L.W., Farace, M.G., et al. Changes in globin synthesis with erythroid cell maturation in sickle thalassemia. *Blood* 41:353–357, 1973.

109. Conconi, F., Bargellesi, A., Del Senno, L., et al. Globin chain synthesis in Sicilian thalassaemic subjects. *Br. J. Haematol.* 19:469–475, 1970.

110. Bank, A., and Marks, P.A. Excess alpha chain synthesis relative to beta chain synthesis in thalassemia major and minor. *Nature* 212:1198–1200, 1966.

111. Friedman, Sh., Schwartz, E., Ahern, V., et al. Globin synthesis in the Jamaican Negro with beta-thalassaemia. *Br. J. Haematol.* 28:505–513, 1974.

112. Gill, F.M., and Schwartz, E. Free $\alpha$-globin pool in human bone marrow. *J. Clin. Invest.* 52:3057–3063, 1973.

113. Yataganas, X., and Fessas, P. The pattern of hemoglobin precipitation in thalassemia and its significance. *Ann. NY Acad. Sci.* 165:270–287, 1969.

114. Clegg, J.B., and Weatherall, D.J. Haemoglobin synthesis during erythroid maturation in $\beta$-thalassaemia. *Nature (New Biol)* 240:190–192, 1972.

115. Singer, K., Singer, L., and Goldberg, S.R. Studies on abnormal hemoglobins: XI. Sickle cell-thalassemia disease in the Negro. The significance of the S+A+F and S+A patterns obtained by hemoglobin analysis. *Blood* 10:405–415, 1955.

116. Robinson, M.G. Clinical aspects of sickle cell disease. Edited by Richard D. Levere. In *Sickle Cell Anemia and Other Hemoglobinopathies.* New York: Academic Press, 1975.

117. Hurwitz, D., and Roth, H. Sickle cell-thalassemia presenting as arthritis of the hip. *Arthritis Rheum.* 13:422–425, 1970.

118. Golding, J.S.R., MacIver, J.E., and Went, L.N. The bone changes in sickle cell anemia and its genetic variants. *J. Bone Joint Surg.* 41-B:711–718, 1959.

119. Goldberg, M.F., Charache, S., and Acacio, I. Ophthalmologic manifestations of sickle cell thalassemia. *Arch. Intern. Med.* 128:33–39, 1971.

120. Henderson, A.B., Potts, E.B., Burgess, D., et al. Sickle-cell thalassemia disease and pregnancy: A case study. *Am. J. Med. Sci.* 244:605–611, 1962.

121. Kim, H.C., Weierbach, R.G., Friedman, Sh., et al. Detection of sickle $\alpha$- or $\beta^0$-thalassemia by studies of globin biosynthesis. *Blood* 49:785–792, 1977.

122. Benz, E.J., Jr., Swerdlow, P.S., and Forget, B.G. Absence of functional messenger RNA activity for beta globin chain synthesis in $\beta^0$-thalassemia. *Blood* 45:1–10, 1975.

123. Huisman, T.H.J., Schroeder, W.A., Bouver, N.G., et al. Chemical heterogeneity of fetal hemoglobin in subjects with sickle cell anemia, homozygous Hb-C disease, SC-disease, and various combinations of hemoglobin variants. *Clin. Chim. Acta* 38:5–16, 1972.

246

124. Friedman, Sh., Atwater, J., Gill, F.M., et al. $\alpha$-Thalassemia in Negro infants. *Pediatr. Res.* 8:955–959, 1974.

125. Weatherall, D.J. Abnormal haemoglobins in the neonatal period and their relationship to thalassaemia. *Br. J. Haematol.* 9:265–277, 1963.

126. Kazazian, H.H., Jr. Commentary: Globin synthesis ratios and $\alpha$-thalassemia. *J. Pediatr.* 91:10–20, 1977.

127. Weatherall, D.J., Clegg, J.B., Blankson, J., et al. A new sickling disorder resulting from interaction of the genes for haemoglobin S and $\alpha$-thalassaemia. *Br. J. Haematol.* 17:517–526, 1969.

128. Van Enk, A., Lang, A., White, J.M., et al. Benign obstetric history in women with sickle cell anaemia associated with $\alpha$-thalassaemia. *Br. Med. J.* 4:524–526, 1972.

129. Honig, G.R., Koshy, M., Mason, R.G., et al. Sickle cell anemia-$\alpha$-thalassemia syndrome. *J. Pediatr.* 92:556–561, 1978.

130. Ben-Bassat, I., Mozel, M., and Ramot, B. Globin synthesis in iron-deficiency anemia. *Blood* 44:551–555, 1974.

131. Schwartz, E., and Atwater, J. $\alpha$-Thalassemia in the American Negro. *J. Clin. Invest.* 51:412–418, 1972.

132. Pearson, H.A. Alpha-beta-thalassemia disease in a Negro family. *N. Engl. J. Med.* 275:176–181, 1966.

133. Zelkowitz, L., Torres, C., Bhoopalam, N., et al. Double heterozygous $\beta\delta$-thalassemia in Negroes. *Arch. Intern. Med.* 129:975–979, 1972.

134. Kinney, T.R., Friedman, Sh., Cifuentes, E., et al. Variations in globin synthesis in delta-beta-thalassaemia. *Br. J. Haematol.* 38:15–22, 1978.

135. Russo, G., La Crutta, A., and Mollica, F. Sulla eterogeneita delta talassemia. Contributo casistico ed interpretazione biochimica e genetica. *Riv. Ped. Sicil.* 18:239, 1963.

136. Silvestroni, E., and Bianco, I. Un Caso di malattia microdreparnocitica da Hb S e varieta di microcitemia con quota normale di Hb $A_2$ e quota elevata di Hb F. *Progr. Med. Napoli* 20:509, 1964.

137. Stamatoyannopoulos, G., Sofroniadou, C., and Akkivakis, A. Absence of hemoglobin A in a double heterozygote for F-thalassemia and hemoglobin S. *Blood* 30:772–776, 1967.

138. De Contardi, N.W., and Barros, C.A. Doble heterocigota para beta-delta talasemia Y hemoglobina S. *SNGRA* 20(1):56–62, 1975.

139. Conley, C.L., Weatherall, D.J., Richardson, S.N., et al. Hereditary persistence of fetal hemoglobin: A study of 79 affected persons in 15 Negro families in Baltimore. *Blood* 21:261–281, 1963.

140. Schneider, R.G., Levin, W.C., and Everett, C. A family with S and C hemoglobins and the hereditary persistence of F hemoglobin. *N. Engl. J. Med.* 265:1278–1283, 1961.

141. Makler, M.T., Berthrong, M., Locke, H.R., et al. A new variant of sickle cell disease with high levels of foetal haemoglobin homogeneously distributed within red cells. *Br. J. Haematol.* 26:519–526, 1974.

142. Friedman, Sh., Schwartz, E., Ahern, E., et al. Variations in globin chain synthesis in hereditary persistence of fetal haemoglobin. *Br. J. Haematol.* 32:357–364, 1976.

143. Cifuentes, E. Personal communication, 1976.

144. Serjeant, G.R., Serjeant, B.E., and Mason, K. Heterocellular hereditary persistence of fetal haemoglobin and homozygous sickle cell disease. *Lancet* 1:795–796, 1977.

145. Stamatoyannopoulos, G., and Fessas, P. Observations on hemoglobin "Pylos": The hemoglobin pylos-hemoglobin S combination. *J. Lab. Clin. Med.* 62:193–200, 1963.

146. Silvestroni, E., Bianco, I., and Baglioni, C. Interaction of hemoglobin Lepore with sickle cell trait and microcythemia (thalassemia) in a southern Italian family. *Blood* 25:457–469, 1965.

147. Ahern, E.J., Ahern, V.N., Aarons, G.H., et al. Hemoglobin Lepore Washington in two Jamaican families: Interaction with beta chain variants. *Blood* 40:246–256, 1972.

148. Ashcroft, M.T., Miall, W.E., and Milner, P.F. A comparison between the characteristics of Jamaican adults with normal hemoglobin and those with sickle cell trait. *Am. J. Epidemiol.* 90:236–243, 1969.

149. Steinberg, M.H., Adams, J.G., and Dreiling, B.J. Alpha thalassaemia in adults with sickle cell trait. *Br. J. Haematol.* 30:31–37, 1975.

150. Moo-Penn, W., Bechtel, K., Jue, D., et al. The presence of hemoglobin S and C Harlem in an individual in the United States. *Blood* 46:363–367, 1975.

151. Kinney, T.R. Personal communication, 1978.

152. Aksoy, M., and Lehmann, H. The first observation of sickle cell haemoglobin E disease. *Nature* 179:1248–1250, 1957.

153. Aksoy, M. The hemoglobin E syndromes. II. Sickle-cell-hemoglobin E disease. *Blood* 15:610–613, 1960.

154. Altay, C., Niazi, G.A., and Huisman, T.H.J. The combination of Hb S and Hb E in a black female. *Hemoglobin* 1:100–102, 1977.

155. Schroeder, W.A., Powars, D., Reynolds, R.D., et al. Hb-E in combination with Hb-S and Hb-C in a black family. *Hemoglobin* 1:287–289, 1977.

156. Hill, R.L., Swenson, R.T., and Schwartz, H.C. The chemical and genetic relationships between hemoglobins S and G San Jose. *Blood* 19:573–586, 1962.

157. Beresford, C.H., Clegg, J.B., and Weatherall, D.J. Haemoglobin Ocho Rios ($\beta$ 52 (D 3) aspartic acid→alanine): A new $\beta$-chain variant of haemoglobin A found in combination with haemoglobin S. *J. Med. Genet.* 9:151–153, 1972.

158. Konotey-Ahulu, F.I.D., Kinderlerer, J.L., Lehmann, H., et al. Haemoglobin Osu-Christiansborg: A new $\beta$-chain variant of haemoglobin A ($\beta$52 (D 3) aspartic acid→asparagine) in combination with haemoglobin S. *J. Med. Genet.* 8:302–305, 1971.

159. Efremov, G.D., Huisman, T.H.J., Smith, L.L., et al. Hemoglobin Richmond, a human hemoglobin which forms asymmetric hybrids with other hemoglobins. *J. Biol. Chem.* 244:6105–6116, 1969.

160. Blackwell, R.Q., McCurdy, P.R., Liu, C.S., et al. Double heterozygosity for hemoglobin Camden ($\beta^{131\ Gln \rightarrow Glu}$) and hemoglobin S in an American Negro. *Vox. Sang.* 28:50–56, 1975.

161. Powars, D., Schroeder, W.A., Shelton, J.R., et al. An individual with hemoglobins S and Deer Lodge. *Hemoglobin* 1:97–100, 1976–1977.

162. Steinberg, M.H., Adams, J.G., Thigpen, J.T., et al. Hemoglobin Hope ($\alpha_2\beta_2^{136gly \rightarrow asp}$)-S disease: Clinical and biochemical studies. *J. Lab. Clin. Med.* 84:632–642, 1974.

163. Weatherall, D.J. Hemoglobin J (Baltimore) coexisting in a family with hemoglobin S. *Bull. Johns Hopkins Hosp.* 114:1–12, 1964.

164. Gellady, A.M., and Schwartz, A.D. Hemoglobins S and J coexisting in the same family. *J. Pediatr.* 83:1038–1040, 1973.

165. Gunay, U., Pauli, C., Shamsuddin, M., et al. Sickle hemoglobin in combination with Hb J Bangkok ($\alpha^A_2\beta_2^{56Gly \rightarrow Asp}$). *Blood* 44:683–690, 1974.

166. Allan, N., Beale, D., Irvine, D., et al. Three haemoglobins K: Woolwich, an abnormal, Cameroon and Ibadan, two unusual variants of human haemoglobin A. *Nature* 208:658–661, 1965.

167. O'Gorman, P., Allsopp, K.M., Lehmann, H., et al. Sickle-cell haemoglobin K disease. *Br. Med. J.* 2:1381–1382, 1963.

168. Ringelhann, B., Konotey-Ahulu, F.I.D., Talapatra, N.C., et al. Haemoglobin K Woolwich ($\alpha_2\beta_2$ 132 Lysine→Glutamine) in Ghana. *Acta Haematol.* 45:250–258, 1971.

169. Bookchin, R.M., Nagel, R.M., and Balazs, T. Hemoglobin N Baltimore: Tendency to crystalize and diminished interaction with deoxyhemoglobin S. *Clin. Res.* 22:384A, 1974.

170. Tatsis, B., Sofroniadou, K., and Stergiopoulos, C.I. Hemoglobin Pyrgos $\alpha_2\beta_2^{83}$ (EF7) Gly→Asp: A new hemoglobin variant in double heterozygosity with hemoglobin S. *Blood* 47:827–832, 1976.

171. Beuzard, Y., Basset, P., Braconnier, F., et al. Haemoglobin Saki $\alpha_2\beta_2^{14}$ Leu→Pro($A_{11}$) Structure and Function. *Biochim. Biophys. Acta* 393:182–187, 1975.

172. Lutcher, C.L., Wilson, J.B., Gravely, M.E., et al. Hb Leslie, an unstable hemoglobin due to deletion of glutaminyl residue $\beta$ 131 (H9) occurring in association with $\beta^0$-thalassemia, Hb C and Hb S. *Blood* 47:99–112, 1976.

173. McCurdy, P.R., Sherman, A.S., Kamuzora, H., et al. Globin synthesis in subjects doubly heterozygous for hemoglobin G-Philadelphia and hemoglobin S or C. *J. Lab. Clin. Med.* 85:891–897, 1975.

174. Wrightstone, R.N., Hubbard, M., and Huisman, T.H.J. Hemoglobin S-G$\alpha$ Georgia disease: A case report. *Acta Haematol.* 51:315–320, 1974.

175. Hall-Craggs, M., Marsden, P.D., Raper, A.B., et al. Homozygous sickle-cell anemia arising from two different haemoglobins S: Interaction of haemoglobin S and Stanleyville-II. *Br. Med. J.* 2:87–89, 1964.

176. Van Ros, G., Wiltshire, B., Renoirte-Monjoie, A.M., et al. Interaction entre les hémoglobines Stanleyville IIet S dans une famille du Zaïre. *Biochimie* 55:1107–1119, 1973.

177. Smith, E.W., and Torbert, J.V. Study of two abnormal hemoglobins with evidence for a new genetic locus for hemoglobin formation. *Bull. Johns Hopkins Hosp.* 102:38–45, 1958.

178. Honig, G.R., Gunay, U., Mason, R.G., et al. Sickle cell syndromes. I. Hemoglobin SC-$\alpha$-thalassemia. *Pediatr. Res.* 10:613–620, 1976.

179. Thompson, R.B., Hewett, B., Jr., Ard, E., et al. A new thalassemic syndrome: Homozygous hemoglobin S disease delta thalassemia. *Acta Haematol.* 36:412–417, 1966.

180. Alter, B.P., Friedman, Sh., Hobbins, J.C., et al. Prenatal diagnosis of sickle cell anemia and alpha G-Philadelphia. *N. Engl. J. Med.* 294:1040–1044, 1976.

181. Friedman, Sh., and Kim, H.C. Unpublished observation, 1978.

# 10 Bacterial Infections in Sickling Disorders*

Arthur J. Provisor, M.D.
Robert L. Baehner, M.D.

Life-threatening bacterial infections are common in children with homozygous sickle cell disease (Hb SS) and are also observed in patients with other sickle hemoglobinopathies, such as Hb SC disease and Hb S-$\beta$ thalassemia.[1,2] Bacteremia and meningitis caused by *Streptococcus pneumoniae* and *Hemophilus influenzae* remain the leading causes of death in children with sickle cell anemia under the age of 3.[1] Beyond the preschool period, the risk of overwhelming bacterial infection decreases sharply, with pneumococcal infections after age 3 usually occurring in patients with a past history of similar infections. Although *H. influenzae* infections are less common than pneumococcal infections, the age-dependent incidence patterns are the same. In contrast, salmonella infections occur throughout life in sickle cell patients, but are not associated with overwhelming sepsis or meningitis. As was first reported in 1925, salmonella infection in sickle cell anemia most commonly presents as osteomyelitis.[3]

*This work was supported by grants from the Indiana State Board of Health and the Riley Memorial Association.

The diminished host resistance to bacterial infection in the patient with sickle cell disease has been the focus of much speculation. The biologic basis for susceptibility to infection includes a possible defect in serum opsonic activity[4] as well as the contribution of the functionally asplenic state.[5,6] The phagocytic function of polymorphonuclear leukocytes from sickle cell patients has also been evaluated in an attempt to explain the extraordinary incidence of infection.[7]

Recent reports have emphasized preventive measures to control infectious complications of sickle cell disease. The use of prophylactic penicillin in children with sickle cell anemia has been advocated. Results of clinical trials with an octavalent pneumococcal vaccine in children with sickle cell anemia appear favorable.[8]

In this chapter, we will review the molecular mechanisms for opsonic activity in patients with sickling disorders, examine evidence for altered splenic reticuloendothelial function and neutrophil phagocytic function in these patients, and review those clinical studies that graphically demonstrate increased morbidity and mortality secondary to bacterial infection in sickle cell disease. In addition, we will discuss preventive measures currently available for control of infectious complications of sickle cell disease.


## OPSONIZATION

### Methods of Opsonization

Opsonization refers to the process whereby bacteria combine with serum components and are made more palatable for ingestion by phagocytes. Specific antibody, nonspecific immunoglobulin, complement, and other serum components all function as opsonins. In a review of opsonization, Winkelstein used the opsonization of pneumococci as a model to demonstrate the variety of opsonic mechanisms.[9] Pneumococci may be opsonized through the effect of type-specific anticapsular antibody. Either $IgG_1$, $IgG_3$, or IgM antibody classes may act in this way. Both neutrophils and monocytes contain regions on their surfaces to bind the Fc portion of the antibody, and this ligand between the bacterium and the phagocyte facilitates ingestion of the microbe.

Pneumococci may also be opsonized through the combined action of specific antibody and complement. The Fc portion of the antibody molecule activates the first component of complement (C1), followed rapidly by the activation of C4 and C2 functioning as a bimolecular complex attached to the bacterial surface. This complex leads to the activation of C3 with the formation of C3B. Receptor sites for C3B have been demonstrated on phagocytic cell membranes.[10]

Type-specific anticapsular antibody is produced during persistent pneumococcal infection and acts with complement as an opsonin via the classical pathway of complement activation to combat infection.

The third mechanism for opsonizing pneumococci is the heat-labile opsonin (HLO) system. This nonspecific mechanism is likely to be operative in the nonimmune individual.[11] Heating the serum to 56°C destroys its activity. Immunoglobulin of the 7S type contributes to the HLO system for pneumococcus in nonimmune animals,[12] but lacks the specificity of anticapsular antibody. However, the HLO system requires activation of C3 and fixation of C3B to the pneumococcal surface.[13] In this system, the activation of C3 does not occur through the C4C2 bimolecular complex or classic pathway of complement activation, but rather through the alternative pathway[14] consisting of properdin, factor B (C3 proactivator), factor D (C3 convertase proactivator), and other early acting factors.

## Defects in Opsonization

Winkelstein and Drachman, in an effort to uncover the etiology for increased susceptibility to infection in sickle cell disease, reported a deficiency of the opsonization of pneumococci in serums from 12 of 14 patients with Hb SS.[4] Specific pneumococcal agglutinin levels were low in both control and Hb SS serums. Heating the serums to 56°C eliminated the difference in opsonizing activity, suggesting a deficiency of heat-labile opsonins in Hb SS. Serum opsonizing activity for salmonella was comparable in patients with sickle cell disease and controls.

Johnston and coworkers have also shown a decrease in pneumococcal serum opsonizing activity in patients with Hb SS.[15,16] The phagocytosis assay used by Johnston quantifies the number of type 2 pneumococci ingested by normal human polymorphonuclear leukocytes. This system depends upon the chemical reduction of nitroblue tetrazolium in direct proportion to the number of type 2 pneumococci ingested. The type 2 pneumococci were previously coated with varying amounts of IgG antibody. When a maximal amount of antibody was used, there was no difference in phagocytosis in the presence of serums from normal and Hb SS patients. However, when the amount of antibody previously fixed to the pneumococci was decreased, the mean level of phagocytosis achieved by Hb SS serums was less than half that of normal serums. Antibody deficiency could not explain this opsonic defect, as there was no significant type 2 pneumococcal agglutinating antibody activity in the serums of either the normal or Hb SS populations. Since sickle cell patients showed normal opsonizing activity in the presence of excess antibody, it is not likely that their serums lack the capacity to fix C3 to the bacterial surface via the classical pathway. On the other hand, phagocytosis of zymosan particles opsonized through the alternative pathway was defective when sickle cell serum was employed. Furthermore, there was a lack of fixation of C3 to the zymosan surface as shown by the inability of monospecific anti-C3 serum to agglutinate zymosan previously incubated with sickle cell serum.

Other investigators have not been able to show a defect in alternative pathway function. In our laboratory, we studied the opsonization of $^{14}$C type 2 pneumococci by serums from normal controls and from 28 patients with Hb SS, ranging in age from 3 months to 16 years. Two of the samples were obtained from children during episodes of fatal pneumococcal sepsis. Serums were treated with ethylene glycol tetra-acetic acid to chelate calcium and block the classical complement pathway, and excessive magnesium was added to ensure alternative pathway function. Using an assay system in which the uptake of $^{14}$C bacteria by neutrophils was quantified directly, we failed to show an opsonic defect with any of the Hb SS serums.[17] Strauss and associates[18] recently studied alternative pathway components in an effort to define the previously postulated abnormality in this system. Concentrations of C3, factor B, total hemolytic activity, properdin, and C3B inactivator were similar to serums from patients and control subjects. The alternative pathway was activated by inulin and cobra venom factor to the same extent in patient and control serums.

## PHAGOCYTE FUNCTION

Recognition of opsonized bacteria by phagocytes requires the directed movement of the neutrophils to the site of the infection by a variety of chemoattractants, including C3a, C5$_a$ and $\overline{C567}$, bacterial products resembling formyl tripeptides, lymphokines, and fibrinopeptides. In Hb SS no specific chemotactic defect has been described. Similar to the results of opsonic studies, metabolic assessment of phagocytic function in Hb SS has given disparate results. Dimitrov and associates[7] have shown that sickle cell patients with a history of recurrent infection have leukocytes that fail to stimulate respiration, hydrogen peroxide ($H_2O_2$) production, and hexose monophosphate shunt activity during phagocytosis adequately.[7] These metabolic aberrations were associated with impaired degranulation and decreased intracellular bacterial killing.

In contrast to these studies, Strauss and coworkers[18] have shown oxidative metabolism to be normal in neutrophils from patients with sickle cell disease. Nitroblue tetrazolium reduction, oxygen consumption, HMP shunt activity, superoxide production, and bacterial killing were all normal in neutrophils from sickle cell patients.[19]

The reasons for these contrasting results are not readily apparent, but may be related to a temporary defect in neutrophil function at the time of infection in patients with sickle cell disease.

## SPLENIC FUNCTION

Splenomegaly is common during the first three or four years of life in patients with sickle cell anemia. Splenic size, however, is not a reflection of function in these children. O'Brien and colleagues[20] have demonstrated a lack of splenic uptake of technetium-labeled sulfur colloid in children as early as 5 months of age. Initially, this lack of function is reversible in some patients by transfusions of normal red cells in quantities sufficient to reduce by half the number of irreversibly sickled cells,[21] but reversibility is gradually lost. As a result of the plugging of splenic sinusoids with sickled cells, and subsequent infarction, autosplenectomy occurs. Pathologically, this state is characterized by a small fibrosed spleen. The increased incidence of overwhelming bacterial infection seen in the splenectomized child[22,23,24] is also seen in the child with sickle cell disease and functional asplenia. In the nonimmune individual, clearance of [125]I pneumococci occurs primarily through the spleen rather than the liver.[25] Thus, the spleen serves as the first line of defense against blood-borne particulate material such as the pneumococcus.

Loss of reticuloendothelial function of the spleen in Hb SS results from the following sequence of events. Blood flow is sluggish in the splenic circulation. The relatively anoxic and acidotic environment stimulates sickling, with a resultant increase in viscosity and further obstruction of blood flow at the presinusoidal level. The spleen contains arteriovenous shunts.[21] Blood flow in the patient with sickling is directed through these channels, bypassing the phagocytic reticuloendothelial elements of the spleen and leading to a functionally asplenic state.

To understand the immunologic impact of functional asplenia in Hb SS, the response of the normal spleen to acute bacterial (i.e., pneumococcal) sepsis should be considered. In general, the spleen responds to acute bacterial infection by enlarging secondary to vascular engorgement. There is increased phagocytic activity with increased numbers of neutrophils in the sinusoids.[26] In the experimental animal, the spleen clears particles, including bacteria, from blood more efficiently than does the liver, even though the liver possesses more reticuloendothelial tissue.[27] The splenic macrophages are better scavengers than the neutrophils in trapping the particles.[28,29]

The spleen also appears to be essential for the production of antibody in response to small doses of intravenously administered particulate antigen. As early as 1950, Rowley[30] reported that a single

intravenous injection of sheep red cells administered to a splenectomized man failed to elicit a significant rise in heterophile antibody
titer. Children with hereditary splenic hypoplasia have also
demonstrated this defect.[31] Schwartz and Pearson[6] showed that
children with sickle cell anemia had abnormally low antibody production in response to intravenously administered sheep erythrocytes. In
contrast, one child with sickle cell anemia had normal antibody production in response to intramuscular injection of antigen. These investigators emphasized that visualization of the spleen by technetium
sulfur colloid following red cell transfusions could not be equated with
return of immunologic function.

The spleen may play an important role in antibody production in
response to bacterial invasion. In the rabbit, the spleen normally processes unencapsulated organisms more effectively than encapsulated
ones.[32] Polysaccharide capsules covering the pneumococcus, men-
ingococcus, and H. influenzae organisms impede phagocytosis.[33] The
intravenous injection of heat-killed pneumococci in the rabbit leads to
antibody formation that is protective eight hours later when these
animals are challenged with a lethal dose of virulent pneumococci.
Asplenic rabbits die from this challenge dose.[34] Splenic macrophages
probably transport the antigen to the splenic lymphoid follicle where
antibody formation occurs. The human spleen is rich in IgM-bearing B
lymphocytes which give rise to immunoglobulin-producing plasma
cells.[35] Following splenectomy in normal children, serum IgM levels
fall, while levels of IgG and IgA remain normal.[36] These studies suggest
that splenic macrophages process and transmit antigenic material to
splenic B lymphocytes for IgM antibody synthesis by plasma cells.
Winkelstein and Lambert[37] have measured pneumococcal serum opsonizing activity in splenectomized children and found it to be normal.
Thus, it would appear that if there is a decrease in serum opsonizing
activity in sickle cell disease, autosplenectomy is not the primary
cause.

In an earlier but related study, Kaye and Hook[38] investigated the
sites of multiplication of a single strain of Salmonella typhimurum in
tissues of mice with hemolysis induced by antimouse erythrocyte
serum or by phenylhydrazine. They found that replication of
salmonella could be detected earlier in pretreated mice than in controls. In animals with hemolysis, it appeared that the normal
mechanisms operating to remove micro-organisms from livers and
spleens were impaired. The reticuloendothelial cells of the liver and
spleen in the mouse pretreated with antierythrocyte serum or
phenylhydrazine were not as effective in killing bacteria as were
reticuloendothelial cells of the normal mouse. In effect, a reticuloendothelial blockade was established by the hemolyzed red cell
fragments, leading to a functionally asplenic state.

The spleen has been thought to be the site of synthesis of a tetrapeptide called tuftsin, which acts directly on phagocytic cells.[39] Deficiency of tuftsin has been shown to be associated with recurrence of severe infections. The splenectomized individual would naturally lack tuftsin. This lack may play a role in the increased susceptibility of the sickle cell patient to bacterial infection.

## INFECTIONS IN Hb SS: BACTEREMIA AND MENINGITIS

Overwhelming bacterial infections (sepsis or meningitis) are frequent complications in patients with Hb SS and are the most common cause of death in children with this disease. In contrast, although salmonella osteomyelitis is commonly observed in Hb SS, it does not cause death.[3,40] Compared to the observations on salmonella infection in Hb SS, the relationship between pneumococcal sepsis or meningitis and Hb SS was not appreciated until relatively recently. Table 10-1 summarizes the experience from five major centers treating large populations of patients with Hb SS and related hemoglobinopathies. Robinson and Watson[41] followed 252 patients with sickle cell disease in Brooklyn, New York. In this population, there were 16 patients with meningitis, an incidence of 6.3%. Meningitis was not seen in any patients with Hb SC disease or Hb S-$\beta$ thalassemia. The group of 16 patients experienced 18 episodes of meningitis, 15 of which proved to be bacterial; 13 or 87% were due to pneumococci. Eighty-five percent of the cases of bacterial meningitis occurred in children under age 3, and 60% occurred in patients 2 years of age or younger.

More recently, Overturf and associates[2] reported a group of 422 patients with various sickle hemoglobinopathies. During the period of observation, 53 episodes of sepsis or meningitis occurred, reflecting an overall risk of 12.5%. Considering only the 325 cases with Hb SS disease the risk increased to 15.2%. Twenty-six of the 27 episodes of meningitis occurred in 24 patients with sickle cell anemia. One patient with Hb SC disease had pneumococcal meningitis at age 11. In this series, 74% of all episodes of meningitis were due to pneumococcus. Eighty percent of the cases of pneumococcal meningitis occurred in children 5 years of age or younger and most were between the ages of 1 and 5 years. Twenty-three of 26 episodes of septicemia occurred among 20 patients with Hb SS. There were seven deaths among these 20 patients. Two of these deaths were secondary to *H. influenzae,* type B, occurring in children ages 2 and 7. Four children died of pneumococcal sepsis before the age of 5. As expected, pneumococcus was the most common organism found, especially in children between ages 1 and 4. Three patients with Hb SC disease developed septicemia secondary to enteric or anaerobic organisms. All of these patients were older than 10 years when they became septic.

Seeler and associates[42] reviewed the experience with pneumococcal infections in children with sickle cell anemia at Cook County Hospital in Chicago. In her series, there were 12 episodes of pneumococcal bacteremia and/or meningitis with two deaths in ten children with sickle cell anemia. Ages ranged from 7 months to 8.25 years, but only three children were older than 2 years of age.

Of interest is a recent report by Ward and Smith from Children's Hospital in Boston.[43] During the preceding three years, ten episodes of bacteremia were documented in children with Hb SS. Six of these episodes were secondary to *H. influenzae* B. There were two pneumococcal bacteremias, and these accounted for the only deaths in the group. There was one episode of *S. aureus* bacteremia and one bout of *E. coli* bacteremia in a 20-year-old girl secondary to pyelonephritis.

Barrett-Connor found that symptomatic urinary tract infection occurred in about 10% of patients, half of whom had bacteremia.[1] *Enterobacter klebsiella* was responsible for a higher proportion of urinary tract infections than expected.

Barrett-Connor's comprehensive review of bacterial infections in sickle cell anemia is the major contribution to our knowledge of this clinical association.[1] During an 11-year period, 166 patients with sickle cell anemia were hospitalized at least once. There were 250 hospitalizations for presumptive bacterial infection, of which 85 were confirmed by appropriate cultures. Sixty-seven patients were hospitalized on 152 occasions for an illness that clinically and radiologically appeared to be bacterial pneumonia. The incidence of bacterial infection was markedly reduced after age 3. Survival past this age without previous bacterial infection signified a reduced chance of subsequent bacterial infection except for those due to coliform bacteria. Bacterial infection accounted for 60% of the fatalities and pneumococcal meningitis and bacteremia accounted for 50% of the fatalities under age 4. A group of 14 patients had a much higher rate of bacterial infection and accounted for over 40% of the hospitalizations for proven bacterial infection. These high risk patients were not distinguished by frequency of crises, severity of anemia, or other complications of sickle cell anemia. Surprisingly, the morbidity and mortality of bacterial meningitis did not vary from that seen in children without sickle cell disease.[1] Painful crises were no more frequent in patients with bacterial infections than in patients without infections. The relationship of bacterial infection to hematologic crises, usually aplastic, was variable. Some patients experienced repeated bacterial infections without an effect on their anemias, while others experienced hematologic crises only in association with bacterial infection.

## OSTEOMYELITIS

Although pneumococcal and staphylococcal bone infections were observed, salmonella was the most common cause of osteomyelitis in all age groups.[1] Multiple sites of involvement and recurrence in the face of appropriate therapy characterized all types of osteomyelitis in patients with sickle cell disease.[40,44] Salmonella osteomyelitis is not an overwhelming fatal infection in patients with sickle cell disease but it is responsible for increased morbidity with a chronic course. The unusual susceptibility to salmonella osteomyelitis in these patients has never been satisfactorily explained. As an initial event, capillary thrombosis may make the gastrointestinal tract less capable of resisting invasion by enteric organisms. Having gained entrance to the circulation, salmonella is known to localize in areas of ischemia and necrosis. Areas of infarcted bone due to the sickling process provide an excellent culture media for salmonella.

## PREVENTION OF INFECTION IN Hb SS

What practical measures can be taken to reduce the incidence of overwhelming septicemia in patients with sickle cell disease? The continuous use of prophylactic penicillin has been advocated by investigators and clinicians alike. More recently, the use of an octavalent pneumococcal vaccine has been shown to be effective in the prevention of fatal pneumococcal disease in these patients.[8]

In a review of overwhelming bacterial infections in children splenectomized for Hodgkin's disease, Chilcote and coinvestigators[45] found 20 episodes of meningitis and septicemia in 18 of 200 children. The pneumococcus was the predominant organism responsible for 50% of the cases. The functionally asplenic state seen in sickle cell disease corresponds to the postsplenectomy state after staging laparotomy in Hodgkin's disease. The prevalence of pneumococcal septicemia is seen in both the children with sickle cell disease and in the Hodgkin's disease patients. The use of prophylactic penicillin in the functionally asplenic sickle cell patient is a rational approach to the prevention of pneumococcal sepsis. As the vast majority of cases occur in children under age 5 years, with a few episodes between ages 5 and 10, the use of prophylactic penicillin would be most effective between infancy and age 10. A guideline for the introduction of prophylactic penicillin may be lack of visualization of the spleen using $^{99m}$Tc-sulfur colloid or the appearance of Howell-Jolly bodies in peripheral blood red cells.

Since patients with sickle cell disease and functional asplenia are able to develop a normal antibody response to antigens not

**Table 10-1**
**Incidence of Sepsis and Meningitis in Sickle Cell Anemia and Related Hemoglobinopathies**

| Center | Age range | Number of patients | Number of patients with meningitis or sepsis | Etiologic agent | Mortality |
|---|---|---|---|---|---|
| State University of New York Downstate Medical Center[41] | 5 mos–5 yrs, 10 mos | 252 Hb SS<br>31 Hb SC<br>22 Hb S-b thalassemia | 16 SS meningitis<br>0 SC<br>0 S thalassemia | 87% *Streptococcus pneumoniae* | 2 |
| Los Angeles County USC Medical Center[2] | 12 mos–32 yrs<br>13 pts. over 5 years | 323 Hb SS<br>99 S-hemoglobinopathy (primarily Hb SC) | 26 SS meningitis<br>1 SC meningitis<br>23 SS sepsis<br>3 SC sepsis | 74% *S. pneumoniae*<br><br>46% *S. pneumoniae*<br>12% *H. influenzae* | 2<br>7 |
| Cook County Hospital, Chicago[42] | 7 mos–8 yrs, 3 mos | not given | 12 SS meningitis or sepsis | 100% *S. pneumoniae* | 2 |
| Children's Hospital Medical Center, Boston[43] | 8 pts. 3 yrs or less<br>1 pt. 9 yrs<br>1 pt. 20 yrs | 37 Hb SS and hemoglobinopathy S- | 10 SS sepsis | 60% *H. influenzae*<br>20% *S. pneumoniae* | 2 |
| Jackson Memorial Hospital, Variety Children's Hospital, Miami[1] | 5 mos–5 yrs | 166 Hb SS | 13 meningitis<br>5 sepsis | 71% *S. pneumoniae*<br>21% *H. influenzae*<br>40% *S. pneumoniae*<br>20% *H. influenzae*<br>40% *E. coli*<br>(2 pts., ages 10 and 27) | 11 |

administered intravenously, the use of a purified polyvalent pneumococcal vaccine might provide protection against pneumococcal sepsis. Ammann, Addiego, and coworkers[8] used an octavalent pneumococcal polysaccharide vaccine containing 50 μg of each of the individual pneumococcal polysaccharides (types 1, 3, 6, 7, 14, 18, 19, and 23) to immunize patients with sickle cell disease, asplenic patients without a hemoglobinopathy, and a group of normal black children. The controls were a group of 106 unimmunized black patients with sickle cell disease. The sickle cell group and the splenectomized group responded to immunization in the same manner as normal controls. Postimmunization antibody titers were still significant one year later. During a two-year follow-up period, eight episodes of systemic pneumococcal infections were observed, all in the unimmunized group. There were two fatalities in this group. All eight infections were documented by blood culture to be pneumococcal types contained in the vaccine. This preliminary study provides the clinical data needed to justify the large scale use of a polyvalent pneumococcal vaccine in children with sickle cell disease and in postsplenectomy patients.

## REFERENCES

1. Barrett-Connor, E. Bacterial infection and sickle cell anemia. *Medicine* 50:97–112, 1971.

2. Overturf, C.D., Powars, D., and Baraff, L.J. Bacterial meningitis and septicemia in sickle cell disease. *Am. J. Dis. Child.* 131:784–787, 1977.

3. Carrington, C.L., and Davison, W.C. Multiple osteomyelitis due to bacillus paratyphosus B: Demonstration of bacillus in fresh blood preparation. *Bull. Johns Hopkins Hosp.* 36:428, 1925.

4. Winkelstein, J.A., and Drachman, R.H. Deficiency of pneumococcal serum opsonizing activity in sickle-cell disease. *N. Engl. J. Med.* 279:459–466, 1968.

5. Pearson, H.A., Spencer, R.P., and Cornelius, E.A. Functional asplenia in sickle cell anemia. *N. Engl. J. Med.* 281:925–926, 1964.

6. Schwartz, A.D., and Pearson, H.A. Impaired antibody response to intravenous immunization in sickle cell anemia. *Pediatr. Res.* 6:145–149, 1972.

7. Dimitrov, N.V., Downes, F.R., Bartolotta, B., et al. Metabolic activity of polymorphonuclear leukocytes in sickle cell anemia. *Acta Haematol.* 47:283–291, 1972.

8. Ammann, A.J., Addiego, J., Wara, D.W., et al. Polyvalent pneumococcal polysaccharide immunization of patients with sickle cell anemia and patients with splenectomy. *N. Engl. J. Med.* 297:897–900, 1977.

9. Winkelstein, J.A. Opsonins: Their function, identity, and clinical significance. *J. Pediatr.* 82:747–753, 1973.

10. Lay, W.H., and Nussenzweig, V. Receptors for complement on leukocytes. *J. Exp. Med.* 128:991, 1968.

11. Smith, M.R., and Wood, W.B., Jr. Heat labile opsonins to pneumococcus. I. Participation of complement. *J. Exp. Med.* 130:1209, 1969.

12. Winkelstein, J.A., Shin, H.S., and Wood, W.B., Jr. Heat labile opsonins

to pneumococcus. III. The participation of immunoglobulin and of the alternate pathway of $C_3$ activation. *J. Immunol.* 108:1681, 1972.

13. Shin, H.S., Smith, M.R., and Wood, W.B., Jr. Heat labile opsonins to pneumococcus. II. Involvement of $C_3$ and $C_5$. *J. Exp. Med.* 130:1229, 1969.

14. Phillemer, L., Blum, L., and Lepow, I. The properdin system and immunity. I. Demonstration and isolation of a new serum protein, properdin, and its role in immune phenomena. *Science* 120:279, 1954.

15. Johnston, R.B., Jr., Newman, S.L., and Struth, A.G. An abnormality of the alternate pathway of complement activation in sickle-cell disease. *N. Engl. J. Med.* 288:803–808, 1973.

16. Johnston, R.B., Jr. Increased susceptibility to infection in sickle cell disease. *South Med. J.* 67:1342–1348, 1974.

17. Provisor, A.J., Allen, J.M., and Baehner, R.L. Utilization of a functional phagocytic assay system in the evaluation of opsonic activity in sera from patients with sickle cell anemia. *Pediatr. Res.* 10:380, 1976.

18. Strauss, R.G., Asbrock, T., Forristal, J., et al. Alternative pathway of complement in sickle cell anemia. *Pediatr. Res.* 11:285–289, 1977.

19. Strauss, R.G., Johnston, R.B., Jr., Asbrock, T., et al. Neutrophil oxidative metabolism in sickle cell disease. *J. Pediatr.* 89:391–394, 1976.

20. O'Brien, R.T., McIntosh, S., Aspnes, G.T., et al. Prospective study of sickle cell anemia in infancy. *J. Pediatr.* 89:205–210, 1976.

21. Pearson, H.A., Cornelius, E.A., Schwartz, A.D., et al. Transfusion reversible functional asplenia in young children with sickle cell anemia. *N. Engl. J. Med.* 243:334, 1970.

22. Diamond, L.K. Splenectomy in childhood and the hazard of overwhelming infection. *Pediatrics* 43:886, 1969.

23. Eraklis, A.J., Kevy, S.V., Diamond, L.K., et al. Hazard of overwhelming infection after splenectomy in childhood. *N. Engl. J. Med.* 276:1125, 1967.

24. King, H., and Schumacher, H.B. Susceptibility to infection after splenectomy performed in infants. *Ann. Surg.* 136:234, 1952.

25. Schulkind, M.L., Ellis, E.F., and Smith, R.T. Effect of antibody upon clearance of $I^{125}$ labelled pneumococci by the spleen and liver. *Pediatr. Res.* 1:178, 1967.

26. Robbins, S.L. *Pathology.* 3rd Ed. Philadelphia: W.B. Saunders Co., 1967.

27. Drinker, C.K., and Shaw, L.A. Quantitative distribution of particulate material (manganese dioxide) administered intravenously to the cat. *J. Exp. Med.* 33:77, 1921.

28. Burke, J.S., and Simon, G.T. Electron microscopy of the spleen. I. Anatomy and microcirculation. *Am. J. Pathol.* 58:127, 1970.

29. Simon, G.T., and Burke, J.S. Electron microscopy of the spleen. II. Erythroleukophagocytosis. *Am. J. Pathol.* 58:451, 1970.

30. Rowley, D.A. The formation of circulating antibody in the splenectomized human being following intravenous injection of heterologous erythrocytes. *J. Immunol.* 65:515, 1950.

31. Kevy, S.V., Tefft, M., Vawter, G.F., et al. Hereditary splenic hypoplasia. *Pediatrics* 42:752. 1968.

32. Rogers, D.E. Host mechanisms which act to remove bacteria from the blood stream. *Bacteriol. Rev.* 24:50, 1960.

33. Krause, R.M., and Davie, J. Edited by P.A. Miescher and H.J. Muller-Eberhard. *Textbook of Immunopathology.* New York: Grune and Stratton, Inc., 1968.

34. Ellis, E.F., and Smith, R.T. The role of the spleen in infants. *Pediatrics* 37:111, 1966.

35. Neiburger, J.B., Neiburger, R.G., Richardson, S.T., et al. Distribution of

T and B lymphocytes in lymphoid tissue of infants and children. *Infect. Immun.* 14:118-121, 1976.

36. Schumacher, M.J. Serum immunoglobulin and transferrin levels after childhood splenectomy. *Arch. Dis. Child.* 45:114-117, 1970.

37. Winkelstein, J.A., and Lambert, G.H. Pneumococcal serum opsonizing activity in splenectomized children. *J. Pediatr.* 87:430-433, 1975.

38. Kaye, D., and Hook, E.W. The influence of hemolysis on susceptibility to salmonella infection: Additional observations. *J. Immunol.* 91:518, 1963.

39. Constantopoulos, A., Najjar, V.A., and Smith, J.W. Tuftsin deficiency: A new syndrome with defective phagocytosis. *J. Pediatr.* 80:564-572, 1972.

40. Hook, E.N., Campbell, C.G., Weens, H.S., et al. Salmonella osteomyelitis in patients with sickle cell anemia. *N. Engl. J. Med.* 257:403-407, 1957.

41. Robinson, M.G., and Watson, R.J. Pneumococcal meningitis in sickle cell anemia. *N. Engl. J. Med.* 274:1006-1008, 1966.

42. Seeler, R.A., Metzger, W., and Mufson, M.A. Diplococcus pneumoniae infections in children with sickle cell anemia. *Am. J. Dis. Child.* 123:8-10, 1972.

43. Ward, J., and Smith, A.L. Hemophilus influenzae bacteremia in children with sickle cell disease. *J. Pediatr.* 88:261, 1976.

44. Hughes, J.G., and Carroll, D.S. Salmonella osteomyelitis complicating sickle cell disease. *Pediatrics* 19:184, 1957.

45. Chilcote, R.R., Baehner, R.L., Hammond, D., et al. Septicemia and meningitis in children splenectomized for Hodgkin's disease. *N. Engl. J. Med.* 295:798, 1976.

# 11 The National Sickle Cell Disease Program

Clarice D. Reid, M.D.

The National Sickle Cell Disease Program was initiated in 1971 following the President's health message to Congress in which he targeted sickle cell anemia as a major health problem. Early in 1970, however, the Hematology Study Section of the National Institutes of Health (NIH) had begun deliberations on problems of sickle cell disease and had sponsored a conference in 1971 to formulate broad proposals on avenues to explore in sickle cell disease. Although the conference was primarily concerned with research, it was found that many areas of patient care were related to research. The conference described what were considered to be (1) optimal approaches for providing delivery of patient care, (2) improved opportunities for clinical research, (3) priorities in basic research, and (4) coordinated programs of education, screening, and counseling.[1] This conference played a significant role in the final structure of the National Program.

Prior to the initiation of the National Program, at the NIH approximately $1 million was being distributed annually among several institutes for research in sickle cell disease. These institutes included the National Institute of Arthritis, Metabolism and Digestive Diseases, the National Institute of General Medical Sciences, the National Institute of Child Health and Human Development, and the National Heart and Lung Institute. The President's budget added $5 million to this base, which was later increased to $10 million in 1972 for research and service activities. Subsequent years have seen this support increased annually, to approximately $16 million in fiscal 1977.

Of the estimated 22 to 23 million blacks who comprise the major at risk population in the United States, one of 600 persons may have sickle cell anemia.[2] Sickle cell anemia is the most commonly occurring genetic blood disorder of clinical significance in this country. The cost of patient care, loss of time from school and employment, and the sequelae of psychological and educational problems for persons with sickle cell anemia and their families place sickle cell anemia among the diseases of major psychological, educational, and economic importance. The number of persons affected and the seriousness of the disorder justify the need for a national effort to focus on all aspects of sickle cell disease.

## NATIONAL SICKLE CELL DISEASE ADVISORY COMMITTEE

The National Sickle Cell Disease Advisory Committee was established by the Secretary of the Department of Health, Education and Welfare to make recommendations to implement the National Program. This committee consists of eleven members: seven scientific experts in appropriate fields of science and four prominent lay members. In addition, the Secretary augmented the committee with four ex officio members: the Director, National Institutes of Health; the Administrator, Health Services Administration; the Administrator, Veterans' Administration; and an Assistant Secretary of Defense; or their respective designees. More recently, the Director, Center for Disease Control, has been appointed an ex officio member.

At its first meeting in August 1971, the committee recommended a program of research and service to meet the overall goal of reducing the frequency, morbidity, and mortality of sickle cell anemia.[3] Further recommendations included the fostering of research and development both at the fundamental and clinical level; the initiation and expansion of community education, screening, and counseling programs with voluntary participation; the strengthening and expansion of the base of black professional and technical personnel; and the improvement of clinical care for individuals with sickle cell anemia, including the application of current technical knowledge. This committee continues to provide overall guidance to the National Program in program planning, implementation, and evaluation consistent with its basic objectives. In many instances, it has served as a catalyst for translating new ideas into program initiatives.

## LEGISLATION

The legislative history of the National Program is important in that a congressional mandate was expressed for efforts in controlling sickle cell disease in the sociopolitical environment of the early seventies.

In May 1972, the National Sickle Cell Anemia Control Act (P.L. 92-294) provided for a national program of research, training, education, screening, and counseling in sickle cell disease. This enactment authorized a three-year program with authorized appropriations of $25, $40, and $50 million for fiscal years 1973, 1974, and 1975, respectively. Appropriations were never made under this authorizing legislation, which expired in June 1975. Program funding has been through the existing authority of the National Heart, Lung, and Blood Institute for research and demonstration services. The Act further assured that services must be used voluntarily by clients and that all test results, medical records, and other information regarding services for sickle cell anemia be kept strictly confidential. Paradoxically, many states, in their zeal to express concern about this health problem, enacted laws for the compulsory screening of individuals in the at risk population. Most were never implemented and were subsequently repealed.

The most recent federal legislation, Title IV (P.L. 94-278), the National Sickle Cell Anemia, Cooley's Anemia, Tay-Sachs, and Genetic Diseases Act, was enacted on April 22, 1976. This act provided an "authorization" of $30 million annually for fiscal years 1976, 1977, and 1978 for testing, counseling, information, and education programs. While no funds were appropriated for fiscal years 1976 or 1977, $4 million were appropriated for fiscal year 1978 to provide support for service activities administered by the Health Services Administration. Legislation for further support for another three years is pending.

## NATIONAL PROGRAM

The National Heart, Lung, and Blood Institute of NIH is responsible for implementing the National Program and coordinating the activities of the Health Services Administration and other federal agencies (Figure 11-1). The long-range goal of the National Sickle Cell Disease Program is to decrease the frequency, morbidity, and mortality of sickle cell disease through a program of research, development, and service demonstrations. Programs initiated in 1972 to carry out these goals and objectives included the establishment of Comprehensive

# National Sickle Cell Disease Program

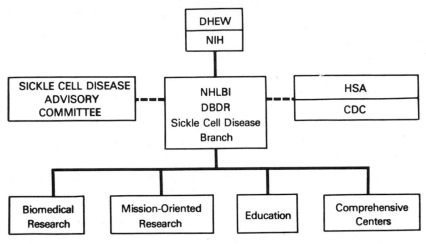

**Figure 11-1.** Organization of the National Sickle Cell Disease Program.

Sickle Cell Centers, Screening and Education Clinics, Mission-Oriented Research and Development Programs, Biomedical Research Programs, and an Information and Education Program. The Hemoglobinopathy Training Program at the Center for Disease Control was added in 1973.

## Comprehensive Sickle Cell Centers

These centers bring together research (basic, clinical, clinical trials, clinical application, research training) and community demonstration services (education, screening, and counseling). Resources, facilities, and manpower are concentrated in a coordinated approach to solving the many problems related to sickle cell disease, to bridging the gap between scientific investigations and service efforts, and to bringing findings in one area into practical use in others. Investigator-initiated research projects on a wide spectrum of subjects related to Hb S and sickle cell disease are juxtaposed with educational, diagnostic, and counseling programs with significant mutual benefits. This mechanism is most effective for the expeditious incorporation of research findings into medical education and health care delivery systems and it provides knowledgeable patients for participation in research protocols. Fifteen centers were initially established in geographic areas serving large black populations. Currently there are ten such centers. These centers are funded through the grant mechanism and provide support for research investigations as well as service demonstration programs with community involvement.

## Screening and Education Clinics

These clinics are administered by the Bureau of Community Services, Health Services Administration. They were designed to determine methods for conducting service activities, such as fostering public awareness of sickle cell disease and trait, education, screening, counseling, and patient referral, in various settings. These clinics do not provide for patient care and are funded under the contract mechanism to health departments, neighborhood health centers, hospitals, medical schools, and free-standing institutions. Currently, there are 22 projects providing quality service at the community level.

## The Mission-Oriented Research and Development Program

This program supports projects related to specific problems in sickle cell disease. It is a contract-supported component and has as one of its objectives the study of mechanisms for the prevention and reversal of sickling of red blood cells. It is based on the concept that if sickling of red cells could be impaired or prevented, perhaps by a pharmacologic agent, the quality and duration of life for patients with sickle cell disease would be markedly improved. In fiscal year 1972, approximately 27 investigators were supported by contracts under this program, including those involved in the last phase of the clinical trials of urea for the treatment of vaso-occlusive crises. Currently, there are twenty projects supported, sixteen of which are directly involved in the multicenter Cooperative Study of the Clinical Course of Sickle Cell Disease initiated in September 1977.

## The Biomedical Research Program

This program supports research projects initiated by individual investigators through the traditional grant mechanism. Grants have increased from eight in fiscal year 1972 to more than fifty in fiscal year 1977, in addition to three program project grants. Additional grant-related research in sickle cell disease is funded by the National Institute of Arthritis, Metabolism and Digestive Diseases and the National Institute of General Medical Sciences.

## The Information and Education Program

This was established in the wake of the sudden publicity about sickle cell disease which generated not only an increase in public interest but also fostered many myths and misconceptions about this disease. The lack of a clear understanding of and differentiation between sickle cell disease and sickle cell trait among health professionals as well as laymen further aggravated existing fears and confusion. Although centrally administered by the Sickle Cell Disease Branch, the education effort is an integral part of every component of the National Program. Varied approaches have been used to accomplish the objectives of the Information and Education Program, including regional workshops and an Information Center.

### The Hemoglobinopathy Training Program

This is an interagency agreement with the Hematology Division, Bureau of Laboratories, Center for Disease Control, to train laboratory personnel in the detection and identification of abnormal hemoglobins with an emphasis on sickle hemoglobin. This program provides bench training at the Center for Disease Control as well as basic courses at the regional level throughout the country. Additionally, a proficiency testing program has been instituted to provide quality control in hemoglobin identification by federally-supported funded projects. A number of federal, state, and local laboratories participate in this program.

### ADMINISTRATIVE STRUCTURE

The National Program's administrative structure has remained essentially unchanged during the past five years, although there has been a shift in emphasis. The initial outcry for mass screening rapidly subsided in recognition of the potential hazards of such screening in the absence of extensive and continuous education. A large number of early issues, including the purpose of screening programs, goals of genetic counseling, social implications of detecting trait carriers, and relative importance of sickle cell disease as compared with other health problems, all contributed to reshaping the direction of the National Program. Recent technologic advances have ushered in new issues related to the legal and ethical concerns in prenatal diagnosis and informed consent for newborn screening. While the unprecedented attention to the problems of sickle cell disease created an atmosphere of skepticism in the early seventies, there appears to be a consensus today that programs of service and of basic and clinical research are clearly desirable.

## PROJECTIONS

There have been significant milestones in the areas of research and services during the past five years, resulting in improved care and higher quality of life for many persons with sickle cell anemia. Although research advances have been made, answers to major clinical problems remain elusive. Fundamental studies of the complex structure and function of Hb S, a systematic approach to drug development, and research in other areas of potential yield will be expanded. While dramatic "breakthroughs" are intrinsically more newsworthy than new concepts of model approaches to health problems, a program of coordinated activities at the community level, integrated with the pursuit of opportunities in research, can be effective. It is within this framework that the National Sickle Cell Disease Program may serve as a prototype for research into other blood disorders.

## REFERENCES

1. Report of the Working Conference on Sickle Cell Disease. Bethesda, Maryland, April 5-6, 1971.
2. Motulsky, A.C. Frequency of sickling disorders in U.S. blacks. *N. Engl. J. Med.* 288:31-33, 1973.
3. First Annual Report of the National Sickle Cell Disease Advisory Committee, 1973.

# PART III

# Thalassemia

# 12 Molecular Biology of Thalassemia*

Gary F. Temple, M.D.
Yuet Wai Kan, M.D.

During the past decade, discoveries made in the field of molecular biology have been rapidly applied to the investigation of the molecular mechanism of the thalassemia syndromes. Unlike the abnormal hemoglobin syndromes in which the molecular defects are usually the result of a mutation affecting one or more nucleotides within globin structural genes, the imbalance in $\alpha$ and non-$\alpha$ globin synthesis in thalassemia involves many stages of gene expression.[1] These include deletion of the globin structural genes, unequal crossover, defective transcription and metabolism of globin mRNA, and single nucleotide mutations producing aberrant termination of protein synthesis.[2-8] A single clinical syndrome can result from several different types of molecular defects.[6-8] As such, these disorders provide opportunities to study the effects of various kinds of mutations upon gene expression in higher animals, and, in particular, in man.

*We thank Jennifer Gampell for editorial assistance. This work is supported by NIH grant, AM 16666, National Foundation-March of Dimes, and a contract from the Department of Health, State of California, Maternal and Child Health Branch. Dr. Kan is an investigator of the Howard Hughes Medical Institute.

## NORMAL GLOBIN CHAIN SYNTHESIS

### The Globin Genes

The normal human hemoglobins are listed in Table 12-1. Each of the polypeptide chains is controlled by separate globin structural genes. It is generally agreed that in most populations there are two loci for the $\alpha$ globin structural genes.[2-5,8-11] The strongest evidence for the duplication was the finding of two separate $\alpha$ globin chain mutants, each comprising 25% of the total hemoglobin, together with 50% normal Hb A in the same individual.[12] Also, individuals homozygous for Hb Constant Spring, an elongated $\alpha$ globin chain mutant due to a terminator codon mutuation, also have Hb A.[13] In addition, the number of $\alpha$ globin chains deleted in Hb H disease also indicates that a normal individual has at least four $\alpha$ globin structural genes.[10] On the other hand, in certain populations, there is some evidence to support the theory of a single $\alpha$ structural locus.[4,11] For example, Hb A is absent in Melanesians homozygous for the $\alpha$ mutant, Hb J Tongariki,[14,15] Likewise, patients with the $\alpha$ globin mutant, Hb Q, in combination with $\alpha$ thalassemia, have no Hb A.[2,4,16] Individuals with Hb G Philadelphia have different amounts of Hb G and an individual homozygous for this mutant has no Hb A.[17] However, as these $\alpha$ globin mutants occur in populations in which a significant incidence of $\alpha$-thalassemia is present, the existence of the $\alpha$-thalassemia lesion on the same chromosome as the structural mutation cannot be ruled out.

**Table 12-1**
**Normal Human Hemoglobins**

| Hemoglobin | Polypeptide chain |
|---|---|
| Adult | |
| Hemoglobin A | $\alpha_2\beta_2$ |
| Hemoglobin A$_2$ | $\alpha_2\delta_2$ |
| Fetal | |
| Hemoglobin F | $\alpha_2\gamma_2$ |
| Embryonic | |
| Hemoglobin Portland | $\zeta_2\gamma_2$ |
| Hemoglobin Gower I | $\zeta_2\varepsilon_2$ |
| Hemoglobin Gower II | $\alpha_2\varepsilon_2$ |

Recent studies using restriction mapping (page 144) have shown that the two $\alpha$ globin structural loci are about 4000 nucleotides apart.[18] By using heterokaryons of mouse cells which carry specific human chromosomes, and radioactive probes for human globin structural genes, the $\alpha$ globin structural genes have been localized to chromosome 16.[19] Earlier reports on the location of $\alpha$ globin genes on other chromosomes using in situ hybridization of chromosomes are probably erroneous.

There is little information on the $\zeta$ globin chain, an embryonic $\alpha$-like chain, which resembles the $\alpha$ globin chain in amino acid sequence.[20] During fetal development it combines with the $\gamma$ chain to form Hb Portland ($\zeta_2\gamma_2$), which functions normally in oxygen transport.[21] In normal fetuses Hb Portland disappears almost totally by the twelfth gestational week,[1,22] but in fetuses affected by homozygous $\alpha$ thalassemia, it persists at a level of 7% to 15% of the total hemoglobin at time of delivery.[23,24] A $\beta$-like embryonic chain, $\varepsilon$ chain, is present in both forms of Hb Gower in early fetal life.[1] The chromosomal location of the $\zeta$ and $\varepsilon$ globin genes and their relationship to the other globin genes is not known.

The $\delta$ and $\beta$ structural genes are not duplicated.[11] There are at least two $\gamma$ globin structural genes. This was demonstrated when two $\gamma$ globin chains differing in amino acid sequence at position 136 were found.[25] The chain containing glycine in this position is called $^G\gamma$, and that containing alanine is $^A\gamma$. There could be additional loci for the $\gamma$ chain. For example, a $\gamma$ chain was found recently wherein isoleucine is replaced by threonine in position 75.[26,27] The exact relationship of the chain, called $^T\gamma$, to the $^G\gamma$ and $^A\gamma$ chains is not known.

The structural genes for the $\beta$, $\gamma$, and $\delta$ globins are located on the same chromosome.[11] Recent heterokaryon studies have located the $\beta$, $\gamma$, and presumably the $\delta$ structural genes on chromosome 11.[28] Genetic analysis and examination of globin chains resulting from unequal crossover suggests that the arrangement of these genes on the chromosome is $^G\gamma$, $^A\gamma$, $\delta$, and $\beta$.[11] The exact distance between the $\gamma$ and the $\beta$ structural loci is not certain, but recent studies indicate that the $\delta$ and $\beta$ loci are 5.4 thousand bases apart.[29]

## Messenger RNA

The control mechanisms by which the structural genes are transcribed into mRNA are not fully understood.[30] Recently, studies of mouse, rabbit, and human globin structural genes show that they are not continuous; sequences of nucleotides not represented in the globin chains interrupt the continuity of the structural gene.[29,31,32,32a,32b,32c] More than one such intervening sequence may be present in a structural gene. In the $\beta$ globin genes, for example, there are two intervening sequences of about 100 and 600–900 base pairs.[29,31,32d] Studies in the mouse indicate that when the $\alpha$ and $\beta$ globin mRNAs are first transcribed they include sequences homologous to the intervening sequences.[33a,33b] These sequences subsequently are excised and the processed mRNA reaches the cytoplasm, now 600–780 nucleotides in length.[33a,33b,34] Intervening sequences have recently been found in other structural genes,[35] such as ovalbumin[36,37] and immunoglobulin.[38]

Other modifications of the mRNA occur. A stretch of polyadenylic acids [poly(A)] of approximately 100 to 200 nucleotides in length is added at the 3' end of the molecule.[39] The poly(A) sequence is gradually shortened during the maturation of erythroblasts to reticulocytes.[40] It probably serves to stabilize the mRNA against degradation.[41] At the 5' end, a 5' cap structure containing 7-methylguanosine ($m^7G$) in a 5' to 5' pyrophosphate linkage is added and specific nucleotides are methylated.[42] The cap structure promotes efficient binding of the globin mRNAs to ribosomes during initiation of protein synthesis, but is probably not absolutely required for this activity.[42-45]

Cytoplasmic globin mRNA contains a translated region starting with the sequence AUG and ending with a terminator codon.[42] This coding region is 429 nucleotides in length for the $\alpha$ globin, and 444 for the $\beta$ and $\gamma$ globins.[46] Preceding the AUG sequence is a 5' untranslated region containing 38 nucleotides for $\alpha$,[47,48] 51 for $\beta$,[47,48] and 54 for $\gamma$ globin.[49] Following the terminator codon and before the poly(A), there is a region of nucleotides which is normally untranslated. Their lengths are 109 for $\alpha$,[50,51] 132 for $\beta$,[52,53] and 87 for $\gamma$.[54] The 5' and 3' untranslated sequences of $\alpha$ and $\beta$ mRNAs appear to be conserved between rabbit and human species.

The process of translation of globin mRNA into globin polypeptides involves other components apart from the mRNAs.[42] A defect in one of these could produce globin chain deficiencies. However, examination of the function of thalassemia ribosomes, transfer RNAs, and soluble factors has detected no abnormalities.[1,4] Furthermore, in $\beta^+$ thalassemic cells, the rates of initiation, elongation, and termination of the polypeptide chains, as well as the assembly of the completed chains into their hemoglobin tetramers, appear to be normal.[1,4] An exception to this is the possible deficiency of a postulated $\beta$ mRNA specific factor in cells from patients with homozygous $\beta^0$ thalassemia of the Ferrara type.[55,56]

## METHODS USED IN THE INVESTIGATION OF THALASSEMIA

### Globin Chain Synthesis

The presence of specific globin chain deficiencies in the different thalassemias is demonstrated by protein synthesis experiments using intact erythroid cells.[57] Whole blood or enriched reticulocytes are incubated with radioactive amino acids, and the rate of incorporation of these radioactive amino acids into the different globin chains is measured after separation of the chains on carboxymethyl cellulose column chromatography.[57] These studies have confirmed that indeed $\alpha$ globin chain synthesis is deficient in $\alpha$ thalassemia and $\beta$ chain synthesis is impaired in $\beta$ thalassemia.

## Cell-Free Synthesis Studies

To characterize the lesion in thalassemia further, globin mRNA extracted from the blood of thalassemic patients is assayed in a number of heterologous systems, including the rabbit reticulocyte lysate,[58] ascites tumor cells,[59] and wheat germ.[60] Translation can also be studied after injection of mRNA into Xenopus oocytes.[42] The protein synthesis directed by the added messenger in these heterologous systems can then be analyzed. Since the globin chain defect in thalassemia is reproducible in these heterologous systems, it is clear that the defect lies in the mRNA.[58-60] Whether this defect is due to the lack of a specific globin mRNA or to the presence of a defective mRNA can be distinguished by methods that quantitate the specific globin mRNAs.

## mRNA Quantitation

The rapid advances in the study of thalassemia owe a great deal to the discovery of RNA-dependent DNA polymerase, or reverse transcriptase.[61,62] With this enzyme, a DNA copy complementary to mRNA sequences (cDNA) can be synthesized and used to quantitate the amount of mRNA.[63] Specific cDNAs complementary to $\alpha$ and $\beta$ globin mRNA sequences can be synthesized and used for hybridization analysis to compare the amount of $\alpha$ and $\beta$ globin mRNA in the erythroid cell.[64] When a globin cDNA is incubated with a preparation of mRNA to be analyzed, the rate and extent to which the cDNA anneals to complementary globin mRNA sequences depends on the concentration of globin RNA sequences in the reaction.[65]

Globin mRNA can also be separated by electrophoresis under specific conditions, as the $\alpha$ globin mRNA is shorter than the $\gamma$, which in turn is shorter than the $\beta$.[64] Using this technique, a specific deficiency in one species of globin mRNA can be detected. However, as the resolution of the different species on electrophoresis is not complete, this method is not as quantitative as the hybridization analysis.

## Measurement of Globin Genes

A globin mRNA could be absent as a result of a defect in the transcription process, or as a result of the absence of that globin structural gene due to deletion. To distinguish between these possibilities, two methods of hybridization analysis can be applied to the genomic DNA.

**Liquid Hybridization**     In this method, cellular DNA is reannealed in the presence of globin cDNA. If the globin gene is present, the rate of annealing of cDNA to globin genes is related to the number of globin genes present.[65] If the globin gene is absent, the cDNA will not be annealed to any cellular DNA. Thus, measurement of the rate and quantity of cDNA converted into double stranded DNA would indicate the presence or absence of a structural gene, as well as the number of globin genes.[65]

**Gene Mapping**     Cellular DNA is digested with restriction endonucleases, enzymes that cleave DNA only at specific sequences.[66] The DNA fragments are then separated according to size by agarose gel electrophoresis and transferred to a nitrocellulose filter.[67] The immobilized DNA fragments are hybridized with specific radioactive cDNA probes, and the bands containing globin cDNA are identified by autoradiography. Through the use of different restriction enzymes it is possible to map and detect many genes, including the globin genes.[18,29]

## MOLECULAR MECHANISM OF THALASSEMIA

Table 12-2 lists those thalassemia syndromes in which the molecular mechanisms are known.

**Table 12-2**
**The Thalassemias and Related Syndromes**

---

I.   α Thalassemia
　　a. Deletion defects
　　　　Silent carrier state (α thalassemia-2)
　　　　Heterozygous α thalassemia (α thalassemia-1)
　　　　Hemoglobin H disease
　　　　Homozygous α thalassemia (hydrops fetalis)

　　b. Nondeletion defects
　　　　Terminator codon mutation (hemoglobin Constant Spring)
　　　　Nondeletion α thalassemia-1 and hemoglobin H disease

II.  β Thalassemia
　　a. Deletion defects
　　　　Hemoglobin Lepore syndromes (unequal crossover)
　　　　$\delta^0\beta^0$ thalassemia

　　b. β thalassemia with elevated $A_2$
　　　　　$\beta^+$ thalassemia
　　　　　$\beta^0$ thalassemia

III. Hereditary persistence of fetal hemoglobin (HPFH)
　　a. Deletion
　　　　HPFH of the African type
　　　　HPFH with hemoglobin Kenya (unequal crossover)

---

## α Thalassemia

The molecular mechanisms of α thalassemia have been best defined in the Asian population. The four syndromes can be classified by globin chain synthesis studies. In homozygous α thalassemia, no α globin chain is synthesized; in Hb H disease, the α/β ratio is around 0.3; in heterozygous α thalassemia, this ratio is 0.75, and in the silent carrier state it is 0.85.[2,68,69] Cell-free synthesis studies [9,70-73] as well as hybridization experiments[9,71,73,74] with mRNA isolated from reticulocytes of patients with various α-thalassemia syndromes have demonstrated that α mRNA is deficient and that its concentration correlates with the amount of α globin chain synthesized. Thus, in homozygous α thalassemia, no globin mRNA is present,[73] whereas in Hb H disease the concentration of α globin mRNA is approximately 10% to 30% of β mRNA.[9,10,71,74] When the DNA from these patients was studied by molecular hybridization, it was found that there are no α globin structural genes in homozygous α thalassemia.[9,73,75] Detailed analysis of the kinetics of hybridization shows that the structural gene deletion is complete.[76] In Hb H disease, only one of the four normally present α globin genes is present.[9,10,77] This provides additional evidence for the duplication of α globin structural genes. Hybridization showed that two α globin structural genes are present in α thalassemia-1.[77] Recent gene mapping studies have confirmed these findings.[18,78] For example, in homozygous α thalassemia, the DNA restriction fragment containing α globin structural genes was absent, and in Hb H disease, the DNA fragment containing the α globin loci appeared to be shortened.[78]

Another mechanism producing α thalassemia is Hb Constant Spring and related syndromes, in which mutation results in the production of an elongated α globin chain.[1,79] In this disease, there is a mutation of the DNA in the region of the terminator codon. In the human α globin mRNA, the terminator codon is UAA.[49] In Hb Constant Spring disease, this is presumably mutated to CAA, which is a codon for glutamine. Instead of terminating, glutamine is inserted and the globin chain continues for an additional 31 amino acids until another terminator codon is reached. For reasons not yet understood the elongated α chain is produced in small amounts and may also be degraded more rapidly.[80] The clinical effect is similar to that of α thalassemia-2, in which one α globin structural gene is deleted. Hence, in combination with the α thalassemia-1 gene, the Hb Constant Spring defect results in Hb H disease.[2,79] This is diagnosed by detecting the Constant Spring component, which migrates much more slowly than Hb $A_2$ on electrophoresis.[2] Single nucleotide mutations of the terminator codon UAA could theoretically give rise to six different types of terminator codon mutations, each producing elongated α chains. In fact, four have been found.[3,79]

Recently, a nondeletion type of $\alpha$ thalassemia defect has been detected.[81] Here, although both structural genes are present on the same chromosome, $\alpha$ globin chain synthesis directed by this chromosome is reduced. A carrier of this nondeletion lesion phenotypically resembles $\alpha$ thalassemia-1. However, the defect is not complete because the combination of this gene with the deletion type of $\alpha$ thalassemia-1 gene produces some $\alpha$ globin chain and results in Hb H disease instead of homozygous $\alpha$ thalassemia.[81]

The distribution of $\alpha$ thalassemia in the world populations varies according to ethnic origin (Table 12-3).[3] While all types of $\alpha$ thalassemia are common in people of Asian origin, in the Mediterranean population, although Hb H disease is found not infrequently, only one case of homozygous $\alpha$ thalassemia has ever been described.[82] In people of African origin, cord blood screening has demonstrated the incidence of $\alpha$ thalassemia-1 and $\alpha$ thalassemia-2 to be approximately 3% to 5% each.[2] However, Hb H is extremely rare in this population, and homozygous $\alpha$ thalassemia associated with hydrops fetalis has never been described.

**Table 12-3**
**The Distribution of $\alpha$-Thalassemia Syndromes in Different Populations**

|  | Asian | Mediterranean | African |
|---|---|---|---|
| $\alpha$ Thalassemia | Present | Present | Present |
| Hemoglobin H disease | Present | Present | Rare |
| Homozygous $\alpha$ thalassemia | Present | 1 case reported | Absent |

The reasons for the peculiar ethnic distribution of $\alpha$ thalassemia are unclear. Recent data indicate that $\alpha$ thalassemia-1 in the African population is most commonly due to deletion.[83] Study of one black patient with Hb H disease revealed the presence of only one $\alpha$ globin structural gene, as is found in Asian patients with Hb H disease.[83a] It has been suggested and recent evidence confirms[83b] that in the black, the phenotype of $\alpha$ thalassemia-1 is most often due to homozygous $\alpha$ thalassemia-2; that is, deletion of the two $\alpha$ globin genes occurs in transposition. The notable lack of hydrops fetalis in Africans is probably due to the very low incidence of cis deletion of two $\alpha$ genes in this population.[83b].

In the Mediterranean population, the reason for the lack of homozygous $\alpha$ thalassemia is not known, but a preliminary study indicates that the nondeletion defect appears to be more common than in the Asian population.[84] However, whether or not this accounts for the distribution of the different syndromes requires further study.

## β Thalassemia

In the common type of β thalassemia, δ globin chain synthesis is not impaired, and the Hb $A_2$ level is elevated.[2] In heterozygous β thalassemia, study of the peripheral blood reticulocytes showed that the β/α ratio is 0.5.[85-88] On the other hand, the ratio in the bone marrow is very close to unity.[85-88] The explanation for this is unclear. It has been postulated that there is a contaminating protein in the bone marrow which migrates in the same area as the $β^A$ chain on carboxymethyl cellulose chromatography.[87,88] However, the same phenomenon is also found in patients with sickle cell β thalassemia, making this explanation unlikely.[89] It has also been proposed that there is a compensatory decrease in α globin chain synthesis.[1,90] as well as an increase in proteolysis of the excess α globin chain.[87,88,91] Probably both mechanisms are responsible for the equalization of the β/α ratio in the bone marrow.

Study of globin chain synthesis in the homozygous state reveals two types of β thalassemia, one with some residual β chain ($β^+$ type) and another with no β chain ($β^0$ type).[7,92] Molecular hybridization studies have demonstrated that β globin structural genes are present in both types of diseases.[9,93-94] In $β^+$ thalassemia, the amount of β globin chain synthesized varies from a trace to about 10% of the α chain synthesis. The globin mRNA content appears to correlate with the amount of globin chain produced.[9,71,74] The molecular structure of the β globin mRNA in $β^+$ thalassemia has not been investigated. Recently, a study comparing the nuclear and cytoplasmic content of β globin mRNA showed a relatively larger amount of the β chain in the nuclear fraction as compared to the cytoplasmic fraction.[95] This study suggested that there is an increased turnover of this mRNA. However, further studies which follow the life span of labeled mRNA are needed to support this conclusion. Studies on the assembly of the β chain show that the rates of initiation, elongation, and termination of the β chain are normal in $β^+$ thalassemia.[1]

There is disagreement concerning the presence or absence of the β globin mRNA in $β^0$ thalassemia.[7,93,94,96-98] In fact, the molecular pathology may be heterogeneous. A difficulty with the use of β globin cDNA for detecting a small amount of β globin mRNA in hybridization analysis is that crosshybridization between the β globin cDNA and δ globin mRNA probably occurs. In one type of patient with homozygous $β^0$ thalassemia, a small amount of β globin mRNA-like material has been detected by hybridization.[74,93,96,97] This could be due to the presence of a small amount of β globin mRNA. Alternatively, β globin mRNA could be absent and the RNA sequences detected by the β globin cDNA could be δ globin mRNA. These findings are variable in some patients. One patient who had trace amounts of $\beta$-like globin mRNA in one study had 15% as much $\beta$ as $\alpha$ globin mRNA on a separate occasion.[97] In some other patients, the bone marrow contained more $\beta$ mRNA relative to $\alpha$ than in the reticulocytes. Recently, in a study using 3' and 5' probes, there was a suggestion of a loss of part of the $\beta$ mRNA in some patients.[98] However, more investigation is needed before this can be clarified.

In another type of $\beta^0$ thalassemia, hybridization studies have conclusively demonstrated the presence of $\beta$ globin mRNA at about one-fifth to one-half the concentration of $\alpha$ globin mRNA.[94,98,99] RNA as well as cDNA sequence analysis has also revealed authentic $\beta$ globin mRNA sequences.[100,101] This mRNA does not direct $\beta$ globin synthesis in heterologous cell-free systems.[99] Sequence analysis of defective $\beta$ globin mRNA in one patient demonstrated a single base mutation in the codon for amino acid 17, lysine (AAG), producing a terminator codon (UAG).[101a] Addition of an amber suppressor tRNA (which inserts serine at UAG) to a cell-free system programmed with $\beta^0$ mRNA allowed the synthesis of full length $\beta$ globin chains.[101b]

A third type of $\beta^0$ thalassemia is the Ferrara type. In this syndrome, although there is no $\beta$ globin chain synthesis, study in homologous cell-free systems has demonstrated some $\beta$ globin chain synthesis upon the addition of an undefined factor from the cells of normal individuals.[56] In addition, in some of these patients, $\beta$ globin chain synthesis could be induced in vivo by blood transfusion.[102] Molecular hybridization experiments show that there may be some $\beta$-like material in such patients.[94,103] However, the exact molecular mechanism is not understood.

Thus, unlike the $\alpha$ thalassemia syndromes in which in most cases the defects are fairly well characterized, the exact molecular mechanism in most of the $\beta$ thalassemias is still not known. In $\beta^+$ thalassemia, the decrease in $\beta$ globin mRNA could be due to defective transcription of the $\beta$ globin gene or to a defective processing of the mRNA, or to both. Such mRNA could have a shortened life span and would turn over prematurely. In $\beta^0$ thalassemia, there may be patients who have no $\beta$ globin mRNA due to absence of transcription, or a defect in the $\beta$ globin RNA transcript may result in its rapid turnover and destruction in the nucleus during processing. In $\beta^0$ thalassemia with nonfunctional $\beta$ globin mRNA, an abnormality in a structural or intervening sequence may result in abnormal processing so that the mRNA does not direct normal protein synthesis. One known mechanism is a mutation which results in an early terminator codon so that synthesis of the globin chain terminates prematurely. Such short peptides may be destroyed rapidly and escape detection.

## Hereditary Persistence of Fetal Hemoglobin and $\delta^0\beta^0$ Thalassemia

Both these disorders are due to deletion of the $\beta$ and $\delta$ globin structural genes.[94,104-107] In the homozygous states, only Hb F is synthesized; Hbs A and A$_2$ are absent. The $\gamma/\alpha$ ratios are unbalanced in $\delta^0\beta^0$ thalassemia, but are almost balanced in hereditary persistence of fetal hemoglobin.[1,3,104] Recent hybridization and gene restriction mapping studies show that the amount of $\beta$ and $\delta$ structural genes deleted varies. These studies indicate that in HPFH there is a greater length of DNA sequence deleted than in $\delta^0\beta^0$ thalassemia.[108a,108b] It is possible that the difference between these two syndromes depends on whether or not a critical region of DNA is involved. If one assumes that this region is essential for initiating the switch from fetal to adult hemoglobin synthesis, its deletion may result in the loss of the signal to switch to adult hemoglobin and fetal hemoglobin synthesis would persist. If this region is not involved, then the switching from $\gamma$ to adult hemoglobin synthesis could be attempted. And, in the absence of intact $\delta$ and $\beta$ genes, the $\delta^0\beta^0$ thalassemia condition would ensue.

## Hemoglobin Lepore Syndromes and Hemoglobin Kenya

These diseases are examples of unequal crossover of the DNA.[109] In Hb Lepore, the non-$\alpha$ chain is made up of $\delta$ globin near the amino end and $\beta$ globin at the carboxyl end.[109] The several types of Hb Lepore are due to the differences in the points at which the crossover occurs.[4] These hemoglobins are synthesized in decreased amounts.[110] Hybridization studies show that in the homozygous states, the Lepore mRNA to $\alpha$ mRNA ratio is decreased to 0.1.[111] Whether this is due to defective production or to increased turnover has not yet been established. The reduced amount of Hb Lepore results in non-$\alpha$ globin chain deficiency. Thus, the homozygous state of Hb Lepore and the double heterozygosity of Hb Lepore and $\beta$ thalassemia result in syndromes similar to homozygous $\beta$ thalassemia.[1,4]

Hemoglobin Kenya is also the result of a crossover. In this syndrome a hybrid globin chain is made up of $\gamma$ chain at the amino end and $\beta$ chain at the carboxyl end.[112] Presumably, by a crossover mechanism, deletion starts from the sequences encoding for the 3' end of the $^A\gamma$ gene, includes the $\delta$ gene, and extends to the 5' end of the $\beta$ globin genes. It is interesting to note that the clinical manifestation of this disease is hereditary persistence of fetal hemoglobin. The fetal hemoglobin present is the $^G\gamma$ type.[113] Thus, the postulated region essential for the switch may be contained somewhere within the deleted region.

## CONCLUSION

The thalassemias are an extremely complex group of syndromes, with large numbers of molecular alterations which commonly result in imbalanced $\alpha$ and non-$\alpha$ globin chain synthesis. The exact defects in many of these disorders are not known. For example, in the $\alpha$ thalassemias, although the number of $\alpha$ globin genes deleted in each syndrome can be estimated, the extent of the deletion and its effect on the sequences surrounding the structural genes are not known. In the $\beta$ thalassemias, we have some idea as to the presence or absence of the $\beta$ globin mRNA; however, the reasons for the reduction in quantity or the failure of this mRNA to function are not known in most cases.

The advances made in molecular biology are providing new insights into normal and abnormal mechanisms of gene expression. For example, the discovery of intervening sequences within the globin genes suggests a possible explanation for some thalassemia syndromes. With the advent of the technology of cloning mammalian genes in bacteria, it is now possible to obtain large quantities of purified globin genes for detailed analysis. As these and future developments are applied to the thalassemia syndromes, the basic molecular defects will be further defined.

## REFERENCES

1. Bunn, H.F., Forget, B.G., and Ranney, H.M. *Human Hemoglobins.* Philadelphia: W.B. Saunders Co., 1977.

2. Weatherall, D.J., and Clegg, J.B. *The Thalassemia Syndromes.* 2nd Ed. Oxford: Blackwell Scientific Publications, 1972.

3. Weatherall, D.J., The thalassemias. Edited by W.J. Williams, E. Beutler, A.J. Erslev, and R.W. Rundles. In *Hematology.* 2nd Ed. New York: McGraw Hill Book Company, 1977.

4. Benz, E.J., and Forget, B.G. The molecular genetics of the thalassemia syndromes. *Prog. Hematol.* 9:107–155, 1975.

5. Bank, A. The thalassemia syndromes. *Blood* 51:369–384, 1978.

6. Nienhuis, A., and Benz, E.J. Regulation of hemoglobin synthesis during the development of the red cell. Part 2. *N. Engl. J. Med.* 297:1371–1381, 1977.

7. Benz, E.J., Jr. Molecular heterogeneity of the $\beta^0$ thalassemias. *Nature* 263:635–636, 1976.

8. Orkin, S.A., and Nathan, D.G. The thalassemias. *N. Engl. J. Med.* 295:710–714, 1976.

9. Ramirez, F., Natta, C., O'Donnell, J.V., et al. Relative numbers of human globin genes assayed with purified $\alpha$ and $\beta$ complementary DNA. *Proc. Natl. Acad. Sci. USA* 72:1550–1554, 1975.

10. Kan, Y.W., Dozy, A.M., Varmus, H.E., et al. Deletion of $\alpha$-globin genes in hemoglobin-H disease demonstrates multiple $\alpha$-globin structural loci. *Nature* 255:255–256, 1975.

11. Weatherall, D.J., and Clegg, J.B. Molecular genetics of human hemoglobin. *Annu. Rev. Genet.* 10:157–178, 1976.

12. Hollan, S.R., Szelenyi, J.G., Brimhall, G., et al. Multiple α chain loci for human hemoglobin: Hb J-Buda and Hb G-Pest. *Nature* 235:47–50, 1972.

13. Lie-Injo, L.E., Ganesan, J., Clegg, J.B., et al. Homozygous state for Hb Constant Spring. *Blood* 43:251–259, 1974:

14. Abramson, R.K., Rucknagel, D.L., Shreffler, D.C., et al. Homozygous Hb J Tongariki: Evidence for only one alpha chain structural locus in Melanesians. *Science* 169:194–196, 1970.

15. Beaven, G.H., Hornabrook, R.W., Fox, R.H., et al. Occurrence of heterozygotes and homozygotes for the α-chain haemoglobin variant Hb J (Tongariki) in New Guinea. *Nature* 235:46–47, 1972.

16. Forget, B.G., and Kan, Y.W. Thalassemia and the genetics of hemoglobin. Edited by D.G. Nathan and F.A. Oski. In *Hematology of Infancy and Childhood*. Philadelphia: W.B. Saunders Co., 1974.

17. Baine, R.M., Rucknagel, D.L., Dublin, P.A., et al. Trimodality in the proportion of hemoglobin G Philadelphia in heterozygotes: Evidence for heterogeneity in the number of human α chain loci. *Proc. Natl. Acad. Sci. USA* 73:3633–3636, 1976.

18. Orkin, S.A. The duplicated human α globin genes lie close together in cellular DNA. *Proc. Natl. Acad. Sci. USA* 75:5950–5954, 1978.

19. Deisseroth, A., Nienhuis, A., and Turner, P. Localization of the human alpha globin structural gene to chromosome 16 in somatic cell hybrids by molecular hybridization assay. *Cell* 12:205–218, 1977.

20. Kamuzora, H., and Lehmann, H. Human embryonic haemoglobins including a comparison by homology of the human ζ and α chains. *Nature* 256:511–513, 1975.

21. Huehns, E.R., and Farooqui, A.M. Oxygen dissociation studies of red cells from chicken, mouse, and human embryos. Ciba Foundation Symposium. In *Congenital Disorders of Erythropoiesis*. New York: Elsevier, 1976.

22. Pataryas, H.A., and Stamatoyannopoulos, G. Hemoglobins in human fetuses: Evidence for adult hemoglobin production after the 11th gestational week. *Blood* 39:688–696, 1972.

23. Todd, D., Lai, M.C.S., Beaven, G.H., et al. The abnormal hemoglobins in homozygous α-thalassaemia. *Br. J. Haematol.* 19:27–31, 1970.

24. Weatherall, D.J., Clegg, J.B., and Knox-Macaulay, A.H.M. The haemoglobin constitution of infants with the haemoglobin Bart's hydrops fetalis syndrome. *Br. J. Haematol.* 18:357–367, 1970.

25. Huisman, T.H.J., Schroeder, W.A., Bannister, W.H., et al. Evidence for four nonallelic structural genes for γ-chain of human fetal hemoglobin. *Biochem. Genet.* 7:131–139, 1972.

26. Ricco, G., Mazza, U., Turi, R.M., et al. Significance of a new type of human fetal hemoglobin carrying a replacement isoleucine→threonine at position 75 (E19) of the γ chain. *Hum. Genet.* 32:305–313, 1976.

27. Huisman, T.H.J., Schroeder, W.A., Reese, J.B., et al. The $^T$γ chain of human fetal hemoglobin at birth and in several abnormal hematological conditions. *Pediatr. Res.* 11:1102, 1977.

28. Deisseroth, A., Nienhuis, A., Lawrence, J., et al. Chromosomal localization of human β-globin gene on human chromosome 11 in somatic cell hybrids. *Proc. Natl. Acad. Sci. USA* 75:1456–1460, 1978.

29. Lawn, R.M., Fritsch, E.C., Packer, R.C., et al. The isolation and characterization of linked δ- and β-globin genes from a cloned library of human DNA. *Cell* 15:1157–1174, 1978.

30. Nienhuis, A., and Benz, E.J. Regulation of hemoglobin synthesis during the development of the red cell. Part 1. *N. Engl. J. Med.* 297:1318–1328, 1977.

31. Tilghman, S.M., Tiemeier, D.C., Seidman, J.G., et al. Intervening

sequence of DNA identified in the structural portion of a mouse β-globin gene. *Proc. Natl. Acad. Sci. USA* 75:725–729, 1978.

32a. Jeffreys, A.J., and Flavell, R.A. The rabbit β-globin gene contains a large insert in the coding sequence. *Cell* 12:1097–1108, 1977.

32b. Mears, J.G., Ramirez, F., Leibowitz, D., et al. Organization of human δ- and β-globin genes in cellular DNA and the presence of intragenic inserts. *Cell* 15:15–23, 1978.

32c. Flavell, R.A., Kooter, J.M., DeBoer, E., et al. Analysis of β-δ-globin gene loci in normal and Hb Lepore DNA: Direct determination of gene linkage and intergene distance. *Cell* 15:25–41, 1978.

32d. Van den Berg, J., Van Ooyen, A., Mantei, N., et al. Comparison of cloned rabbit and mouse β-globin genes showing strong evolutionary divergence of two homologous pairs of introns. *Nature* 276:37–44, 1978.

33a. Tilghman, S.M., Curtis, P.J., Tiemeier, D.C., et al. The intervening sequence of a mouse β-globin gene is transcribed within the 15s β-globin mRNA precursor. *Proc. Natl. Acad. Sci. USA* 75:1309–1313, 1978.

33b. Curtis, P.J., Mantei, N., Van den Berg, J., et al. Presence of a putative 15s precursor to β globin mRNA but not to α globin mRNA in Friend cells. *Proc. Natl. Acad. Sci. USA* 74:3184–3188, 1977.

34. Bastos, R.N., and Aviv, H. Globin RNA precursor molecules: Biosynthesis and processing in erythroid cells. *Cell* 11:641–650, 1977.

35. Williamson, R. DNA insertions and gene structure. *Nature* 270:295–297, 1977.

36. Breathnack, R., Mandel, J.L., and Chambon, P. Ovalbumin gene is split in chicken DNA. *Nature* 270:314–319, 1977.

37. Weinstock, R., Sweet, R., Weiss, M., et al. Intragenic DNA spacers interrupt the ovalbumin gene. *Proc. Natl. Acad. Sci. USA* 75:1299–1303, 1978.

38. Brack, C., and Tonegawa, S. Variable and constant parts of the immunoglobin light chain gene of a mouse myeloma cell are 1250 non-translated bases apart. *Proc. Natl. Acad. Sci. USA* 74:5652–5656, 1977.

39. Merkel, C.G., Kwan, S-P, and Lingrel, J.B. Size of the polyadenylic acid region of newly synthesized globin messenger ribonucleic acid. *J. Biol. Chem.* 250:3725–3728, 1975.

40. Merkel, C.G., Wood, T.G., and Lingrel, J.B. Shortening of the poly(A) region of mouse globin messenger RNA. *J. Biol. Chem.* 251:5512–5515, 1976.

41. Huez, G., Marbaix, G., Hubert, E., et al. Readenylation of polyadenlate-free globin messenger RNA restores its stability in vivo. *Eur. J. Biochem.* 59:589–592, 1975.

42. Lodish, H.F. Translational control of protein synthesis. *Ann. Rev. Biochem.* 45:39–72, 1976.

43. Kowalczewska, M.Z., Bretner, M., Sierakowska, A., et al. Removal of 5′-terminal m⁷G from eucaryotic mRNAs by potato nucleotide pyrophosphatase and its effect on translation. *Nucleic Acids Res.* 4:3065–3080, 1977.

44. Held, W.A., West, K., and Gallagher, J.P. Importance of initiation factor preparations in the translation of reovirus and globin mRNAs lacking a 5′-terminal 7-methylguanosine. *J. Biol. Chem.* 252:8489–8497, 1977.

45. Kaempfer, R., Rosen, H., and Israeli, R. Translational control: Recognition of the 5′ methylated end and an internal sequence in eucaryotic mRNA by the initiation factor that binds methionyl-tRNA$_f^{Met}$. *Proc. Natl. Acad. Sci. USA* 75:650–654, 1978.

46. Dayhoff, M.O. *Atlas of Protein Sequence and Structure.* Vol. 5. Washington, D.C.: National Biomedical Research Foundation, 1972.

47. Chang, J.C., Temple, G.F., Poon, R.P., et al. The nucleotide sequences

of the untranslated 5' regions of human α- and β-globin mRNAs. *Proc. Natl. Acad. Sci. USA* 74:5145–5149, 1977.

48. Baralle, F.E. Complete nucleotide sequence of the 5' noncoding region of human α- and β-globin mRNA. *Cell* 12:1085–1095, 1977.

49. Change, J.C., Poon, R., Neumann, K.H., and Kan, Y.W. The nucleotide sequence of the 5' untranslated region of human γ-globin mRNA. *Nucleic Acids Res.* 5:3515–3522, 1978.

50. Wilson, J.T., de Riel, J.K., Forget, B.G., et al. Nucleotide sequence of 3' untranslated portion of human alpha globin mRNA. *Nucleic Acids Res.* 4:2353–2368, 1977.

51. Proudfoot, N.J., and Longley, J.I. The 3' terminal sequences of human α and β globin messenger RNAs: Comparison with rabbit globin messenger RNA. *Cell* 9:733–746, 1976.

52. Marrotta, C.A., Wilson, J.T., Forget, B.G., et al. Human β globin messenger RNA. III. Nucleotide sequences derived from complementary DNA. *J. Biol. Chem.* 252:5040–5053, 1977.

53. Proudfoot, N.J. Complete 3' noncoding region sequences of rabbit and human β globin messenger RNAs. *Cell* 10:559–570, 1977.

54. Poon, R., Kan, Y.W., and Boyer, H.W. Sequence of the 3'-noncoding and adjacent coding regions of human γ-globin mRNA. *Nucleic Acids Res.* 5:4625–4630, 1978.

55. Conconi, F. and Del Senno, L. The molecular defect of the Ferrara β-thalassemia. *Ann. NY Acad. Sci.* 232:54–64, 1974.

56. Conconi, F., Rowley, P.T., Del Senno, L., et al. Induction of β-globin synthesis in the β thalassaemia of Ferrara. *Nature (New Biol.)* 238:83–87, 1972.

57. Kan, Y.W., Nathan, D.G., Cividalli, G., et al. Intrauterine diagnosis of thalassemia. *Ann. NY Acad. Sci.* 232:145–151, 1974.

58. Nienhuis, A.W., and Anderson, W.F. Isolation and translation of hemoglobin messenger RNA from thalassemia, sickle sell anemia and normal human reticulocytes. *J. Clin. Invest.* 50:2458–2460, 1971.

59. Dow, L.W., Terada, M., Natta, C., et al. Globin synthesis of intact cells and activity of isolated mRNA in β thalassemia. *Nature (New Biol.)* 243:114–116, 1973.

60. Pritchard, J., Longley, J., Clegg, J.B., et al. Assay of thalassaemic messenger RNA in the wheat germ system. *Br. J. Haematol.* 32:473–485, 1976.

61. Baltimore, D. Viral RNA dependent DNA polymerase. *Nature* 226:1209–1211, 1970.

62. Temin, H.M., and Mizutani, S. RNA-dependent DNA polymerase in virions of Rous sarcoma virus. *Nature* 226:1211–1213, 1970.

63. Verma, I.M., Temple, G.F., Fan, H., et al. In vitro synthesis of DNA complementary to rabbit globin mRNA. *Nature (New Biol.)* 235:163–167, 1972.

64. Forget, B.G., Housman, D., Benz, E., et al. Synthesis of DNA complementary to separate human α and β globin messenger RNAs. *Proc. Natl. Acad. Sci. USA* 72:984–988, 1975.

65. Wetmur, J.G. Hybridization and renaturation kinetics of nucleic acids. *Annu. Rev. Biophys. Bioeng.* 5:337–361, 1976.

66. Roberts, R.J., The role of restriction endonucleases in genetic engineering. Edited by R.F. Beerks, Jr., and E.G. Basselt. In *Recombinant Molecules: Impact on Science and Society*. New York: Raven Press, 1977.

67. Southern, E.M. Detection of specific sequences among DNA fragments separated by gel electrophoresis. *J. Mol. Biol.* 98:503–517, 1975.

68. Schwartz, E., Kan, Y.W., and Nathan, D.G. Unbalanced globin chain synthesis in alpha-thalassemia heterozygotes. *Ann. NY Acad. Sci.* 165:288–294, 1969.

69. Kan, Y.W., Schwartz, E., and Nathan, D.G. Globin chain synthesis in the α-thalassemia syndromes. *J. Clin. Invest.* 47:2515–2522, 1969.

70. Benz, E.J., Jr., Swerdlow, P.S., and Forget, B.G. Globin messenger RNA in hemoglobin H disease. *Blood* 42:825–833, 1973.

71. Kacian, D.L., Gambino, R., Dow, L.W., et al. Decreased globin messenger RNA in thalassemia detected by molecular hybridization. *Proc. Natl. Acad. Sci. USA* 70:1886–1890, 1973.

72. Grossbard, E., Terada, M., Dow, L.W., et al. Decreased α globin messenger RNA activity with polyribosomes in α thalassemia. *Nature (New Biol.)* 241:209–211, 1973.

73. Taylor, J.M., Dozy, A., Kan, Y.W., et al. Genetic lesion in homozygous α thalassemia (hydrops fetalis). *Nature* 251:392–393, 1974.

74. Housman, D., Forget, B.G., Skoultchi, A., et al. Quantitative deficiency of chain specific globin mRNA in the thalassemia syndromes. *Proc. Natl. Acad. Sci. USA* 70:1809–1813, 1973.

75. Ottolenghi, S., Lanyon, W.G., Paul, J., et al. Gene deletion as the cause of α-thalassaemia. *Nature* 251:389–392, 1974.

76. Meehan, J., Ramirez, F., Mears, J.G., et al. Extent of deletion of α globin genes in homozygous α thalassemia. *Clin. Res.* 26:330A, 1978.

77. Kan, Y.W., Dozy, A.M., Varmus, H.E., et al. The molecular basis of the α-thalassemia syndromes. *Clin. Res.* 23:398A, 1975.

78. Embury, S.H., Dozy, A.M., and Kan, Y.W. Heterogeneity between Hb H deletion and non-deletion syndromes further defined by restriction endonuclease gene mapping. *Blood* 52:111, 1978.

79. Weatherall, D.J., and Clegg, J.B. The α-chain termination mutants and their relationship to α-thalassaemia. *Philos. Trans. R. Soc. Lond. (Biol.)* 271:411–455, 1975.

80. Kan, Y.W., Todd, D., and Dozy, A.M. Haemoglobin Constant Spring synthesis in red cell precursors. *Br. J. Haematol.* 28:103–107, 1974.

81. Kan, Y.W., Dozy, A.M., Trecartin, R., et al. Identification of a nondeletion defect in α-thalassemia. *N. Engl. J. Med.* 297:1081–1084, 1977.

82. Diamond, M.P., Cotgrove, I., and Parker, A. Case of intrauterine death due to α-thalassaemia. *Br. Med. J.* 2:278–279, 1965.

83a. Davis, J.R., Dozy, A.M., Lubin, B., et al. The molecular mechanism of α thalassemia in the black. *Blood* 50:105, 1977.

83b. Dozy, A.M., Kan, Y.W., Koenig, H.M., et al. Alpha globin gene organization in Blacks precludes the severe form of α thalassemia. *Clin. Res.* In press, 1979.

84. Kan, Y.W., Dozy, A.M., and Stamatoyannopoulos, G. Heterogeneity in the molecular pathology of α-thalassemia. *Clin. Res.* 26:500A, 1978.

85. Schwartz, E. Heterozygous beta thalassemia: Balanced globin synthesis in bone marrow cells. *Science* 67:1512–1214, 1970.

86. Kan, Y.W., Nathan, D.G., and Lodish, H.F. Equal synthesis of α and β globin chains in erythroid precursors in heterozygous β thalassemia. *J. Clin. Invest.* 51:1906–1909, 1972.

87. Clegg, J.B., and Weatherall, D.J. Haemoglobin synthesis during erythroid maturation in β-thalassaemia. *Nature (New Biol.)* 240:190–192, 1972.

88. Chalevelakis, G., Clegg, J.B., and Weatherall, D.J. Imbalanced globin chain synthesis in heterozygous β-thalassemia bone marrow. *Proc. Natl. Acad. Sci. USA* 72:3853–3857, 1975.

89. Gill, F.M., and Schwartz, E. Synthesis of globin chains in sickle β-thalassemia. *J. Clin. Invest.* 52:709–714, 1973.

90. Nathan, D. Thalassemia: A progress report in applied molecular biology. *N. Engl. J. Med.* 288:1122–1123, 1973.

91. Wood, W.G., and Stamatoyannopoulos, G. Globin synthesis in fractionated normoblasts of β-thalassemia heterozygotes. *J. Clin. Invest.* 55:567-578, 1975.

92. Fessas, P., and Loukopoulos, D., The β thalassaemias. Edited by D.J. Weatherall. In *Clinics in Haematology.* Vol. 3. Philadelphia: W.B. Saunders Co., 1974.

93. Tolstoshev, P., Mitchell, J., Lanyon, G., et al. Presence of gene for β globin in homozygous β⁰ thalassaemia. *Nature* 259:95-98, 1976.

94. Ramirez, F., O'Donnell, J.V., Marks, P.A., et al. Abnormal or absent β mRNA in β⁰ Ferrara and gene deletion in δβ thalassaemia. *Nature* 263:471-475, 1976.

95. Nienhius, A.W., Turner, P., and Benz, E.J., Jr. Relative stability of alpha and beta mRNA in homozygous beta⁺ thalassemia. *Proc. Natl. Acad. Sci. USA* 74:3960-3964, 1977.

96. Forget, B.G., Benz, E.J., Jr., Skoultchi, A., et al. Absence of messenger RNA for beta globin chain in β⁰ thalassaemia. *Nature* 247:379-381, 1975.

97. Forget, B.G., Hillman, D.G., Cohen-Solal, M., et al. β globin messenger RNA in beta⁰ thalassemia. *Blood* 48:998, 1976.

98. Old, J.M., Proudfoot, N.J., Wood, W.G., et al. Characterization of β globin messenger RNA in the β⁰ thalassemias. *Cell* 14:289-298, 1978.

99. Kan, Y.W., Holland, J.P., Dozy, A.M., et al. Demonstration of nonfunctional β globin mRNA in homozygous β⁰ thalassemia. *Proc. Natl. Acad. Sci. USA* 72:5140-5144, 1975.

100. Temple, G.F., Chang, J.C., and Kan, Y.W. Authentic β globin sequences in homozygous β⁰ thalassemia. *Proc. Natl. Acad. Sci. USA* 74:3047-3051, 1977.

101a. Chang, J.C., and Kan, Y.W. The sequence of the 5' untranslated region of a β⁰ mRNA inactive in protein synthesis. In preparation, 1979.

101b. Chang, J.C., Temple, G.F., Trecartin, R., et al. Suppressor tRNA allows synthesis of β globin chains in β⁰ thalassemia. In preparation, 1979.

102. Conconi, F., Del Senno, L., Ferarrese, P., et al. Appearance of β globin synthesis in erythroid cells of Ferrara β⁰-thalassaemic patients following blood transfusion. *Nature* 254:256-259, 1975.

103. Ottolenghi, S., Comi, P., and Giglioni, G. Direct demonstration of β-globin mRNA in homozygous Ferrara β⁰-thalassaemia patients. *Nature* 266:231-234, 1977.

104. Weatherall, D.J., and Clegg, J.B. Hereditary persistence of fetal haemoglobin. *Br. J. Haematol.* 29:191-198, 1975.

105. Forget, B.G., Hillman, D.G., Lazarus, H., et al. Absence of messenger RNA and gene DNA for β globin chains in hereditary persistence of fetal hemoglobin. *Cell* 7:323-239, 1976.

106. Kan, Y.W., Holland, J.P., Dozy, A.M., et al. Deletion of the β globin structural gene in hereditary persistence of foetal hemoglobin. *Nature* 258:162-163, 1975.

107. Ottolenghi, S., Comi, P., Giglioni, B., et al. δβ thalassemia is due to a gene deletion. *Cell* 9:71-80, 1976.

108a. Mears, J.G., Ramirez, F., Leibowitz, D., et al. Organization of human globin genes in normal and thalassemic DNA. *Clin. Res.* 26:506A, 1978.

108b. Mears, J.G., Ramirez, F., Leibowitz, D., et al. Changes in restricted human cellular DNA fragments containing globin gene sequences in thalassemias and related disorders. *Proc. Natl. Acad. Sci. USA* 75:1222-1226, 1978.

109. Baglioni, C. The fusion of two peptide chains in hemoglobin Lepore and its interpretation as a genetic deletion. *Proc. Natl. Acad. Sci. USA*

48:1880–1886, 1962.

110. White, J.M., Lang, A., Lorkin, P.A., et al. Synthesis of haemoglobin Lepore. *Nature (New Biol.)* 235:208–210, 1972.

111. Ramirez, F., Mears, G., Nudel, U., et al. Decreased Lepore globin mRNA content in homozygous hemoglobin Lepore disease. *Blood* 50:117, 1978.

112. Huisman, T.H.J., Wrightstone, R.N., Wilson, J.B., et al. Hemoglobin Kenya, the product of fusion of γ and β polypeptide chains. *Arch. Biochem. Biophys.* 153:850–853, 1972.

113. Nute, P.E., Wood, W.G., Stamatoyannopoulos, G., et al. The Kenya form of hereditary persistence of fetal haemoglobin: Structural studies and evidence for homogeneous distribution of haemoglobin F using fluorescent antihaemoglobin F antibodies. *Br. J. Haematol.* 32:55–63, 1976.

# 13 Varieties of Beta Thalassemia*

Thomas R. Kinney, M.D.
Shlomo Friedman, M.D.

The thalassemia syndromes are genetic disorders characterized by reduced synthesis of one or more of the normal polypeptide globin chains of human hemoglobin. Genetic classification of the thalassemic disorders is derived from the name of the globin chain(s) synthesized at a reduced rate, and they may be divided into two main categories: $\alpha$ thalassemia and $\beta$ thalassemia.

The inheritance of thalassemia is autosomal, and although the defect is expressed in both the heterozygous and homozygous states, this expression is more pronounced in the homozygote. Homozygous disease is called thalassemia major and heterozygous disease, thalassemia minor. The severity of the defect in $\beta$ thalassemia major, however, is influenced by a variety of factors, including race and interaction with other thalassemia genes. For example, homozygous $\beta$ thalassemia usually results in a chronic, transfusion-dependent anemia

*The authors are indebted to Sandra Termini for her secretarial assistance and to Janet Fithian for editorial assistance. The work was supported in part by NIH AM 16691 and The Cooley's Anemia Fund.

292

in Caucasians while blacks with the same disorder often are not dependent on transfusions until the second decade of life or later. The mildness of $\beta$ thalassemia minor is also influenced by genetic and acquired factors. For example, high Hb $A_2$ $\beta$ thalassemia trait is associated with microcytosis and hypochromia while the silent carrier for $\beta$ thalassemia has no hematologic abnormalities.

This chapter discusses the clinical, hematologic, and globin synthesis findings in varieties of $\beta$ thalassemia, the Hb Lepore syndromes, hereditary persistence of fetal hemoglobin, less common forms of thalassemia, and disorders produced by the interaction of different thalassemia genes (Table 13-1). Genetic counseling for thalassemic disorders is also discussed.

**Table 13-1**
**Varieties of Beta Thalassemia**

---

Disorders of $\beta$ chain synthesis
    High Hb $A_2$ $\beta$ thalassemia
    $\beta$-thalassemia trait of unusual severity
    $\beta$-thalassemia trait with normal Hb $A_2$ and Hb F and hypochromia
    Silent carrier for $\beta$ thalassemia
    $\alpha\beta$ thalassemia
Disorders of $\beta$ and $\delta$ chain synthesis
    $\delta\beta$ thalassemia (F thalassemia)
    Hb Lepore syndromes

Hereditary persistence of fetal hemoglobin syndromes
    Pancellular HPFH
        Greek type
        Black type
        HPFH with $\beta^A$ chain production in cis position
        Hb Kenya
    Heterocellular HPFH
Rare thalassemic disorders
    $\gamma\beta$ thalassemia
    $\delta$ thalassemia

---

## DISORDERS OF $\beta$ CHAIN SYNTHESIS

### High Hb $A_2$ $\beta$ Thalassemia

The most common variety of $\beta$ thalassemia is high Hb $A_2$ $\beta$ thalassemia, a disorder prevalent in people of Italian, Greek, African, and Oriental heritage. It has also been observed occasionally in individuals of northern European stock.[1] There are two major types of genes that produce high Hb $A_2$ $\beta$ thalassemia. One type ($\beta O$) is associated with total absence of $\beta$ globin chain synthesis directed by the affected chromosome. The other ($\beta^+$) is associated with reduced $\beta$ chain production by the affected chromosome. The $\beta O$-thalassemia gene is commonly observed in people from the Ferrara region of Italy and in Greeks, but it also occurs in people of African, Arab, Jewish, and Asian ancestry.[2-9]

**Heterozygous High Hb $A_2$ $\beta$ Thalassemia**   The clinical and hematologic expression of high Hb $A_2$ $\beta$ thalassemia in the heterozygote is similar for both the $\beta^+$ and $\beta O$ types of genes.[8-10] Clinical symptoms are usually absent or minimal, with findings from the physical examination normal except for occasional mild splenomegaly. Women with this disorder become more anemic during pregnancy than do normal women but blood transfusion is usually not required.[11] The hemoglobin concentration is usually normal or minimally to moderately reduced. In a series of 45 persons of Greek or Italian origin with $\beta$-thalassemia trait, the mean corpuscular volume (MCV) as determined by electronic measurement was 64.7 ± 4.35 femtoliters (fl) (1 SD) and the MCV in 239 normal controls was 88.67 ± 5.3 fl.[12] The average mean corpuscular hemoglobin (MCH) in these same groups was 20.26 ± 2.23 picograms (pg) and 28.82 ± 2.87 pg, respectively.

The reticulocyte count may be slightly elevated. Red cell morphology is abnormal, with microcytosis, anisocytosis, poikilocytosis, hypochromia, target cells, and basophilic stippling being the most commonly identified findings. (See Chapter 4 for a photograph of a typical peripheral smear.) The osmotic fragility of the red cells is usually decreased. The measurement of free erythrocyte porphyrin (FEP) will usually distinguish $\beta$-thalassemia trait from iron deficiency in persons with microcytosis. In patients with iron deficiency anemia the FEP is elevated, while in individuals with $\beta$-thalassemia trait the FEP is usually normal.[13] The bone marrow examination reveals a normal marrow or mild erythroid hyperplasia. Methyl violet stained inclusions of precipitated $\alpha$ chain are usually not found in marrow polychromatophilic or orthochromatic normoblasts. Hemoglobin electrophoresis demonstrates a predominance of Hb A, normal to minimally increased levels of Hb F, and increased levels of Hb $A_2$. Hemoglobin $A_2$ comprises about 3.5% to 8% of the total hemoglobin.[14] Hemoglobin F is increased in approximately half of the individuals with $\beta$-thalassemia trait.[15] The reason for the variability of Hb F levels in $\beta$-thalassemia trait is not known.

Globin synthesis studies in high Hb $A_2$ $\beta$-thalassemia trait reveal a reduced rate of $\beta$ chain production compared to $\alpha$ chain production in the peripheral blood of Caucasians and Orientals with this disorder. In both these racial groups, $\beta$ chain synthesis is about one-half that of $\alpha$

chain synthesis, with a mean $\beta/\alpha$ ratio in Caucasians of 0.57 ± 0.08 (1 SD),[16] in Orientals with $\beta^+$-thalassemia trait 0.49 ± 0.10 (1 SD), and in Orientals with $\beta^0$-thalassemia trait 0.44 ± 0.07 (1 SD).[9] In blacks with high Hb $A_2$ $\beta$-thalassemia trait, however, a wide range of peripheral blood $\beta/\alpha$ ratios is observed, and approximately 50% of patients have normal ratios.[17] The cause of this wide range of $\beta/\alpha$ ratios in blacks is not known.

Globin synthesis studies performed on bone marrow from individuals with high Hb $A_2$ $\beta$-thalassemia trait have produced conflicting results. Normal $\beta/\alpha$ ratios have been obtained in the bone marrow by some workers.[18-20] Other workers have consistently obtained reduced $\beta/\alpha$ ratios in the marrow, with a greater imbalance in the peripheral blood than in the bone marrow,[21,22] suggesting that contamination of the $\beta$ globin peak by nonheme white cell proteins was responsible for the normal marrow $\beta/\alpha$ ratios observed in some laboratories. However, this explanation cannot account for the finding of normal $\beta/\alpha$ ratios in bone marrow of some patients with sickle-$\beta$ thalassemia,[16] since the $\beta^s$ globin elutes in a different position from $\beta^A$ globin and the white cell proteins, nor does it account for the normal ratios observed using methods which minimize liberation of white cell proteins.[18] An alternate explanation is that $\alpha$ globin proteolysis occurring after $\alpha$ chain is synthesized could account in part for normal $\beta/\alpha$ bone marrow ratios, perhaps with more $\alpha$ chain proteolysis in the marrow than in the peripheral blood responsible for the greater degree of globin chain imbalance observed in the peripheral blood compared to the marrow.[21,22]

In normal individuals, there is a small excess of $\alpha$ chains in the red cells. In the bone marrow of seven nonthalassemic controls, 3.7% to 9.8% of the newly synthesized radioactive $\alpha$ chain was found in the free $\alpha$ chain pool.[23] In the bone marrow in six patients with $\beta$-thalassemia trait or Hb S $\beta^+$ thalassemia, the free radioactive $\alpha$ chain pools ranged from 14% to 43.4%, higher than those observed in normal controls.[24,25] In the peripheral blood, the mean standard deviation and range of 20 nonthalassemic controls was 14.1 ± 3.6% (1 SD) and 6.1% to 18.6%, respectively.[25] In three patients with Hb S $\beta^0$ thalassemia, the peripheral blood radioactive $\alpha$ chain pools ranged from 35.1% to 53%, higher than those observed in normal controls.[25]

Despite the similarity of clinical and hematologic data in $\beta^+$ and $\beta^0$ heterozygotes for high Hb $A_2$ $\beta$ thalassemia, globin synthesis ratios appear to be useful in distinguishing between these two types of high Hb $A_2$ $\beta$-thalassemia trait.[9]

Family studies are also of major help in making this distinction. If both parents are heterozygous for high Hb $A_2$ $\beta$ thalassemia and no Hb A is synthesized by the offspring, the $\beta^0/\beta^0$ genotype can be assigned to the child and heterozygous $\beta^0$ thalassemia to each parent. If the child produces Hb A and both parents are heterozygous for high Hb $A_2$

$\beta$ thalassemia, the genotype of the child may be $\beta^+/\beta^+$ or $\beta^0/\beta^+$ thalassemia. Distinction between these genotypes may be possible by analysis of pretransfusion hemoglobin composition.[3] Patients with $\beta^+/\beta^0$ thalassemia appear to have lower levels of Hb A, ranging from 4.1% to 11.7% of the total hemoglobin concentration, than patients with $\beta^+/\beta^+$ thalassemia, who have levels of Hb A ranging from 23.5% to 31.3%. In the case of one parent having a $\beta$ chain variant and the other being heterozygous for high Hb $A_2$ $\beta$ thalassemia, the thalassemic genotype may be determined by analysis of an offspring who has inherited a $\beta$-thalassemia gene in association with a $\beta$ chain variant. If this child produces Hb A, the thalassemic genotype is $\beta^+$ in the child and the thalassemic parent, but if no Hb A is produced the thalassemic genotype is $\beta^0$.

**Homozygous $\beta$ Thalassemia**   Homozygous $\beta$ thalassemia, or Cooley's anemia, results from the inheritence of two high Hb $A_2$ $\beta$-thalassemia genes. Three genotypes produce the clinical features of $\beta$ thalassemia major. These are $\beta^0/\beta^0$, $\beta^+/\beta^0$, or $\beta^+/\beta^+$ thalassemia.

In the homozygote for $\beta$ thalassemia, hemoglobin analysis reveals a predominance of Hb F and variable amounts of Hb $A_2$.[1] In $\beta^0$ thalassemia, Hb F constitutes about 95% of the total hemoglobin and no Hb A is found. In untransfused patients with $\beta^+/\beta^+$ or $\beta^0/\beta^+$ thalassemia, variable amounts of Hb A may be present but there are always lesser amounts of Hb A than Hb F. In the latter two disorders, the Hb F is heterogeneously distributed among the red cells. Hemoglobin $A_2$ levels may be normal, decreased, or increased in homozygous $\beta$ thalassemia.[26,27] In 13 untransfused patients with homozygous $\beta^0$ thalassemia, Hb $A_2$ levels ranged from 1.0% to 5.9% with a mean value of 1.7%.[3] In six untransfused patients with homozygous $\beta^+$ thalassemia, the Hb $A_2$ ranged from 2.4% to 8.7% with a mean of 4.1%.[3] In $\beta^+/\beta^0$ thalassemia, the Hb $A_2$ in 11 untransfused patients ranged from 0.6% to 3.4% with a mean of 1.8%.[3]

In all cases of $\beta$ thalassemia major studied to date, two types of Hb F, differing only in one amino acid at position 136 of the $\gamma$ chain, are found[28]; either alanine ($^A\gamma$) or glycine ($^G\gamma$) is found at position 136 of the $\gamma$ chain. This presence of both $^A\gamma$ and $^G\gamma$ chains suggests that both $^A\gamma$ and $^G\gamma$ loci are functional despite the $\beta$-thalassemia gene. A third type of $\gamma$ globin chain has recently been identified in some patients with homozygous $\beta$ thalassemia and in some normal individuals. This $\gamma$ chain contains threonine rather than isoleucine at position 75 ($^T\gamma$).[29,30] The clinical and genetic significance of this abnormality is not known.

In Italians, Greeks, Kurdish Jews, and a black homozygous for $\beta^0$ thalassemia, $\gamma/\alpha$ peripheral blood ratios ranged from 0.15 to 0.53.[2,5,6,31,32,33] In Greeks, blacks, Orientals, Jews, Arabs, and Italians with $\beta^+$ thalassemia major, the $\beta/\alpha$ ratio ranged from 0.07 to 0.43.[7,20,32-36] The lower $\beta/\alpha$ ratios and high Hb F levels in patients with $\beta^+$

thalassemia major help to distinguish these patients from most individuals with high Hb A$_2$ β-thalassemia trait, who usually have higher β/α ratios and lower Hb F levels. Patients with β⁰ thalassemia major are easily distinguished from heterozygotes by the absence of Hb A in the former.

In the bone marrow of three patients homozygous for β thalassemia, the free radioactive α chain pool ranged from 42.4% to 70.9%, overlapping the bone marrow α chain pool values observed in high Hb A$_2$ β-thalassemia trait.[23] The range of the free radioactive α chain pool in marrows of normal controls is 3.7% to 9.8%,[25,37] while in β thalassemia heterozygotes or homozygotes it is higher. Measurement of the free radioactive α chain pool appears useful in confirming β thalassemia but does not differentiate heterozygous from homozygous β thalassemia.

### β-Thalassemia Trait of Unusual Severity

The clinical and hematologic features observed in β-thalassemia trait are variable. The majority of individuals are asymptomatic. Symptomatic β-thalassemia trait is a rare disorder which has been described in individuals of Swiss-French, Italian, Irish, and English-German extraction.[23,38] Symptoms include fatigue, pallor, and leg ulcers. Hepatosplenomegaly and gallstones are common abnormalities. Frequent transfusions are not required, but occasional transfusions may be necessary as dictated by symptoms of anemia. The hemoglobin concentration is variable, ranging from 7.7 to 12.6 g/dl in reported cases. Red cell morphologic abnormalities include anisocytosis, poikilocytosis, target cells, hypochromia, microcytosis, and nucleated red cells. The concentration of Hb A$_2$ is elevated in all cases and the Hb F ranges from 1.5% to 12.2% of the total hemoglobin.

Bone marrow examination reveals erythroid hyperplasia. Methyl violet stained inclusions composed of precipitated α chain have been identified in the erythroid cells of the marrow in most patients.[23,38] Methyl violet inclusions are not found in the bone marrow or peripheral blood erythrocytes of patients with the asymptomatic form of heterozygous β thalassemia.

In 15 patients studied, a reduced β/α globin synthesis ratio was observed in the peripheral blood, ranging from 0.47 to 0.81 with a mean of 0.65 ± 0.12 (1 SD).[23,38] These ratios are similar to those observed in Caucasians with the usual form of β-thalassemia trait. In four patients with unusually severe β-thalassemia trait, the free α chain pool in the bone marrow ranged from 37.7% to 91.6% of the radioactive α globin.[23] These values were well above the range of the α chain pool observed in the bone marrow of nonthalassemic controls and were similar to the values in individuals with the usual form of β-thalassemia trait and some patients with thalassemia major.[23,24]

The β/α ratio in the bone marrow of eight patients ranged from 0.66 to 0.88,[23,38] generally lower than values found in asymptomatic heterozygotes when studied with identical methods.[23]

In the three families described by Friedman et al,[23] there were members with high Hb A$_2$ β-thalassemia trait who were symptomatic and others with β-thalassemia trait who were asymptomatic. In contrast, all of the members of the French-Canadian family were symptomatic.[38] These differences suggest the modifying influence of undefined acquired or hereditary factors on the expression of β thalassemia.


### β-Thalassemia Trait with Normal Concentrations of Hb A$_2$ and Hb F and Red Cell Hypochromia

Persons of Turkish and Greek extraction have been described with β-thalassemia trait in association with normal concentrations of Hb A$_2$ and Hb F.[39] These heterozygotes are asymptomatic. The hemoglobin concentration is normal or minimally reduced and the concentrations of Hb A$_2$ and Hb F are normal. There is anisocytosis, poikilocytosis, and hypochromia in this disorder, similar to some red cell abnormalities observed in the usual form of β-thalassemia trait. These morphologic abnormalities distinguish this condition from the silent carrier of β thalassemia, as the red cell morphology is normal in the silent carrier. The diagnosis in heterozygotes for β-thalassemia trait with normal levels of Hb A$_2$ and Hb F and hypochromia is established by family studies. Some offspring of these heterozygotes and individuals with high Hb A$_2$ β thalassemia have been described.[39] Pertinent physical abnormalities included hepatosplenomegaly and x-ray abnormalities of the bone typical of β thalassemia major. These patients rarely required transfusion as the hemoglobin concentration ranged between 5.2 to 7.3 g/dl and their growth and development were satisfactory. Hemoglobin analysis revealed a predominance of Hb A, and Hb A$_2$ and Hb F levels ranged between 1.9% to 5.8% and 11% to 30%, respectively.

Two homozygous offspring of heterozygotes for β thalassemia with normal concentrations of Hbs A$_2$ and F have been described.[39] Pallor, hepatosplenomegaly, and widening of the diploic space were present. Chronic transfusion therapy was not required, as the hemoglobin ranged between 7 and 8 g/dl. The morphologic abnormalities of the red cells included anisocytosis, poikilocytosis, hypochromia, and nucleated red cells. Hemoglobin analysis revealed an elevated concentration of Hb A$_2$ (5.8%, 6.0%) and Hb F (10.5%, 10.0%).

## Silent Carrier of β Thalassemia

The silent carrier for β thalassemia has been noted in three members of one family.[40] Hematologic features for the silent carrier include a normal hemoglobin concentration, normal levels of Hbs $A_2$ and F, and essentially normal red cell morphology. The diagnosis of the silent carrier abnormality was established by peripheral blood globin synthesis studies. The β/α specific activity ratios in the three affected individuals were reduced, ranging from 0.60 to 0.63, similar to the ratios observed in Caucasians with high Hb $A_2$ β-thalassemia trait.[16] The proband and his sister in the family described were heterozygous for both the silent carrier abnormality and for typical high Hb $A_2$ β-thalassemia trait. Both children had normal growth and development, hepatosplenomegaly, and anemia, but did not require blood transfusions. The concentration of the proband's hemoglobin was 6.9 g/dl, and his sister's was 8.3 g/dl. The red cell morphology of these children was similar to that observed in Caucasians with homozygous β thalassemia and included anisocytosis, poikilocytosis, hypochromia, target cells, microcytosis, and nucleated red cells. Methyl violet positive inclusions of precipitated α chain were observed in the nucleated and non-nucleated erythroid cells of the marrow in the proband. Both children had an increase in the concentration of Hb $A_2$ (3.9%, 4.8%) and Hb F (11.8%, 6.2%). Hemoglobin F was heterogeneously distributed in the red cells of the proband and his sister.

This family illustrates the need for globin synthesis studies in patients in whom the diagnosis cannot be established by routine hematologic investigations.

## αβ Thalassemia

Four syndromes involving the interaction of α and β thalassemia, including $α_1$/β-, $α_2$/β-, $α_1α_2$/β-thalassemia trait, and $α_1$/homozygous β thalassemia,[24,41-44] have been recognized. Heterozygotes for both α and β thalassemia have been described in Italians, Cypriots, Orientals, and American blacks.[22,41-44] Hematologic data in Caucasians, blacks, Cypriots, and Orientals with $α_1$/β thalassemia include a hemoglobin concentration ranging from 9.6 to 13.9 g/dl, MCV from 67 to 77.5 fl, and MCH from 18.0 to 24.4 pg. The red cell morphology is similar to high Hb $A_2$ β-thalassemia trait. The Hb $A_2$ level ranges from 3.2% to 5.7% of the total hemoglobin. In 13 of 15 patients, the Hb $A_2$ level was above 3.5%, a clearly elevated level. In four of the 15 patients, the Hb F was greater than 2%, with the highest level being 2.7%.

Four persons with $α_2$/β thalassemia have been described.[42-44] Two had normal MCV, with the remaining hematologic data similar to those of patients with $α_1$/β thalassemia.

Two Oriental patients and two Cypriots with the genotype of $\alpha_1\alpha_2$ thalassemia in association with $\beta$-thalassemia trait have been identified.[42-44] The clinical picture was that of thalassemia of intermediate severity. Hemoglobin H was not identified in either Oriental patient but was detected in both Cypriots. All patients had severe hypochromia and microcytosis with mild anemia. Hemoglobin $A_2$ was elevated in both Oriental patients but normal in the two Cypriots.

One Italian and one Cypriot with $\alpha_1$-thalassemia trait and homozygous $\beta$ thalassemia have been described.[42-44] Clinically, the patients had thalassemia of intermediate severity. The hemoglobin was 10.0 g/dl in the Italian and 8.4 g/dl in the Cypriot, and the indices were severely reduced in both. Hemoglobin F levels were 39% and 40%, within the range of homozygous $\beta$ thalassemia.

Peripheral blood globin synthesis studies appear to be able to distinguish between these four $\alpha/\beta$-thalassemia syndromes.[24,42-44] In $\alpha_1/\beta$-thalassemia trait, globin synthesis is balanced. In $\alpha_2/\beta$-thalassemia trait, the $\beta/\alpha$ ratio is reduced (0.68, 0.83). In $\alpha_1\alpha_2/\beta$-thalassemia trait, the $\beta/\alpha$ ratio was increased (1.23, 1.31). In two patients with homozygous $\beta$ thalassemia and $\alpha_1$-thalassemia trait, the $\beta/\alpha$ ratios were 0.32 and 0.45, ratios higher than the usual ratio found in Italians with homozygous $\beta$ thalassemia.[16] One person heterozygous for both $\alpha_1$ and $\beta$ thalassemia had 14.1% radioactivity in the $\alpha$ chain pool, a lower value than in simple $\beta$-thalassemia trait but higher than normal, reflecting the modifying effect of $\alpha_1$-thalassemia trait on the expression of $\beta$ thalassemia.[24] One black with Hb S-$\beta^+/\alpha$ thalassemia and with a reduced non-$\alpha/\alpha$ ratio of 0.66 had a radioactive free $\alpha$ chain pool in peripheral blood of 18.9%, below the expected range for Hb S-$\beta^+$ thalassemia.[25] Measurement of the $\alpha$ chain pool may help confirm the diagnosis of combined $\alpha\beta$ thalassemia.


## DISORDERS OF $\beta$ AND $\delta$ CHAIN SYNTHESIS

### $\delta\beta$ Thalassemia

This thalassemia is characterized by a reduction in synthesis of both $\delta$ and $\beta$ globin. The disorder is not common, but it has been observed in Greeks, Italians, American blacks, and Arabs.[45-51] In the heterozygous state, clinical symptoms usually are absent. Anemia is mild or absent, and there is hypochromia, anisocytosis, poikilocytosis, and microcytosis. The concentration of Hb $A_2$ is normal or reduced, and Hb F comprises approximately 10% of the total hemoglobin. Hemoglobin F is heterogeneously distributed in the red cells of these individuals. Globin synthesis studies in heterozygotes for $\delta\beta$ thalassemia show a wide range of peripheral blood $\beta/\alpha$ specific activity ratios (0.58

to 1.04).[49] A normal $\beta/\alpha$ specific activity ratio does not exclude a diagnosis of $\delta\beta$-thalassemia trait. Therefore, the definitive diagnosis of $\delta\beta$-thalassemia trait is based on a normal or reduced concentration of Hb $A_2$, an increased amount of Hb F, a heterogeneous distribution of Hb F in the red cells, and abnormal red cell morphology, including hypochromia and microcytosis.

Only Hb F is produced in homozygotes with $\delta\beta$ thalassemia. There is total absence of Hb A and Hb $A_2$ due to deletion of the $\beta$ chain and, presumably, $\delta$ structural genes.[52] The clinical findings in homozygous $\delta\beta$ thalassemia are of intermediate severity (Table 13-2). Although homozygotes for $\delta\beta$ thalassemia usually have pallor, hepato-splenomegaly, and bone changes on x-ray, the anemia is less pronounced than in most homozygotes for $\beta$ thalassemia. The hemoglobin concentration in homozygous $\delta\beta$ thalassemia usually ranges from 9 to 12 g/dl and chronic red cell transfusion is not required. The peripheral smear reveals anisocytosis, poikilocytosis, hypochromia, microcytosis, and nucleated red cells. Bone marrow examination reveals red cell hyperplasia, and precipitates of $\alpha$ globin can be detected in the nucleated erythroid precursors by methyl violet staining.[53] The $\gamma/\alpha$ globin synthesis ratios in three homozygotes were reduced, with values of 0.56, 0.66, and 0.72.[48] One patient, an Arab, had a ratio of 1.28.[50]

The diagnosis of homozygous $\delta\beta$ thalassemia is best made by careful evaluation of family members. Both parents of the patient have the findings of $\delta\beta$-thalassemia trait. Homozygous $\delta\beta$ thalassemia must be distinguished from homozygous HPFH, where Hb A and Hb $A_2$ are also absent and only Hb F is present (Table 2). Homozygous HPFH does not cause clinical symptoms and has a benign prognosis. Homozygous $\delta\beta$ thalassemia can be distinguished from homozygous HPFH by evaluating the distribution of Hb F in the red cells of the parents. In heterozygotes for HPFH, variable amounts of Hb F are present in every, or almost every, red cell, while in $\delta\beta$-thalassemia heterozygotes many red cells lack Hb F.

Persons heterozygous for $\delta\beta$ and high Hb $A_2$ $\beta$ thalassemia have been described. In Greeks,[45,54] an Oriental,[55] Italians,[47,56] and in a black[49] with the genotype $\delta\beta/\beta^O$ thalassemia, the clinical manifestations were less severe than those observed in homozygotes for $\beta^O$ thalassemia (Table 2). Although all except the black had pallor, hepatosplenomegaly, and bone changes of thalassemia on x-ray, transfusions were rarely needed. The black was asymptomatic with no abnormal findings on physical examination. The hemoglobin concentration for the patients with $\delta\beta/\beta^O$ thalassemia ranged between 6.8 to 12.6 g/dl. Abnormalities of red cell morphology included anisocytosis, poikilocytosis, hypochromia, microcytosis, and nucleated red cells. The hemoglobin composition in these patients included Hb F and Hb $A_2$, the latter ranging from 0.3% to 2.4% of the total hemoglobin.

Patients with δβ/β⁺ thalassemia usually have between 20% to 30% Hb A.⁴⁵ Peripheral blood globin synthesis studies have been reported in only one Chinese and one black with δβ/β⁰ thalassemia.⁴⁹,⁵⁵ The γ/α ratio for the Chinese was 0.38, while the black had a ratio of 0.54. In two Greeks, a mixture of ᴳγ and ᴬγ was present, while in one Chinese, only glycine was present at position 136 of the γ chain (Table 13-2).⁵⁵,⁵⁷

## Hemoglobin Lepore Syndromes

The Hb Lepore syndromes have many features that are similar to β thalassemia, including the production of hypochromic, microcytic red cells and a reduced rate of synthesis of β globin. Three types of Hb Lepore have been identified: (1) Hb Lepore Hollandi, (2) Hb Lepore Baltimore, and (3) Hb Lepore Washington-Boston, which is identical to Hb Lepore Bronx, Cyprus, Augustus, and Pylos.⁵⁸ Each type of Lepore hemoglobin is composed of two normal α chains and two identically abnormal Lepore globin chains. Lepore globin has an N-terminal amino acid sequence similar to that of normal δ chain and a C-terminal amino acid sequence similar to that of normal β chain. The hybrid Lepore globin is thought to be a product of a δβ fusion gene arising from a crossing-over during meiosis between misaligned δ and β globin structural genes residing on different chromosomes.⁵⁹ The three types of Lepore hemoglobins have different amino acid sequences, reflecting different sites of crossover.⁶⁰

Hemoglobin Lepore has been described in Italians, Greeks, Yugoslavs, and American blacks. Approximately 250 individuals with Hb Lepore have been identified.⁶¹ The highest incidence of Hb Lepore is found in individuals from the Campania region of Italy. The clinical and hematologic features of disorders associated with the production of Hb Lepore are similar, regardless of the type of Hb Lepore. Therefore, the different Lepore hemoglobins will not be discussed individually.

Heterozygotes for Hb Lepore are usually asymptomatic, similar to individuals with β-thalassemia trait. Splenomegaly has been noted occasionally.⁶² The hemoglobin concentration is usually normal or minimally reduced. Red cell morphologic abnormalities are found in Hb Lepore trait, including hypochromia, microcytosis, anisocytosis, poikilocytosis, and target cells.⁶²,⁶³

Heterozygotes for Hb Lepore have normal to reduced concentrations of Hb A₂, normal to increased levels of Hb F, and 5% to 15% of Hb Lepore. Hemoglobin F has been noted to be as high as 14% of the total hemoglobin in occasional patients, but usually is in the range of 2% to 4%.⁶²

Lepore globin is synthesized primarily in the bone marrow normoblasts, and there is little or no Lepore globin synthesized by the reticulocytes of the peripheral blood.[59,60,61,64-66] The radioactive ratio of ($\beta$ + Lepore)/$\alpha$ in the peripheral blood of heterozygotes with Hb Lepore ranged from 0.39 to 0.55.[64,67] In one study, the bone marrow globin synthesis ($\beta$ + Lepore)/$\alpha$ ratios after a 2-hour incubation ranged from 0.85 to 1.07, suggesting balanced total synthesis.[67] Other workers have obtained reduced $\beta/\alpha$ ratios after a 2-hour incubation of bone marrow,[65] but a $\beta/\alpha$ ratio closer to unity (0.84) when the marrow was incubated for only 10 minutes.

A possible explanation for differences in marrow and peripheral blood ratios is preferential destruction of $\alpha$ chain in the marrow as compared to the peripheral blood.[65] The free radioactive $\alpha$ chain pool in the bone marrow of three patients heterozygous for Hb Lepore ranged from 29.1% to 59.5%, close to the values observed in $\beta$ thalassemia.[24]

The homozygous condition for Hb Lepore has many of the clinical and hematologic features of $\beta$ thalassemia major. These include growth retardation, thalassemic facies, pallor, hepatosplenomegaly, and x-ray evidence of expansion of the intramedullary cavities of bone as a consequence of ineffective erythropoiesis. Some patients require transfusion therapy[68] while others are able to maintain

**Table 13-2**
**Hb F Syndromes: Clinical Features**

| Genotype | Ethnic group | Number of patients | Age (years) | Signs | Transfusion | Reference |
|---|---|---|---|---|---|---|
| $\beta^o/\beta^o$ Thalassemia | Italian Jew Greek Arab | 80 | 3/12-17 | Pallor, facial changes, H-S, growth failure, bone changes on x-ray | Majority transfusion-dependent after age 3 | 2,3,7,26, 28,31,32,33 |
| | Black | 2 | 2,7 | Pallor, H-S, bone changes on x-ray | Intermittent, one patient transfused regularly after age 12 | 4,5,6 |
| $\delta\beta/\beta^o$ Thalassemia | Greek | 12 | 1-26 | Pallor, H-S, bone changes on x-ray | None | 45,54,57 |
| | Italian | 2 | 18,37 | Icterus, S | None | 47,56 |
| | Chinese | 1 | 8/12 | Pallor, H-S | Several | 55 |
| | Black | 1 | 2 | None | None | 49 |
| $\delta\beta/\delta\beta$ Thalassemia | Italian | 7 | 2-31 | H-S, bone changes on x-ray | None | 48,51,52,57,100 |
| | Greek | 2 | 22 | Facial changes, H-S | None | 46,57 |
| | Arab | 3 | 25 | S | Rare | 50,52 |
| HPFH/$\beta^o$ Thalassemia | Turk | 1 | 6 | Pallor | None | 87 |
| | Black | 1 | 69 | S | None | 88 |
| HPFH/HPFH | Black | 8 | 7-54 | S in one patient who also had hereditary elliptocytosis | None | 52,73,76-85 |
| | Indian | 1 | 7 | Pallor, jaundice, H-S | Rare | 84,86 |

A: anisocytosis, P: poikilocytosis. H: hypochromia. T: target cells. NRBC: nucleated red blood cells. H-S: heptosplenomegaly.
S: splenomegaly. +: performed in a cell-free system.

# Table 13-2 (Continued)
## Hb F Syndromes: Hematologic and Biochemical Features

| Genotype | Ethnic group | Number of patients | Hb concentration (g/dl) | Retics (%) | MCV (fl) | MCH (pg) | Red cell morphology | Hb A$_2$ (%) | Globin synthesis ratio γ/α | Glycine composition G$_\gamma$ | Reference |
|---|---|---|---|---|---|---|---|---|---|---|---|
| β°/β° Thalassemia | Italian Jew Greek Arab | 80 | — | — | — | — | A,P,H,T,NRBC | 0.80-5.9 | 0.15-0.53 | 0.35-0.66 | 2,3,7,26, 28,31,32,33 |
| | Black | 2 | 4.8,9.0 | 3.2,7.9 | — | 29 | A,P,H,T,NRBC | 2.6,1.6 | 0.18 | — | 4,5,6 |
| | Greek | 12 | 6.8-12.6 | 3.5-4.0 | 64-85 | 19-28 | A,P,H,T,NRBC | 0.3-2.4 | — | 0.59,0.61 | 45,54,57 |
| δβ/β° Thalassemia | Italian | 2 | 9.5,12.5 | 1.2 | 80,86 | 26,26.5 | A,P,H,T,NRBC | 1.2,1.5 | 0.32+ | — | 47,56 |
| | Chinese | 1 | 7.4 | 6.0 | — | — | A,P,H,T,NRBC | 1.8 | 0.38 | 0.94-1.09 | 55 |
| | Black | 1 | 10.6 | 3.0 | 56 | 21.2 | A,P,H,T, occ NRBC | 0.7 | 0.54 | — | 49 |
| | Italian | 7 | 10-12.7 | — | 58-82 | 20.4-23.9 | A,P,H,T,NRBC | None | 0.56-0.72 | 0.49-0.64 | 48,51,52,57,100 |
| δβ/δβ Thalassemia | Greek | 2 | 9 | 8.0 | 88 | 23 | A,P,H,T | None | — | 0.50,0.51 | 46,57 |
| | Arab | 3 | 12.3 | 3.5 | 85 | — | A,P,T | None | 1.28 | 0.59 | 50,52 |
| HPFH/β° Thalassemia | Turk | 1 | 9.0 | 0.4 | — | — | mild A,P,H,T | 1.75 | — | — | 87 |
| | Black | 1 | 12.4 | 4.4 | 64 | 19.7 | mild A,P,H,T | 1.9 | — | 0.77 | 88 |
| | Black | 8 | 14.8-18.2 | 0.8-5.3 | 68-84 | 24-28 | minimal A,P,T | None | 0.30-0.66 | 0.52-0.65 | 52,73,76-85 |
| HPFH/HPFH | Indian | 1 | 7.5 | 10.0 | 69.0 | 21.0 | A,P,H,T,NRBC | None | 0.33 | 1.01 | 84,86 |

A: anisocytosis, P: poikilocytosis. H: hypochromia. T: target cells. NRBC: nucleated red blood cells. H-S: heptosplenomegaly. S: splenomegaly. +: performed in a cell-free system.

hemoglobins in the range of 6.5 to 10.2 g/dl without transfusions, particularly after splenectomy.[62-68] In the homozygote for Hb Lepore, Hb F predominates and Hb Lepore comprises 10% to 20% of the total hemoglobin.[1] No Hb A or Hb $A_2$ is found, supporting the concept that functioning structural $\delta$ and $\beta$ genes are absent in cis due to a Hb Lepore fusion gene. The $\gamma/\alpha$ globin synthesis ratio in the peripheral blood of a homozygote for Hb Lepore was 0.24,[66] in the range of $\gamma/\alpha$ ratios observed in homozygotes for $\beta$ thalassemia.

Hemoglobin Lepore in association with $\beta$ thalassemia has been described in several ethnic groups, including Greeks, Italians, and Yugoslavs.[1] The clinical course does not appear to differ whether the patient has inherited the $\beta^+$ or $\beta^0$ type of thalassemia in association with Hb Lepore.[1] The clinical and hematologic features are similar to those of $\beta$ thalassemia major or thalassemia of intermediate severity. Hemoglobin electrophoresis reveals Hb F and Hb Lepore, the latter constituting about 10% of the total hemoglobin. If the patient has inherited a $\beta^+$ gene, Hb A will be detected in addition to Hb F and Hb Lepore. Although many patients have severe clinical disease, chronic transfusion is not needed in some patients and splenectomy may reduce the frequency of transfusion in others.[62] Genetic studies are helpful in the diagnosis of double heterozyotes for Hb Lepore and $\beta$ thalassemia. One parent has the finding of Hb Lepore trait and the other has high Hb $A_2$ $\beta$-thalassemia trait.

One patient who was heterozygous for both Hb Lepore and $\delta\beta$ thalassemia has been described.[69] The clinical features in this individual were similar to those of homozygotes for $\delta\beta$ thalassemia. Hemoglobin electrophoresis revealed only Hb F and Hb Lepore, the latter comprising 8% of the total hemoglobin. No Hb $A_2$ was identified, supporting the belief that there are no functioning $\delta$ structural genes in cis position to the Lepore gene or $\delta\beta$ thalassemia defects.

## HEREDITARY PERSISTENCE OF FETAL HEMOGLOBIN SYNDROMES

Hereditary persistence of fetal hemoglobin (HPFH) refers to a group of uncommon genetic disorders characterized by a failure of the affected chromosome to switch from $\gamma$ to $\beta$ chain synthesis. This failure results in the continued synthesis of Hb F, but it is not associated with any severe clinical or hematologic abnormalities in either homozygous or heterozygous states. The most commonly observed types of HPFH are the Greek type and the black type. Two other types of HPFH also have been described—the HPFH type with Hb A production in cis position to the HPFH determinant and the HPFH type with production of Hb Kenya. In these types, Hb F is found in every, or almost every red cell (pancellular distribution), as determined by the acid elution technique of Kleihauer. A second type of HPFH is associated with a heterocellular distribution of Hb F. In this disorder, there is a small increase in Hb F, but the individuals are otherwise hematologically normal. Examples of heterocellular HPFH include Swiss HPFH and British HPFH.

## Greek HPFH

Heterozygotes for the Greek type of HPFH are asymptomatic and have normal concentrations of hemoglobin, normal red cell indices, and normal red cell morphology.[70] Hemoglobin analysis reveals normal to reduced concentrations of Hb $A_2$ and an increased amount of Hb F. Hemoglobin F constitutes 10% to 19.4% and Hb $A_2$ 1.2% to 2.8% of the total hemoglobin. Hemoglobin F can be identified in each red cell by the acid elution technique. Homozygotes for the Greek type of HPFH have not been identified, nor has the heterozygous condition been described in association with the production of an abnormal $\beta$ chain.

Globin synthesis studies in heterozygotes with the Greek type of HPFH are limited. Sofronidou et al[71] studied three individuals in one family and observed a mean $(\beta + \gamma + \delta)/\alpha$ peripheral blood ratio of 1.03, reflecting balanced synthesis in this disorder.

Biochemical analysis of the $\gamma$ chains of Hb F in heterozygotes for the Greek type of HPFH reveals that only chains containing alanine at position 136 are produced.[72] This biochemical finding appears unique to the Greek type of HPFH and has not been recognized in any other disorder. These data suggest that the $^G\gamma$ locus in Greek HPFH is inactive, possibly being deleted.

The Greek type of HPFH in association with high Hb $A_2$ $\beta$-thalassemia trait has been described on several occasions.[70-72] These double heterozygotes usually have pallor and splenomegaly. The hemoglobin concentrations range from 8.2 to 12.4 g/dl and chronic transfusion is not required. Morphologic abnormalities of the red cells include hypochromia, microcytosis, anisocytosis, and poikilocytosis. Hemoglobin A is the predominant hemoglobin in all cases. The concentration of Hb $A_2$ ranges from 3.65% to 5.2%, and Hb F from 20.9% to 49.3% of the total hemoglobin. Hemoglobin F is found in each red cell, similar to the distribution of Hb F in the heterozygote for Greek HPFH. Globin synthesis data have been reported for only one patient in whom the $(\beta + \gamma + \delta)/\alpha$ ratio was 0.47,[71] similar to that observed in Caucasians with high Hb $A_2$ $\beta$-thalassemia trait. Hemoglobin F in this disorder is a mixture of $^G\gamma$ and $^A\gamma$ chains. The fact that no patients with Greek HPFH/$\beta$ thalassemia have a complete absence of $\beta$ chain synthesis suggests that the $\beta$ gene cis to the HPFH determinant is functional.[72]

## Black HPFH

Black persons heterozygous for HPFH are asymptomatic. The hemoglobin concentration is normal. The red cell indices, including

MCV and MCH, may be reduced to normal.[73,74] Red cell morphology is usually normal, although target cells may be present.[73] Hemoglobin electrophoresis reveals a predominance of Hb A, normal to reduced amounts of Hb $A_2$, and increased amounts of Hb F. The mean value of Hb $A_2$ in 37 heterozygotes was 1.6%, significantly lower than in a group of controls.[73] Individuals, however, had an $A_2$ value within the range observed for normals.[73] The Hb F in the same 37 patients ranged from 17.3% to 33%, with a mean value of 26% of the total hemoglobin. The Hb F is present in all, or almost all, of the red cells, a characteristic feature of this disorder similar to that observed in the Greek type of HPFH.

Peripheral blood globin synthesis studies in heterozygotes for the black variety of HPFH have shown a variable degree of globin chain imbalance.[74,75] The $\beta/\alpha$ ratios may be reduced or normal, ranging from 0.63 to 1.10. Globin synthesis studies do not reliably differentiate HPFH heterozygotes from individuals with $\delta\beta$-thalassemia trait, who also have normal or reduced concentrations of Hb $A_2$, increased concentrations of Hb F, and normal to reduced $\beta/\alpha$ synthesis ratios.[49] Differentiation of blacks with HPFH from those with $\delta\beta$-thalassemia trait is based upon the distribution of Hb F, with relatively even distribution in the HPFH heterozygote and fewer than 50% of the red cells containing Hb F in $\delta\beta$-thalassemia trait.

The homozygous condition for HPFH has been recognized in eight blacks (Table 13-2).[52,73,76-85] All were asymptomatic and splenomegaly was noted in only one patient, who also had hereditary elliptocytosis.[78] No patient required transfusion; the hemoglobin concentrations ranged from 14.8 to 18.2 g/dl. Minimal abnormalities of red cell morphology were observed, including anisocytosis, poikilocytosis, target cells, and microcytosis. Erythrocytosis was present in all patients. The MCV of the red cells ranged from 68 to 84 fl and MCH from 25 to 28 pg. Hemoglobin $A_2$ and Hb A were absent. Globin synthesis $\gamma/\alpha$ ratios in six patients ranged from 0.30 to 0.68, reflecting unbalanced globin chain synthesis. One patient had a ratio of 0.30, in the range usually observed in $\beta$ thalassemia major, while the remaining five patients had ratios above 0.50. Analysis of $\gamma$ chains of Hb F has revealed a mixture of glycine- and alanine-containing chains in all instances.

A 7-year-old Indian, homozygous for HPFH abnormality, had pallor, hepatosplenomegaly, severe anemia (Hb 6.1 g/dl), reduced red cell indices, and marked red cell morphologic abnormalities, including nucleated red cells.[84,86] This patient differs on two counts from all other HPFH homozygotes: he has required occasional red cell transfusions, and he has only $\gamma$ chains which contain glycine at 136. The $\gamma/\alpha$ globin synthesis ratio was 0.33, in the range observed in $\beta$ thalassemia major.

HPFH has been described in association with $\beta^0$ thalassemia in a black and a Turk.[87,88] The black patient was asymptomatic, with splenomegaly, a hemoglobin level of 12.4 g/dl, and mild thalassemic abnormalities of red cell morphology. The Hb $A_2$ level was 1.9%. The other patient was a 6-year-old Turk who had a hemoglobin concentration of 9.0 g/dl and morphologic abnormalities of the red cells and a concentration of Hb $A_2$ similar to that of the black patient. Globin synthesis studies were not done. Analysis of γ chains of Hb F revealed a mixture of glycine and alanine at position 136 in the black patient, with a glycine composition of 0.77. Neither of the two patients required red cell transfusions, suggesting that HPFH/$β^0$ thalassemia is a mild disorder, similar to β-thalassemia trait.

HPFH in association with $β^+$ thalassemia has also been described in blacks.[75,76,79] Five patients were asymptomatic and one icteric. Hepatosplenomegaly was present in one patient. None of the individuals required transfusions. The mean hemoglobin level in this group was 13.2 g/dl. Hypochromia and microcytosis were observed in the red cells of all patients. The mean concentrations of Hb F and Hb $A_2$ were 73.2% and 3.4%, respectively. In all cases, both glycine- and alanine-containing γ chains were found.[79] The $(β + γ)/α$ synthesis ratio in one patient was 0.59,[75] similar to β-thalassemia trait. Definitive diagnosis of this condition can be established by family studies.

## HPFH with $β^A$ Chain Production in Cis Position

An unusual type of HPFH with production of Hb A has been described in two black families.[89,90] The probands produced Hbs S, A, F, and $A_2$. Each red cell contained Hb F, the Hb A presumably being synthesized by a β globin structural gene in cis position to the HPFH determinant. In addition, only $^Gγ$ was detected in the fetal hemoglobin, and Hb $A_2$ was decreased. In this rare form of black HPFH, β chain synthesis is present in cis to the HPFH determinant, but $^Aγ$ synthesis and, probably, δ chain synthesis are absent.

## Hb Kenya

In several black families, a pancellular distribution of Hb F has been described in association with an abnormal hemoglobin, Hb Kenya.[91-95] Hemoglobin Kenya is composed of two normal α chains and two abnormal chains. The Kenya globin chain has an N-terminal amino acid sequence similar to γ chain and a C-terminal amino acid sequence similar to normal β chain. The hybrid Kenya globin is thought to be a product of fusion of γ and β genes produced from crossing-over during meiosis.

Heterozygotes for Hb Kenya are asymptomatic. The hemoglobin levels ranged from 9.9 to 15.8 g/dl. Values of MCV were 71 to 95 fl and MCH were 22.0 to 30.5 pg. Mild microcytosis, hypochromia, and poikilocytosis have been noted in some heterozygotes while others have had normal red cell morphology. Hemoglobin $A_2$ levels were 1.1% to 2.3%, while Hb Kenya comprised 6.9% to 23.4% of the total hemoglobin. The reduced levels of Hb $A_2$ in some patients suggest absent $\delta$ chain synthesis in cis position to the $\gamma\beta$ fusion gene. Hemoglobin F levels were 4.7% to 9.8%; Hb F was identified in all the red cells and was of the $^G\gamma$ type. Hemoglobin Kenya is synthesized in both reticulocytes and marrow normoblasts, in contrast to Hb Lepore, a $\delta\beta$ fusion gene product, which is synthesized almost entirely in the marrow normoblasts.[95]

Hemoglobin Kenya has been described in association with Hb S in several individuals.[93] The hemoglobin concentration was 11.8 to 13.9 g/dl and the red cell indices were normal. Target cells were the only morphologic abnormality noted in the red cells. These individuals produced Hb S, Hb F, Hb Kenya, and Hb $A_2$; they did not produce Hb A. Hemoglobin S was the predominant hemoglobin. The absence of Hb A indicates that no normal $\beta$ globin is produced in cis position to the Kenya fusion gene. No homozygotes for Hb Kenya have been described.

The production of only $^G\gamma$ chains in heterozygotes for Hb Kenya suggests that the fusion occurred between the $^A\gamma$ and $\beta$ genes, resulting in absence of $^A\gamma$, $\delta$, and $\beta$ structural genes in cis position to the Hb Kenya fusion gene.[91] Hemoglobin Kenya also provides evidence for the close linkage of $\gamma$, $\delta$, and $\beta$ genes. Similarly, the $\delta\beta$ fusion genes of Lepore globins provide evidence for close linkage of $\delta$ and $\beta$ genes.

## Heterocellular HPFH

In the British type of heterocellular HPFH,[96] both heterozygotes and homozygotes were asymptomatic and had no hematologic abnormalities except for increased levels of Hb F. The levels of Hb F ranged from 3.9% to 13% with a mean of 8.9% $\pm$ 3.1 (1 SD) in the heterozygote and from 19.4% to 20.4% in the homozygote. In both, the $\gamma$ chains of Hb F were composed of a mixture of $^G\gamma$ and $^A\gamma$ and globin synthesis $\beta/\alpha$ ratios in the peripheral blood were in unity. The concentration of Hb $A_2$ ranged from 1.6% to 1.7% in homozygotes, significantly lower than in normal controls. The British type of HPFH is characterized by heterogeneous distribution of Hb F and the production of $\beta$ and $\delta$ chains cis to the heterocellular HPFH determinant in both heterozygotes and homozygotes.

Heterocellular HPFH has been described in association with $\beta$-thalassemia trait in three individuals of two families of Italian and African ancestry.[97] These persons were asymptomatic. The hematologic findings were similar to β-thalassemia trait with normal to minimally reduced hemoglobin concentrations, reduced red cell indices, and increased levels of Hb A$_2$ and Hb F. The Hb F level ranged from 6.1% to 16.8%. In the one patient studied, the glycine composition at position 136 of the γ chain was 0.77 and the β/α peripheral blood globin synthesis ratio was 0.62. In each of these persons, the Hb F was heterogeneously distributed among the red cells by the acid elution technique. In one of the three persons, 47.7% of the red cells contained Hb F as determined by fluorescent labeled antibody against Hb F. The range of Hb F cells in normal individuals determined by this immunofluorescent technique is 1.2% to 7.0%, while the range in heterozygotes for heterocellular HPFH is 12.1% to 16.9%.[97] The interaction of heterocellular HPFH and β thalassemia results in an increased level of Hb F and in an increased number of Hb F cells.

## RARE THALASSEMIC DISORDERS

### γβ Thalassemia

This thalassemia is associated with a decreased production of γ and β chains. A heterozygote for γβ thalassemia has been described.[98] This patient was a newborn who presented with hypochromic and microcytic hemolytic anemia, reticulocytosis, and hepatosplenomegaly. The patient was shown to be heterozygous both for γ and β thalassemia. The diagnosis was established by a peripheral blood globin synthesis study. The (β + γ)/α ratio was 0.39, well below the (β + γ)/α ratio of two newborns with β-thalassemia trait (0.68, 0.71).

No homozygote with γ thalassemia has been described, and it is thought that this condition, in which no Hb F (α$_2$γ$_2$) could be synthesized, would be incompatible with intrauterine growth and development past early fetal life.

### δ Thalassemia

This thalassemia is characterized by a decreased production of δ chain. There are no clinical symptoms in either the heterozygote or homozygote.[99] In the homozygote, there is a total absence of Hb A$_2$, while in the heterozygote there is a mild reduction in the concentration of Hb A$_2$.

## GENETIC COUNSELING FOR THALASSEMIA

In order that affected persons may make informed decisions concerning reproduction, an understanding of the mode of inheritance of thalassemia and the natural history of thalassemic disorders is essential for both the counselor and the counselee. A complete hematologic and, if necessary, biochemical evaluation should be performed to determine the thalassemia variant in an individual before genetic counseling is initiated. The benign nature of the heterozygous condition for $\beta$ or $\alpha$ thalassemia should be stressed, and the serious nature of the homozygous condition emphasized. The chances of a couple producing an affected offspring should be explained.

If one parent is normal and the other parent carries a thalassemia gene, no homozygous offspring will be produced, but there will be a 50% chance with each pregnancy that the child will have thalassemia trait. If one parent is a homozygote and the other normal, all offspring will have the trait. If both parents are heterozygotes for $\beta$ thalassemia or $\alpha_1$ thalassemia, the risk of producing a child with homozygous disease is one in four with each pregnancy. If a person is heterozygous for both $\alpha$ and $\beta$ thalassemia genes, these genes are transmitted independently as they are located on different chromosomes.

Once a couple is identified as being at risk for producing a child with thalassemia major, the following possibilities are open to the couple: (1) refraining from having children, (2) prenatal diagnosis, (3) artificial insemination, or (4) having children despite the risk. The ultimate decision concerning childbearing should be made by the informed couple.

## REFERENCES

1. Weatherall, D.J., and Clegg, J.B. *The Thalassemia Syndromes*. 2nd Ed. Oxford: Blackwell Scientific Publications, 1972.

2. Conconi, F., Bargellesi, A., and Pontremoli, S. Absence of $\beta$-globin synthesis and excess of $\alpha$-globin synthesis in homozygous $\beta$-thalassemia subjects from Ferrara region. *Nature* 217:259–260, 1968.

3. Kattamis, C., Karambula, K., Metaxotou-Mavromati, A., et al. Prevalance of $\beta^0$ and $\beta^+$ thalassemia in Greek children with homozygous $\beta$-thalassemia. *Hemoglobin* 2:29–46, 1978.

4. Scott, R.B., Ferguson, A.D., and Jenkins, M.B. Thalassemia major (Mediterranean or Cooley's anemia). Report of two cases in Negro children. *Am. J. Dis. Child.* 140:106–113, 1962.

5. Ringlehaun, B., and Rudwick, A.L. Thalassemia major with complete suppression of Hb A production in a Ghanaian girl. *Acta Haematol.* 47:118–126, 1972.

6. Braverman, A.S., McCurdy, P.R., Manos, O., et al. Homozygous beta thalassemia in American blacks: The problem of mild thalassemia. *J. Lab. Clin. Med.* 81:857–866, 1973.

7. Cividalli, G., Kerem, H., and Rachmilewitz, E.A. Homozygous $\beta^0$ and $\beta^+$-thalassemia in Kurdish Jews and Arabs. *Hemoglobin* 1:333–347, 1977.

8. Pootrakul, S., Wasi, P., and Na-Nakorn, S. Haematological data in 312 cases of $\beta$-thalassemia trait in Thailand. *Br. J. Haematol.* 24:703–712, 1973.

9. Pootrakul, S., Assawamunkong, S., and Na-Nakorn, S. $\beta^+$-Thalassemia trait: Hematologic and hemoglobin synthesis studies. *Hemoglobin* 1:75–83, 1976–1977.

10. Mazza, U., Saglio, G., Cappio, C.C., et al. Clinical and haematological data in 254 cases of beta-thalassemia in Italy. *Br. J. Haematol.* 33:91–99, 1976.

11. Schuman, J.E., Tanser, C.L., Peloquin, R., et al. The erythropoetic response to pregnancy in $\beta$-thalassemia minor. *Br. J. Haematol.* 25:249–260, 1973.

12. Pearson, H.A., O'Brien, R.T., and McIntosh, S. Screening for thalassemia trait by electronic measurement of mean corpuscular volume. *N. Engl. J. Med.* 288:351–353, 1973.

13. Stockman, J.A., Weiner, L.S., Sinor, G.E., et al. The measurement of free erythrocyte porphyrin (FEP) as a simple means of distinguishing iron deficiency from beta-thalassemia trait in subjects with microcytosis. *J. Lab. Clin. Med.* 85:113–119, 1975.

14. Kunkle, H.G., Ceppellini, R., Müller-Eberhard, U., et al. Observation on the micro-basic hemoglobin component in the blood of normal individuals and patients with thalassemia. *J. Clin. Invest.* 36:1615–1625, 1957.

15. Beaver, G.H., Ellis, M.J., and White, J.C. Studies of human foetal haemoglobin. III. The hereditary haemoglobinopathies and thalassemia. *Br. J. Haematol.* 7:169–186, 1961.

16. Schwartz, E. Abnormal globin synthesis in thalassemic red cells. *Semin. Hematol.* 11:549–567, 1974.

17. Friedman, Sh., Hamilton, R.W., and Schwartz, E. $\beta$-Thalassemia in the American Negro. *J. Clin. Invest.* 52:1453–1459, 1973.

18. Schwartz, E. Heterozygous beta thalassemia: Balanced globin synthesis in bone marrow cells. *Science* 167:1513–1514, 1970.

19. Kan, Y.W., Nathan, D.G., and Lodish, H.F. Equal synthesis of $\alpha$- and $\beta$-globin chains in erythroid precursors in heterozygous $\beta$-thalassemia. *J. Clin. Invest.* 51:1906–1909, 1972.

20. Nienhuis, A.W., Canfield, P.H., and Anderson, W.F. Hemoglobin messenger RNA from human bone marrow. Isolation and translation in homozygous and heterozygous $\beta$-thalassemia. *J. Clin. Invest.* 52:1735–1745, 1973.

21. Clegg, J.B., and Weatherall, D.J. Haemoglobin synthesis during erythroid maturation in $\beta$-thalassaemia. *Nature (New Biol.)* 240:190–192, 1972.

22. Chalevelakis, G., Clegg, J.B., and Weatherall, D.J. Imbalanced globin chain synthesis in heterozygous $\beta$-thalassemia bone marrow. *Proc. Natl. Acad. Sci. USA* 72:3853–3857, 1975.

23. Friedman, Sh., Özsoylu, S., Luddy, R., et al. Heterozygous beta thalassemia of unusual severity. *Br. J. Haematol.* 32:65–77, 1976.

24. Gill, F.M., and Schwartz, E. Free $\alpha$-globin pool in human bone marrow. *J. Clin. Invest.* 52:3057–3063, 1973.

25. Kim, H.C., Weierbach, R.G., Friedman, Sh., et al. Detection of sickle $\alpha$- or $\beta^0$-thalassemia by studies of globin biosynthesis. *Blood* 49:785–791, 1977.

26. Silvestroni, E., Bianco, I., and Grazioni, G. The haemoglobin picture in Cooley's disease. *Br. J. Haematol.* 14:303–308, 1968.

27. Aksoy, M., and Erdem, S. Some problems of hemoglobin patterns in different thalassemic syndromes showing the heterogeneity of beta-thalassemia genes. *Ann. NY Acad. Sci.* 165:13–24, 1969.

28. Huisman, T.H.J., Schroeder, W.A. , Efremov, G.A., et al. The present status of the heterogeneity of fetal hemoglobin in $\beta$-thalassemia: An attempt to unify some observations in thalassemia and related conditions. *Ann. NY Acad. Sci.* 232:107–122, 1974.

312

29. Ricco, G., Mazza, U., Turi, R.M., et al. Significance of a new type of human fetal hemoglobin carrying a replacement isoleucine→threonine at position 75 (E19) of the γ chain. *Hum. Genet.* 32:305–313, 1976.

30. Huisman, T.H.J., Schroeder, W.A., Reese, J.B., et al. The $^T$γ chain of human fetal hemoglobin at birth and in several abnormal hematological conditions. *Pediatr. Res.* 11:1102–1105, 1977.

31. Bargellesi, A., Pontremoli, S., and Conconi, F. Absence of β globin synthesis and excess of α globin synthesis in homozygous β-thalassemia. *Eur. J. Biochem.* 1:73–79, 1967.

32. Weatherall, D.J.W., and Clegg, J.B. The pattern of disordered haemoglobin synthesis in homozygous and heterozygous β-thalassaemia. *Br. J. Haematol.* 16:251–267, 1969.

33. Braverman, A.S., and Bank, A. Changing rates of globin chain synthesis during erythroid cell maturation in thalassemia. *J. Mol. Biol.* 42:57–61, 1969.

34. Bank, A., and Marks, P.A. Excess α chain synthesis relative to β chain synthesis in thalassemia major and minor. *Nature* 212:1198–1200, 1966.

35. Friedman, Sh., Oski, F.A., and Schwartz, E. Bone marrow and peripheral blood globin synthesis in an American black family with β-thalassemia. *Blood* 39:785–793, 1972.

36. Conconi, F., Bargellesi, A., Del Senno, L., et al. Globin chain synthesis in Sicilian thalassemic subjects. *Br. J. Haematol.* 19:469–475, 1970.

37. Kim, H.C., Weierbach, R.G., Friedman, Sh., et al. Globin biosynthesis in sickle cell, Hb SC, and Hb C diseases. *J. Pediatr.* 91:13–18, 1977.

38. Stamatoyannopoulos, G., Woodson, R., Papayannopoulou, Th., et al. Inclusion-body β-thalassemia trait. A form of β-thalassemia producing clinical manifestations in simple heterozygotes. *N. Engl. J. Med.* 290:939–943, 1974.

39. Askoy, M., Erdem, S., and Dincol, G. β-Thalassemia with normal levels of hemoglobins F and $A_2$. Simple heterozygous and homozygous forms and doubly heterozygous state with β-thalassemia with increased hemoglobin $A_2$. Study in seven families. *International Istambul Symposium on Abnormal Hemoglobins and Thalassemia.* pp. 289–299, Aug. 24–27, 1974. Istanbul, Turkey.

40. Schwartz, E. The silent carrier of beta-thalassemia. *N. Engl. J. Med.* 281:1327–1333, 1969.

41. Pearson, H.A. Alpha-beta thalassemia disease in a Negro family. *N. Engl. J. Med.* 275:176–181, 1966.

42. Kan, Y.W., and Nathan, D.G. Mild thalassemia: The results of interactions of alpha and beta thalassemia genes. *J. Clin. Invest.* 49:635–642, 1970.

43. Knox-MacCaulay, H.H.M., Weatherall, D.J., Clegg, J.B., et al. The clinical and biosynthetic characterization of αβ-thalassemia. *Br. J. Haematol.* 22:497–512, 1972.

44. Bate, C.M., and Humphries, G. Alpha-beta thalassemia. *Lancet* 1:1031–1034, 1977.

45. Stamatoyannopoulos, G., Fessas, Ph., and Papayannopoulou, Th. F-thalassemia. A study of thirty-one families with simple heterozygotes and combinations of F-thalassemia with $A_2$-thalassemia. *Am. J. Med.* 47:194–208, 1969.

46. Tsistrakis, G.A., Amarantos, S.P., and Konkouris, L.L. Homozygous βδ-thalassemia. A report of a case and review of the literature. *Acta Haematol.* 51:185–191, 1974.

47. Gabuzda, T.G., Nathan, D.G., and Gardner, F.H. Thalassemia trait. Genetic combinations of increased fetal and $A_2$ hemoglobins. *N. Engl. J. Med.* 270:1212–1217, 1964.

48. Russo, G., Musumeci, S., Schiliro, G., et al. Haemoglobin synthesis in δβ-thalassemia. Istituto Italiano Di Medicina Sociale Roma. Estratto dagli Atti

del V Congresso Sulle Microcitemie. Cosenza, Ottobre. pp. 101–106, 1973.

49. Kinney, T.R., Friedman, Sh., Cifuentes, E., et al. Variations in globin synthesis in delta beta thalassemia. *Br. J. Haematol.* 38:15–22, 1978.

50. Shchory, M., and Ramot, B. Globin chain synthesis in the marrow and reticulocytes of β-thalassemia, hemoglobin H disease, and beta delta thalassemia. *Blood* 40:105–111, 1972.

51. Brancati, C., and Baglioni, C. Homozygous βδ thalassaemia (βδ-microthaemia). *Nature* 212:262-264, 1966.

52. Ottolenghi, S., Comi, P., Giglioni, G., et al. δβ-Thalassemia is due to a gene deletion. *Cell* 9:71–80, 1976.

53. Yataganas, X., and Fessas, Ph. The pattern of hemoglobin precipitation in thalassemia and its significance. *Ann. NY Acad. Sci.* 165:270–287, 1969.

54. Kattamis, C., Metaxotou-Mavromati, A., Karamboula, K., et al. The clinical and haematological findings in children inheriting two types of thalassaemia: High-$A_2$ type β-thalassaemia, and high-F type or δβ-thalassaemia. *Br. J. Haematol.* 25:375–384, 1973.

55. Mann, J.R., MacNeish, A.S., Bannister, P., et al. δβ-Thalassemia in a Chinese family. *Br. J. Haematol.* 23:393–402, 1972.

56. Ottolenghi, S., Lanyon, W.G., Williamson, R., et al. Human globin gene analysis for a case of β⁰/δβ thalassemia. *Proc. Natl. Acad. Sci. USA* 72:2294–2299, 1975.

57. Stamatoyannopoulos, G., Schroeder, W.A., Huisman, T.H.J., et al. Nature of foetal haemoglobin in F-thalassaemia. *Br. J. Haematol.* 21:633–642, 1971.

58. Quattrin, N., and Ventruto, V. Hemoglobin Lepore: Its significance for thalassemia and clinical manifestations. *Ann. NY Acad. Sci.* 232:65–74, 1974.

59. Baglioni, C. The fusion of two peptide chains in hemoglobin Lepore and its interpretation as a genetic deletion. *Proc. Natl. Acad. Sci. USA* 48:1880–1886, 1962.

60. McDonald, M.J., Nobel, R.W., Sharma, V.S., et al. A comparison of the functional properties of two Lepore hemoglobins with those of hemoglobin A. *J. Mol. Biol.* 94:305–310, 1975.

61. Quattrin, N., and Ventruto, V. Hemoglobin Lepore: Its significance for thalassemia and clinical manifestations. *Blut* 28:327–336, 1974.

62. Fessas, Ph., Stamatoyannopoulos, G., and Karaklis, A. Hemoglobin "Pylos": Study of a hemoglobinopathy resembling thalassemia in the heterozygous, homozygous, and double heterozygous state. *Blood* 19:1–22, 1962.

63. Gerald, P.S., and Diamond, L.K. A new hereditary hemoglobinopathy (the Lepore trait) and its interaction with thalassemia trait. *Blood* 13:835–844, 1958.

64. White, J.M., Lang, A., Lorkin, P.A., et al. Synthesis of haemoglobin Lepore, *Nature (New Biol.)* 235:208–210, 1972.

65. White, J.M., Lang, A., and Lehmann, H. Compensation of β chain synthesis by the β chain gene in Hb Lepore trait. *Nature (New Biol.)* 240:271–273, 1972.

66. Forget, B.G., Cavallesco, C., Benz, E.J., et al. Studies of globin chain synthesis and globin mRNA content in a patient homozygous for hemoglobin Lepore. *Hemoglobin* 2:117–128, 1978.

67. Gill, F., Atwater, J., and Schwartz, E. Hemoglobin Lepore trait: Globin synthesis in bone marrow and peripheral blood. *Science* 178:623–625, 1972.

68. Duma, H., Efremov, G., Sadikario, A., et al. Study of nine families with haemoglobin-Lepore. *Br. J. Haematol.* 15:161–172, 1968.

69. Ventruto, V., Cimino, R., DeRosa, L., et al. Disease due to Hb Lepore

and βδ-microcythemia. The first observation. *Progr. Med.* 23:920-924, 1967.

70. Fessas, Ph., and Stamatoyannopoulos, G. A study and a comparison of hereditary persistence of fetal hemoglobin in Greece. *Blood* 24:223–240, 1964.

71. Sofronidou, K., Wood, W.G., Nute, P.E., et al. Globin chain synthesis in the Greek type ($^A\gamma$) of hereditary persistence of fetal haemoglobin. *Br. J. Haematol.* 29:137–148, 1975.

72. Huisman, T.H.J., Schroeder, W.A., Stamatoyannopoulos, G., et al. Nature of fetal hemoglobin in the Greek type of hereditary persistence of fetal hemoglobin with and without concurrent β-thalassemia. *J. Clin. Invest.* 49:1035-1040, 1970.

73. Conley, C.L., Weatherall, D.J., Richardson, S.N., et al. Hereditary persistence of fetal hemoglobin: A study of 79 affected persons in 15 Negro families in Baltimore. *Blood* 21:261–281, 1963.

74. Friedman, Sh., Schwartz, E., Ahern, E., et al. Variations in globin chain synthesis in hereditary persistence of foetal haemoglobin. *Br. J. Haematol.* 32:357–364, 1976.

75. Natta, C.L., Niazi, G.A., Ford, S., et al. Balanced globin chain synthesis in hereditary persistence of fetal hemoglobin. *J. Clin. Invest.* 54:433–438, 1974.

76. Wheeler, J.T., and Krevans, J.R. The homozygous state of persistent fetal hemoglobin and the interaction of persistent fetal hemoglobin with thalassemia. *Bull. Johns Hopkins Hosp.* 109:217–233, 1961.

77. Siegel, W., Cox, R., Schroeder, W.A., et al. An adult homozygous for persistent fetal hemoglobin. *Ann. Intern. Med.* 72:533–536, 1970.

78. Ringelhaun, B., Konotey-Ahulu, F.I.D., Lehmann, H., et al. A Ghanian adult, homozygous for hereditary persistence of foetal haemoglobin and heterozygous for elliptocytosis. *Acta Haematol.* 43:100–110, 1970.

79. Huisman, T.H.J., Schroeder, W.A., Charache, S., et al. Hereditary persistence of fetal hemoglobin, heterogeneity of fetal hemoglobin in homozygotes and in conjunction with β-thalassemia. *N. Engl. J. Med.* 285:711–716, 1971.

80. Kamuzora, H., Ringelhaun, B., Konotey-Ahulu, F.I.D., et al. The γ-chain in a Ghanaian adult, homozygous for hereditary persistence of foetal haemoglobin. *Acta Haematol.* 51:179–184, 1974.

81. Kamuzora, H., Ringelhaun, B., Konotey-Ahulu, F.I.D., et al. Further investigation of the γ-chain in a Ghanaian adult, homozygous for hereditary persistence of foetal haemoglobin. *Acta Haematol.* 53:315–320, 1975.

82. Charache, S., Clegg, J.B., and Weatherall, D.J. The Negro variety of hereditary persistence of foetal haemoglobin is a mild form of thalassaemia. *Br. J. Haematol.* 34:527–534, 1976.

83. Forget, B.G., Hillman, D.G., Lazarus, H., et al. Absence of messenger RNA and gene DNA for β-globin chains in hereditary persistence of fetal hemoglobin. *Cell* 7:323–329, 1976.

84. Ringelhaun, B., Acquaye, C.T.A., Oldham, J.H., et al. Homozygotes for hereditary persistence of fetal hemoglobin. The ratio of $^G\gamma$ to $^A\gamma$ chain and biosynthesis studies. *Biochem. Genet.* 15:1083–1096, 1977.

85. Acquaye, C.T.A., Oldham, J.H. and Konotey-Ahulu, F.I.D. Blood donor homozygous for hereditary persistence of fetal hemoglobin. *Lancet* 1:796-797, 1977.

86. Sukumaran, P.K., Huisman, T.H.J., Schroeder, W.A., et al. A homozygote for the Hb $^G\gamma$ type of foetal haemoglobin in India: A study of two Indian and four Negro families. *Br. J. Haematol.* 23:403–417, 1972.

87. Yamak, B., Özsylu, S., Altay, C., et al. Hereditary persistence of foetal haemoglobin and β-thalassaemia in a Turkish child. *Acta Haematol.* 50:124–128, 1973.

88. Fogarty, W.M., Jr., Vedvick, T.S., and Itano, H.A. Absence of haemoglobin A in an individual simultaneously heterozygous in the genes for hereditary persistence of foetal haemoglobin and β-thalassaemia. *Br. J. Haematol.* 26:527–533, 1974.

89. Huisman, T.H.J., Miller, A., and Schroeder, W.A. A $^G\gamma$ type of hereditary persistence of fetal hemoglobin with β chain production in cis. *Am. J. Hum. Genet.* 27:765–777, 1975.

90. Friedman, Sh., and Schwartz, E. Hereditary persistence of foetal haemoglobin with β-chain synthesis in cis position ($^G\gamma$-$β^+$-HPFH) in a Negro family. *Nature* 259:138–140, 1976.

91. Huisman, T.H.J., Wrightstone, R.W., and Wilson, J.B. Hemoglobin Kenya, the product of fusion of γ and β polypeptide chains. *Arch. Biochem. Biophys.* 153:850–853, 1972.

92. Clegg, J.B., Weatherall, D.J., and Gilles, H.M. Hereditary persistence of foetal haemoglobin associated with a γβ fusion variant, haemoglobin Kenya. *Nature (New Biol.)* 246:184–186, 1973.

93. Kendall, A.G., Ojwong, P.J., Schroeder, W.A., et al. Hemoglobin Kenya, the product of a γ-β fusion gene: Studies of the family. *Am. J. Hum. Genet.* 25:548–563, 1973.

94. Nute, P.E., Wood, W.G., Stamatoyannopoulos, G., et al. The Kenya form of hereditary persistence of fetal haemoglobin: Structural studies and evidence for homogeneous distribution of haemoglobin F using fluorescent Anti-haemoglobin F antibodies. *Brit. J. Haematol.* 32:55–63, 1976.

95. Wood, W.G., Clegg, J.B., Weatherall, P.J., et al. $^G\gamma$ δβ Thalassaemia and $^G\gamma$ HPFH (Hb Kenya type): Comparison of 2 new cases. *J. Med. Genet.* 14:237–244, 1977.

96. Weatherall, D.J., Cartner, R., and Clegg, J.B. A form of hereditary persistence of foetal haemoglobin characterized by uneven cellular distribution of haemoglobin F and the production of haemoglobins A and $A_2$ in homozygotes. *Br. J. Haematol.* 29:205–220, 1975.

97. Wood, W.G., Weatherall, D.J., Clegg, J.B., et al. Heterocellular hereditary persistence of foetal haemoglobin (Heterocellular HPFH) and its interaction with β-thalassaemia. *Br. J. Haematol.* 36:461–473, 1977.

98. Kan, Y.W., Forget, B.G., and Nathan, D.G. Gamma-beta thalassemia: A cause of hemolytic disease of the newborn. *N. Engl. J. Med.* 286:129–134, 1972.

99. Ohta, Y., Yamaoka, K., Sumida, I., et al. Homozygous delta-thalassemia first discovered in Japanese family with hereditary persistence of fetal hemoglobin. *Blood* 37:706–715, 1971.

100. Silverstroni, E., Bianco, I., and Reitano, G. Three cases of homozygous βδ-thalassaemia (or microcythaemia) with high haemoglobin F in a Sicilian family. *Acta Haematol.* 40:220–229, 1968.

# 14 Beta Thalassemia Major (Cooley's Anemia)*

Frances M. Gill, M.D.
John F. Kelleher, Jr. M.D.

Beta thalassemia major, or Cooley's anemia, is a severe, inherited anemia requiring chronic transfusion therapy in nearly every patient. Decreased synthesis of $\beta$ globin chains leads to the accumulation of an excess of unstable $\alpha$ chains. Some of these are removed by proteolysis, but others precipitate, damaging the red cell membrane and leading to hemolysis of 70% to 85% of proliferative erythroid cells within the bone marrow.[1] Those cells which do circulate have a shortened survival. Because of the ineffective erythropoiesis and severe anemia, there is increased erythropoietic activity in the marrow. Extramedullary hematopoiesis occurs in such sites as the spleen, liver, and lymph nodes. Clinical manifestations are due primarily to chronic hemolysis, the body's attempts to compensate for the anemia, and excess iron that accumulates from blood transfusions. This chapter will

*The authors wish to thank Ruth Cuthbert for the preparation of the manuscript. This work was supported by NIH AM16691, NIH Research Training Grant HL07150, a contract from the Commonwealth of Pennsylvania, and The Cooley's Anemia Fund. Dr. Kelleher is a recipient of a fellowship from the Mainline Chapter of UNICO National.

discuss the clinical aspects of β thalassemia major and forms of intermediate severity.

The β-thalassemia gene is most prevalent in Italian and Greek populations but also occurs in other Mediterranean and in Middle-Eastern peoples, in North and West Africa, and in Asia, including Thailand and India. Although the β-thalassemia gene has been found in people of almost every ethnic background, its frequency is low except in the above-mentioned areas.[2]

## β THALASSEMIA MAJOR

The homozygous form, β thalassemia major or Cooley's anemia, is usually diagnosed in the first year of life. The common findings are pallor, irritability, failure to thrive, diarrhea, and abdominal enlargement. Onset of significant anemia usually occurs by six months of age but may be delayed in some cases until the second year. In three affected children followed prospectively from birth, the hemoglobin levels were below and the percentages of Hb F above the normal ranges by one to two months of age; morphologic abnormalities, reticulocytosis, and circulating nucleated red blood cells were present at six weeks; and splenomegaly was present by one to three months.[3] Physical examination of the infant reveals changes due to the anemia, such as pallor, tachycardia, and systolic ejection murmur. In addition, there is mild scleral icterus and splenomegaly. An occasional child may not have splenomegaly even though anemia is present. If transfusion therapy is delayed, greying of the skin and development of characteristic facies due to intramedullary expansion of the active marrow occur. The progression and severity of facial changes and of hepatic and splenic enlargement vary from child to child and may be prevented to a large degree by early initiation of a transfusion program which maintains the hemoglobin level in a normal or near-normal range.[4]

If no transfusions are given, the anemia becomes severe, as low as 3 to 5 g /dl in most children. Reticulocytosis of about 5% to 15% and the presence of nucleated red cells in the peripheral blood occur. The white cell count is usually elevated, but the platelet count is normal unless hypersplenism is present. The peripheral smear shows microcytic, hypochromic red cells with marked variations in cell size, shape, and hemoglobin content. Basophilic stippling and target cells are present. The most striking finding, however, is the extreme degree of anisocytosis and poikilocytosis.

Diagnosis can be suspected from the results of hemoglobin electrophoresis. Hemoglobin F is elevated, usually comprising 10% to 90% of the hemoglobin.[2] If the child has homozygous β⁰ thalassemia or one of the other variants producing no β chains, no Hb A will be found. If a β⁺-thalassemia allele is present, some Hb A will be synthesized. The Hb A₂ level is normal or slightly elevated but may occasionally be decreased. Confirmation of the diagnosis should include hemoglobin studies in the parents and siblings to determine the exact nature of the thalassemic defect. Globin chain synthesis studies may be necessary in some cases.

The bone marrow has extreme erythroid hyperplasia with predominence of early red cell precursors. Many late red cells show paucity of hemoglobin content. Early erythropoiesis is normoblastic unless there is a complicating folic acid deficiency. Supravital staining with methyl violet reveals purple inclusion bodies containing precipitated α chains in the red cells.[5] Similar precipitates of globin chains are found in some cases of β-thalassemia trait of unusual severity and in Hb H disease. They can be seen in appreciable numbers of circulating red cells only if the spleen is absent or nonfunctioning. Excessive iron is present in the marrow. Dyserythropoietic morphology is often observed.

Some children receiving regular blood transfusions may have such a severe degree of ineffective erythropoiesis that the peripheral blood findings reflect the properties of the transfused blood: normal red cell indices, absence of nucleated red cells, and nearly normal levels of Hb A₂ and Hb F. If confirmation of the underlying diagnosis is needed in these cases, family studies and methyl violet and globin synthesis studies of the marrow cells are helpful.

## β THALASSEMIA OF INTERMEDIATE SEVERITY

Many patients have symptoms intermediate to those of thalassemia trait and Cooley's anemia.[6,7] Anemia is usually moderate, reticulocytosis and the presence of nucleated red cells are more pronounced than in thalassemia trait, and transfusions are rarely required. With a better understanding of the molecular basis of the thalassemias, it has been possible to characterize genetically the assortment of disorders which produce this clinical state (Table 14-1).

Some patients, perhaps 5% to 15%, with β thalassemia major by clinical, laboratory, and globin synthesis studies can maintain their hemoglobin above 7 g/dl without transfusions.[3,6] They nearly always have splenomegaly and bone changes. Since the patients are able to lead an active life at this level of hemoglobin, transfusions should be avoided so that development of hemosiderosis can be prevented or significantly delayed. Occasionally a child with Cooley's anemia who has required regular transfusions may no longer need them after splenectomy. Prognosis is better in this group for sexual maturation and longevity than for the usual child with Cooley's anemia.[3]

**Table 14-1**
**Genetic Classification of β Thalassemia of Intermediate Clinical Severity**

Homozygous β thalassemia (especially in blacks)

Homozygous β thalassemia modified by α thalassemia

β-Thalassemia gene interacting with another thalassemia gene

    Silent carrier gene

    δβ gene

Homozygous δβ thalassemia

β-Thalassemia gene interacting with a gene for a structurally abnormal hemoglobin

    Hb Lepore

    Hb E

    Others

Homozygosity for Hb Lepore

β-Thalassemia trait of unusual severity

     In the American or Jamaican black, β thalassemia major is a milder disease.[7,8,9] Despite elevations of Hb $A_2$ and Hb F and results of globin chain synthesis studies that are similar to those in Italian and Greek patients with Cooley's anemia, black patients are able to maintain acceptable hemoglobin levels without transfusions for a much longer period. Women with this condition have had successful pregnancies. Transfusion therapy becomes necessary as the hemoglobin level decreases, usually in the third or fourth decade. The complications once transfusion therapy has begun are the same, and death usually occurs from cardiac hemosiderosis in the third to fifth decade. In order to delay the development of hemosiderosis, these patients should not be transfused until the hemoglobin level falls sufficiently to cause symptoms and to interfere with a normal life. The reasons for the milder course in blacks are not known.

     The coexistence of an α-thalassemia gene with homozygous β thalassemia may modify the disease.[10,11] It is hypothesized that the decreased production of α chain results in less cell damage and destruction.

     In some patients, a β-thalassemia gene of the high Hb $A_2$ type interacts with another thalassemic gene to produce thalassemia of intermediate severity. Family studies have been helpful in elucidating these interactions. In one family the father was a silent carrier with normal red cell indices and Hb $A_2$ and Hb F levels but with decreased synthesis of β chains by reticulocytes.[12] The two children have the stigmata of thalassemia but do not require transfusions and have grown normally. Other combinations which have been reported to give a milder course are β/δβ thalassemia and homozygous δβ thalassemia.[13,14]

     Interaction of the high Hb $A_2$ gene with a structurally abnormal hemoglobin, such as Hb E, Hb Beograd, or, in some cases, Hb Lepore, results in a milder disease.[15,16] The β-thalassemia gene may also interact with an unstable hemoglobin such as Hb Saki or Hb Leslie to produce clinically important disease.[17,18]

Several families, some of northern European descent, with heterozygous β thalassemia of an unusual severity have been described.[19,20,21] The clinical findings have included anemia of moderate degree, reticulocytosis, circulating nucleated red cells, hepatosplenomegaly, gallstones, mild jaundice, and, in some patients, leg ulcers. The red cells show changes comparable to those in thalassemia major. Elevations of Hb $A_2$ and Hb F, however, are similar to those found in β thalassemia minor. Globin synthesis studies have shown that the decrease in β globin synthesis relative to that of α globin in reticulocytes is comparable to that found in β thalassemia minor.[20,21] The patients with thalassemia trait of unusual severity have shown a greater imbalance of globin synthesis in the bone marrow than have patients with the usual form of β-thalassemia trait.[21,22] This imbalance resulted in hemoglobin inclusion bodies in the red cells and in a larger pool of newly synthesized free α chains. In one family the red cells were not microcytic and hypochromic, and the authors postulated that the disorder was due to increased synthesis of α chains rather than to decreased β chain synthesis.[19]

## CURRENT THERAPY

Before red cell transfusions were available, children with Cooley's anemia had progressive physical deterioration and continued enlargement of the liver and spleen. In one series death occurred within 16 to 45 months in most cases and was due most often to intercurrent infections or congestive heart failure secondary to severe anemia and hypoxia.[23]

### Red Cell Transfusions

The mainstay of current therapy for the child with thalassemia major is a program of regular transfusions of red cells to maintain the hemoglobin at nearly normal levels. Prior to the late 1960's most patients received transfusions only when symptoms developed, usually at hemoglobin levels of 4 to 6 g/dl. However, the benefits of a high-transfusion program, in which the hemoglobin is maintained at levels of greater than 8 to 9 g/dl, have been clearly demonstrated.[24,25,26] This program allows children to participate fully in normal activities with their peers, decreases the degree of hepatosplenomegaly, and prevents or decreases bone changes. To date this program has not been clearly shown either to prolong or to shorten the life span of the children.

Almost all children with β thalassemia major will require transfusion therapy, since the anemia is so severe. It is our policy to give the first transfusion when the hemoglobin level falls below 6 g/dl and the child shows symptoms of irritability or poor growth. An initial series of transfusions is given to raise the hemoglobin to a level of about 10 g/dl. If the child again becomes severely anemic, a program of regular transfusions is begun. Occasionally, a child with either a thalassemic variant or milder homozygous thalassemia is able to maintain his or her hemoglobin above 7 g/dl and does not require transfusions.

Prior to the initial transfusion a complete red cell typing is done, so that unusual red cell antigens may be found and appropriate donor blood selected. The child has scheduled appointments for transfusions at a set interval which is individually determined so that the pre-transfusion level of hemoglobin is 9 to 10 g/dl. Most children require transfusions every two to six weeks. The amount of blood required increases gradually as the child grows. A blood sample is drawn in the morning for blood count and cross-matching, an interval history and complete physical examination are done, and the transfusion is given. The entire procedure requires only about five hours in the outpatient area, and the time spent in the hospital and away from normal activities is minimal.

We use packed red blood cells that are fewer than ten days old and are negative for hepatitis $B_s$ antigen by radioimmunoassay. Common reactions to blood include hives, fever, and chills. Premedication with an antihistamine and/or an antipyretic may help, but the use of washed red cells or frozen red cells is usually necessary to prevent reactions due to leukoagglutinins. Development of red cell antibodies is infrequent but when it occurs requires further screening of donor units to permit selection of compatible units.

Recently a transfusion program has been described in which the hemoglobin level is maintained above 12 g/dl in an attempt to decrease the transfusion requirement and the amount of dietary iron absorbed.[27] It is too early to evaluate this program, but initial results show that the blood volume and the plasma iron turnover, a measure of the amount of erythropoiesis, are decreased.

**Chelation Therapy**

The major complication in thalassemia major is the development of significant iron overload with resultant tissue damage. Although dietary iron absorption is probably inappropriately increased,[28,29] the major source of excessive iron is transfused red cells. The organ damage which results is described in detail below. Death occurs in most cases in the late teens or early twenties and is usually due to cardiac failure.[30] Effective iron chelation should significantly influence the course of the disease and prolong the life of these children. The present status of chelation therapy is described in detail elsewhere (See Chapter 15).

## Splenectomy

Splenectomy may be of major benefit to the patient with thalassemia major or thalassemia of intermediate severity. It may be done to relieve physical discomfort, to reduce the risk of accidental rupture, or to correct hypersplenism, the latter being the most common indication.[31] Splenomegaly results from a combination of extra-medullary hematopoiesis, reticuloendothelial hyperplasia, and hemosiderosis. Massive splenomegaly develops rapidly in untransfused or infrequently transfused patients but also occurs in some patients on adequate transfusion programs. In general, however, the transfusion program designed to keep hemoglobin levels above 8 to 9 g/dl seems to decrease the degree of splenomegaly and may reduce the incidence of hypersplenism.[26,32] Transfusion requirements may increase as the spleen enlarges because the transfused blood is diluted in the larger blood volume and more is pooled in the spleen. In addition, many children develop true hypersplenism with increased hemolysis of transfused cells. Hypersplenism is usually accompanied by thrombocytopenia, granulocytopenia, and an increasing transfusion requirement. Chromium survival studies with scanning for splenic uptake may be useful in documenting hypersplenism. Modell[32] has suggested that a more reliable indicator of hypersplenism is elevation of the patient's actual blood requirement over that predicted from a standard graph. In all of her patients, blood requirements have returned to the expected levels after splenectomy. These findings have been confirmed for patients of Italian extraction in the United States.[33]

Following splenectomy, platelet and granulocyte counts rapidly return to normal levels, and there is almost always a marked improvement in red cell survival.[34] Sustained improvement in transfusion requirements may occur more frequently in those children who have milder forms of the disease and who were therefore started on transfusions at an older age.[35] Increased numbers of nucleated red blood cells, reticulocytes, Howell-Jolly bodies, and methyl violet inclusion bodies may be seen in the peripheral blood following splenectomy. The number of target cells is also increased. Thrombocytosis of greater than $1000 \times 10^9/l$ occurs frequently in the initial days but only rarely has been associated with thrombotic complications. Leukocyte counts of greater than $30 \times 10^9/l$ are frequent. In an occasional patient there will be no significant increase in reticulocytes and nucleated red blood cells following splenectomy.

Splenectomy for any indication and at any age is associated with an increased risk of fatal infection.[36,37] The risk is markedly increased when the operation is performed before 5 years of age[38] or for certain conditions, such as the Wiskott-Aldrich syndrome.[38] Splenectomized children with thalassemia also have a relatively high risk of overwhelming infection. In one series, there were nine serious infections with six deaths in 35 splenectomized patients with thalassemia as compared to three serious infections and no deaths in 23 nonsplenectomized patients.[39] In another group of 18 splenectomized patients there were six fatal infections, while there were none in ten who had their spleens.[38] In a third group, five infections, three of them fatal, occurred in 30 splenectomized patients.[35] Although the pneumococcus is the most frequent cause of serious infections, having been responsible for up to 70% of the cases in one series, infections with *Hemophilus influenzae,* meningococci, and *Escherichia coli* also occur.[31,39]

The mechanisms responsible for the increased risk of fatal infection have not been completely elucidated. The phagocytic function of the spleen is necessary to clear the blood stream of foreign particles or bacteria in the absence of antibodies.[40,41] There is also a suggestion that the spleen has an antibody-producing function early in the course of an infection.[42] Patients with thalassemia have higher levels of all classes of immunoglobulins when compared to normal persons.[43] In one series, significantly lower levels of IgM were found in splenectomized thalassemics than in nonsplenectomized patients, differing from findings in other series.[43,44,45]

The risk of fatal infection is decreased by deferring splenectomy until the patient is at least 5 years of age. Penicillin prophylaxis in the dose of 125 to 250 mg. orally twice a day is used frequently in an attempt to decrease pneumococcal infections after splenectomy. We have placed all our splenectomized patients with thalassemia on oral penicillin V, either 125 mg. or 250 mg. twice daily depending on weight, for an indefinite period. In a small series of patients with Hodgkin's disease, penicillin prophylaxis seems to have been successful in preventing severe infections.[46] Statistically significant data for patients with thalassemia are not available. The new polyvalent pneumococcal vaccine may lessen the risk of fulminant pneumococcal infections. Splenectomized patients should be seen immediately for any fever greater than 101°F. The use of a medical alert bracelet is strongly recommended.

## Other Therapy

The chronic hemolysis and marrow hypertrophy result in an increased requirement for folic acid. Folate deficiency has been found in many patients, and the use of folic acid supplementation has been beneficial.[47,48] Megaloblastic changes are not always seen in the blood cells of these patients. Regular supplementation with 1 mg. of folic acid daily should prevent folic acid deficiency and is particularly important in those patients not requiring regular transfusions.

Children with thalassemia major and their families require emotional support. Although the intelligence of the children is not affected, the stresses of chronic disease may contribute to the development of emotional problems.[49] It is important that physicians spend adequate time explaining the disease to the parents and to the child as he or she matures. The management of the adolescent or young adult who is developing significant organ damage is particularly difficult. At this time, support from ancillary personnel, such as social workers, psychologists, and psychiatrists, as well as from the regular physicians, is particularly important. The financial drain on the family is large, particularly if the family must pay the costs of chelation therapy, and it may be necessary to secure help from social agencies. The establishment of state and federally supported programs should be of major help in this area.

## COMPLICATIONS

The complications of β thalassemia major result primarily from excessive hematopoiesis, chronic hemolysis, and iron overload with resultant organ damage. Children with thalassemia variants such as homozygous δβ thalassemia, β thalassemia/δβ thalassemia, homozygous Hb Lepore, and β thalassemia/Hb Lepore may have a clinical course identical to that of Cooley's anemia.

### Complications Due to Excessive Hematopoiesis

Massive bone marrow hypertrophy and extramedullary hematopoiesis result from the body's attempt to compensate for the profound anemia. Bone changes, particularly cephalofacial deformity, are characteristic findings in most of these children. Radiologic abnormalities of bone appear by the second year of life and are fully developed by the fourth to tenth year.[50] Expansion of the diploic space by marrow hyperplasia causes abnormalities of the skull and interferes with orderly osteogenesis. Rarefaction of the outer table and subperiosteal bone formation contribute to the production of radiating striations, the characteristic "hair on end" appearance of the thalassemic skull on roentgenogram. A typical "rodent facies" develops due to maxillary overgrowth, with resulting overbite, protrusion of the exposed incisor teeth, and separation of the orbits.[4] Slanting of the eyes, malar prominence, and flattening of the nasal bridge produce a "mongoloid facies." Chronic sinusitis is a frequent complication of the skull changes.[2] Hearing may be impaired by extra-medullary hematopoiesis in the ear canal.[51]

Recurrent pathologic fractures are the result of cortical thinning which occurs because of marrow hyperplasia. In one series of 75 patients, 25 developed 47 fractures.[52] These were most common in the long bones of the legs and were frequently associated with poor healing and resultant deformity. The skeletal abnormalities appear to be almost completely preventable by the high hemoglobin transfusion program if it is begun before four years of age.[24,26,53] In cases of pronounced facial deformity and orthodontic problems, surgical treatment may be helpful.[54]

Direct expansion of hematopoietic tissue from the vertebral marrow to the epidural space can cause spinal cord compression and paresis.[55,56,57] Seven cases of spinal cord compression have been described. It is of interest that four of these patients were black, one had thalassemia minor, and all but one were older than 20 years. It is theorized that a prolonged period of marrow hypertrophy, as seen in these milder thalassemic syndromes, may be required for the development of a hematopoietic tumor large enough to cause spinal cord compression. Surgical removal of the hematopoietic tissue, or surgery plus radiation therapy, has led to complete recovery in several cases.[55,56]

Extramedullary hematopoiesis in lymph nodes may cause noticeable enlargement, particularly in the mediastinum. This complication has been noted in patients with thalassemia of intermediate severity,[3] particularly, in our experience, in black patients who have not been receiving regular transfusions. If the physician is not aware of this explanation for mediastinal lymphadenopathy, the patient may be subjected to unnecessary thoracotomy.

Splenomegaly and hepatomegaly are due in part to extramedullary hematopoiesis. In most patients the liver will enlarge further after the spleen is removed.

### Complications Due to Chronic Hemolysis

Multiple pigmentary gallstones are found in two-thirds of patients over 15 years of age.[31] Cholecystectomy has not been recommended unless biliary colic or obstructive jaundice occurs. However, elective cholecystectomy is sometimes done at the time of splenectomy if gallstones are present.

Leg ulcers are not as frequent in thalassemia as in sickle cell disease. Approximately 30 cases have been reported in the literature.[58-62] These ulcers are often chronic or recurrent and usually occur in adolescent or adult patients. A recent report suggests that ulcers occur more frequently if there is an associated G-6-PD deficiency, although the method of measuring G-6-PD was not stated.[59] A controlled series in thalassemic patients demonstrates a promising effect of high doses of vitamin C in healing these chronic ulcers.[62] No complications were noted during the course of therapy.

## Complications Due to Iron Overload

The major cause of morbidity and death in transfused children with thalassemia major is iron overload and organ damage, particularly of the heart. All thalassemic children, even those who have not been transfused, develop some hemosiderosis. Although the contribution of dietary iron, particularly in those patients not receiving regular transfusions, is not clear, the major source of the excessive iron is from red cell transfusions. In animal models it has been extremely difficult to produce organ fibrosis by iron overloading alone.[63,64,65] The question thus arises whether additional pathologic mechanisms, such as hypoxia, must be invoked to explain the pathologic changes seen in thalassemic patients.

**Cardiac Problems**　Two types of cardiac problems are common: acute pericarditis, which appears to be relatively benign; and cardiac failure, arrhythmias, and heart block, which are usually fatal within a few months.[30]

Pericarditis occurred in 19 of 46 patients in one series and was recurrent in many patients.[30] The average age at the time of the initial attack was 11 years. The episodes were preceded by an upper respiratory or gastrointestinal disturbance. Sixteen of the 19 patients had been splenectomized. The illness was self-limited, generally lasting 2 to 3 weeks. Antibiotics were of no value. In an Asian population of splenectomized thalassemics, there was a markedly increased incidence of β-streptococcal infections.[66] The author felt the episodes of pericarditis were probably a manifestation of rheumatic disease. The observation of increased streptococcal disease has also been made in a population of splenectomized Greek thalassemics.[67]

Cardiac arrhythmias and congestive heart failure are the leading causes of death in transfused thalassemic patients. In one series of 25 patients the average age of onset of cardiac failure was 16 years, and the range was from 6 to 31 years of age.[30] Digitalis, diuretics, salt restriction, oxygen, bed rest if needed, and cautious transfusion were employed as therapy. However, 24 of the 25 patients died, 14 within 3 months. Only seven lived more than one year after the appearance of heart failure. Pathologic findings were those of myocardial hemosiderosis. In studies in mice, iron loading alone did not produce myocardial iron deposition, but a combination of hypoxia secondary to anemia and iron loading produced changes comparable to myocardial hemosiderosis.[68] This study suggested that the use of a high transfusion regimen with prevention of hypoxia might prevent cardiac involvement despite the presence of iron overload. However, deaths due to cardiac failure in patients receiving adequate transfusions have been described[69] and have occurred in our own patient population. The efficacy of chelation therapy in preventing or reversing cardiac damage is not yet known.

**Hepatic Problems**    Hepatic fibrosis and cirrhosis develop in transfused patients with thalassemia major, and the pathologic findings are identical to those of idiopathic hemochromatosis.[70] Most patients do not have clinical problems from the hepatic damage. Mild to moderate impairment of the coagulation mechanism due to the decreased production of liver-dependent factors is frequent after 7 years of age, although symptomatic bleeding is rare.[71] Oral vitamin K therapy may be of benefit in patients with early, mild changes. Digital clubbing has been described recently in 10 of 22 Orientals with thalassemia and may be related to liver disease.[72] Liver biopsies in 12 thalassemic patients, ranging in age from 4 to 21 years, showed some evidence of hemosiderosis in all, but only the three who had been previously splenectomized had cirrhosis.[73] The authors felt that the postsplenectomy state rather than age or number of transfusions was the important factor in this association. They hypothesized that splenectomy removes a large reservoir for iron storage and causes subsequent increased hepatic deposition of iron. However, a pathologic study did not find higher total liver iron in splenectomized patients.[70] The advantages of splenectomy in decreasing the transfusion requirement must be weighed against this possible problem.

Histologic evidence of hepatitis was found in 23 of 26 patients biopsied because of liver transaminases which were persistently elevated for more than 6 months.[74] Of the biopsied patients, 77% had serologic evidence of previous exposure to the hepatitis B virus. The authors suggest that hepatitis B infection may be important in the development of thalassemic liver disease.

**Pancreatic Problems**    Abnormal carbohydrate metabolism is a common finding in thalassemic patients. Oral glucose tolerance tests have been reported to be abnormal in 31 of 54 patients tested in several series, and four of these patients had insulin-dependent diabetes.[75-78] There was a definite correlation between age and number of transfusions and the presence of an abnormal glucose tolerance test.[76] The mechanism of this abnormality is not clear. Some investigators have reported a decreased release of insulin,[75] while others have found normal release but insulin resistance.[77] Genetic predisposition also appears to be important, since 75% to 80% of the patients with a positive family history for diabetes have abnormal function.[75,77] Pancreatic glucagon secretion has also been reported to be impaired.[78]

**Growth and Development**    Poor growth and delayed sexual maturation are problems which are distressing to the patient, particularly during adolescent years. Height is significantly decreased from that predicted by parental height.[79] In a series of 229 Greek patients with thalassemia on a relatively infrequent transfusion program, only 14% of children less than 8 years of age were below the tenth percentile, but 69% of children over 12 years of age were less than the tenth percentile.[80] Initially, these patients had a normal or increased height velocity, but this diminished by 6 to 8 years of age. There was no adolescent growth spurt. Bone age lagged behind chronologic age, and the patients continued to grow for up to 21 years. Despite this prolonged growth period, 70% were below the tenth percentile at 21 years of age.[80] It had been hoped that the patients would experience a "catch up" growth spurt when regular transfusions were instituted. However, such a spurt was not observed in 28 patients.[24,81] Even the use of a high hemoglobin regimen from early childhood may not prevent growth failure. In four patients begun on such a program during the first year of life, all were between the 25th and 50th percentile in height at 2 to 6 years of age. Five years later, however, the percentiles for these children were the third, fifth, tenth and 25th.[26,82]

The mechanism of growth failure is not clear. Growth hormone levels have been repeatedly found to be normal or increased.[78,79,83] It has been postulated that hemosiderosis may interfere with the action of growth hormones.[79] Decreased levels of gonadotropins may also contribute to this failure.

Delayed sexual maturation is almost universal in patients with thalassemia major. In girls, breast development and menarche, if they occur, are usually late. Complete or partial failure of sexual development is more common in boys. Gonadotropins appear to be normal during childhood, but the expected rise is not seen at puberty,[78,84] suggesting impaired pituitary or hypothalamic function. Testosterone injections may be of benefit, at least psychologically, to adolescent boys, but the potential risk of hepatocellular cancer must be considered. The effects of chelation therapy on growth and sexual maturation are not yet known.

**Other Organs**    Studies of adrenal cortical function using standard methods have revealed no abnormalities.[75,78,83] Release of cortisol in response to tetracosactrin stimulation is significantly less in patients with thalassemia than in normals, suggesting impaired adrenal cortical function.[75] The author suggests that the very high levels of circulating ACTH found in these patients are necessary to produce normal adrenocortical response. He also suggests that the thalassemic pigmentation is due to the high levels of ACTH, which is similar in structure to melanophore stimulating hormone (MSH).

Thyroid and parathyroid function are generally normal, but acquired hypoparathyroidism has been found in transfused patients.

Epistaxis occurs frequently, but the mechanism is not clear,[71] since it can occur in the presence of a normal platelet count and normal coagulation studies.

Cooley's anemia is a chronic severe disease which at present is incurable. Improvement of bone marrow transplantation techniques may offer the hope of curative therapy in the future. Recent advances in molecular biology suggest that genetic manipulation and reactivation of γ chain synthesis may one day be available. At present the mainstay of therapy is a regular transfusion program to maintain the hemoglobin at normal or near-normal levels. Although this allows the child to lead an active, nearly normal life, it also leads to excessive iron accumulation and eventual death. If effective chelation and prevention of organ damage can be accomplished, then in the near future the useful life of these children should be significantly prolonged.

## REFERENCES

1. Dormer, P., and Betke, K. Erythroblast kinetics in homozygous and heterozygous thalassemia. Br. J. Haematol. 38:5–14, 1978.
2. Weatherall, D.J., and Clegg, J.B. The Thalassemia Syndromes. 2nd Ed. Oxford: Blackwell Scientific Publications, 1972.
3. Erlandson, M.E., Brilliant, R., and Smith, C.H. Comparison of sixty-six patients with thalassemia major and thirteen patients with thalassemia intermedia: Including evaluations of growth, development, maturation, and prognosis. Ann. NY Acad. Sci. 119:727–735, 1964.
4. Logothetis, J., Economidou, J., Constantoulakis, M., et al. Cephalofacial deformities in thalassemia major (Cooley's anemia). Am. J. Dis. Child. 121:300–306, 1971.
5. Fessas, P., Loukipoulos, D., and Kaltsoya, A., Peptide analysis of the inclusions of erythroid cells in beta-thalassemia. Biochim. Biophys. Acta 124:430–432, 1966.
6. Pearson, H.A. Thalassemia intermedia: Genetic and biochemical considerations. Ann. NY Acad. Sci. 119:390–401, 1964.
7. Braverman, A.S., McCurdy, P.R., Manos, O., et al. Homozygous beta thalassemia in American blacks: The problem of mild thalassemia. J. Lab. Clin. Med. 81:857–866, 1973.
8. Friedman, Sh., Hamilton, R.W., and Schwartz, E. Beta-thalassemia in the American Negro. J. Clin. Invest. 52:1453–1459, 1973.
9. Ahern, E., Herbert, R., McIver, C., et al. Beta-thalassemia of clinical significance in adult Jamaican Negroes. Br. J. Haematol. 30:197–201, 1975.
10. Kan, Y.W., and Nathan, D.G. Mild thalassemia: The result of interac-

tions of alpha and beta thalassemia genes. *J. Clin. Invest.* 49:635–642, 1970.

11. Bates, C.M., and Humphries, G. Alpha-beta thalassemia. *Lancet* 1:1031–1033, 1977.

12. Schwartz, E. The silent carrier of beta thalassemia. *N. Engl. J. Med.* 281:1327–1333, 1969.

13. Stamatoyannopoulos, G., Fessas, P., and Papayannopoulou, T. F-thalassemia: A study of thirty-one families with simple heterozygotes and combinations of F-thalassemia with A₂-thalassemia. *Am. J. Med.* 47:194–199, 1969.

14. Kattamis, C., Metaxotou-Mavromati, A., Karamboula, K., et al. The clinical and haematological findings in children with two types of thalassemia: High A₂ type thalassemia, and high F type or δβ-thalassemia. *Br. J. Haematol.* 25:375–384, 1973.

15. Chatterjea, J.B. Some aspects of haemoglobin E and its genetic interaction with thalassaemia. *Indian J. Med. Res.* 53:377–398, 1965.

16. Rudvidić, R., Efremov, G.D., Juricić, D., et al. Hemoglobin Beograd ($\alpha_2\beta_2$ 121 glu→val) interacting with β-thalassemia. *Acta Haematol.* 54:180–184, 1975.

17. Milner, P.F., Corley, C.C., Pomeroy, W.L., et al. Thalassemia intermedia caused by heterozygosity for both β-thalassemia and hemoglobin Saki [β14 (A 11) leu→pro]. *Am. J. Hematol.* 1:283–292, 1976.

18. Lutcher, C.L., Wilson, J.B., Gravely, M., et al. Hb Leslie, an unstable hemoglobin due to deletion of glutaminyl residue β131(H9) occurring in association with β⁰-thalassemia, Hb C, and Hb S. *Blood* 47:99–112, 1976.

19. Weatherall, D.J., Clegg, J.B., Knox-Macauley, H.H.M., et al. A genetically determined disorder with features both of thalassaemia and congenital dyserythropoietic anaemia. *Br. J. Haematol.* 24:681–702, 1973.

20. Stamatoyannopoulos, G., Woodson, R., Papayanopoulou, T., et al. Inclusion-body β-thalassemia trait. A form of β-thalassemia producing clinical manifestations in simple heterozygotes. *N. Engl. J. Med.* 290:939–943, 1974.

21. Friedman, Sh., Ozsoylu, S., Luddy, R., et al. Heterozygous beta thalassemia of unusual severity. *Br. J. Haematol.* 32:65–77, 1976.

22. Schwartz, E., and Gill, F.M. Regulation of hemoglobin synthesis in β-thalassemia. *Ann. NY Acad. Sci.* 232:33–39, 1974.

23. Baty, J.M., Blackfan, K.D., and Diamond, L.K. Blood studies in infants and in children. I. Erythroblastic anemia; a clinical and pathologic study. *Am. J. Dis. Child.* 43:667–704, 1932.

24. Wolman, I.J., and Ortolani, M. Some clinical features of Cooley's anemia patients as related to transfusion schedules. *Ann. NY Acad. Sci.* 165:407–414, 1969.

25. Necheles, T.F., Chung, S., Sabbah, R., et al. Intensive transfusion therapy in thalassemia major: An eight-year followup. *Ann. NY Acad. Sci.* 232:197–185, 1974.

26. Piomelli, S., Karpatkin, M.H., Arzanian, M., et al. Hypertransfusion regimen in patients with Cooley's anemia. *Ann. NY Acad. Sci.* 232:186–192, 1974.

27. Propper, R.D., and Nathan, D.G. Persistent maintenance of normal hematocrits in thalassemia major. *Blood* 50(Suppl. 1):116, 1977.

28. Erlandson, M.E., Walden, B., Stern, G., et al. Studies on congenital hemolytic syndromes. IV. Gastrointestinal absorption of iron. *Blood* 19:359–378, 1962.

29. Bannerman, R.M., Callendar, S.T., Hardisty, R.M., et al. Iron absorption in thalassemia. *Br. J. Haematol.* 10:490–495, 1964.

30. Engle, M.A. Cardiac involvement in Cooley's anemia. *Ann. NY Acad. Sci.* 119:694–702, 1964.

31. Pearson, H.A., and O'Brien, R.T. The management of thalassemia major. *Semin. Hematol.* 12:255–265, 1975.

32. Modell, B. Total management of thalassemia major. *Arch. Dis. Child.* 52:489–500, 1977.

33. Cohen, A.R., Markinson, A., and Schwartz, E. Transfusion requirements and splenectomy in patients with Cooley's anemia. *Pediatr. Res.* 12:462, 1978.

34. Bouroncle, B.A., and Doan, C.A. Cooley's anemia: Indicators for splenectomy. *Ann. NY Acad. Sci.* 119:709–721, 1964.

35. Englehard, D., Cividalli, G., and Rachmilewitz, E.A. Splenectomy in homozygous beta thalassemia: A retrospective study of 30 patients. *Br. J. Haematol.* 31:391–403, 1975.

36. Robinette, C., and Fraumeni, J.W. Splenectomy and subsequent mortality in veterans of the 1939–45 war. *Lancet* 2:127–129, 1977.

37. Krivit, W. Overwhelming postsplenectomy infection. *Am. J. Hematol.* 2:193–201, 1977.

38. Eraklis, A.J., Kevy, S.V., and Diamond, L.K. Hazard of overwhelming infection after splenectomy in childhood. *N. Engl. J. Med.* 276:1225–1229, 1967.

39. Smith, C.H., Erlandson, M.E., Stern, G., et al. Post-splenectomy infection in Cooley's anemia. *Ann. NY Acad. Sci.* 119:748–757, 1964.

40. Benacerraf, B., Sebestyen, M., and Schlossman, S. A quantitative study of the kinetics of blood clearance of $P^{32}$ labelled E. coli and staphylococci by the reticuloendothelial system. *J. Exp. Med.* 110:27–64, 1959.

41. Schulkind, M.L., Ellis, E.F., and Smith, R.T. Effect of antibody upon clearance of $I^{125}$ labelled pneumococci by the spleen and liver. *Pediatr. Res.* 1:178–184, 1967.

42. Johnston, R.B., Newman, S.L., and Struth, A.G. An abnormality of the alternate pathway in complement activation in sickle cell disease. *N. Engl. J. Med.* 288:803–808, 1973.

43. Wasi, C., Wasi, P., and Throngcharoen, P. Serum immunoglobulin levels in thalassemia and the effects of splenectomy. *Lancet* 2:237–239, 1971.

44. Seitanidis, B., Mikas, A., and Angleopoulou, S. Serum immunoglobulins in β-thalassemia after splenectomy. *Acta Haematol.* 46:267–270, 1971.

45. Valissi-Adam, H., Nassika, E., and Kattimis, C. Immunoglobulin levels in children with homozygous beta-thalassemia. *Acta Paediatr. Scand.* 65:23–27, 1976.

46. Lanzkowsky, P., Shander, A., Karayalan, G., et al. Staging laparotomy and splenectomy: Treatment and complications of Hodgkin's disease in children. *Am. J. Hematol.* 1:393–404, 1976.

47. Jandl, J.H., and Greenberg, M.S. Bone-marrow failure due to relative nutritional deficiency in Cooley's hemolytic anemia. Painful "erythropoietic crises" in response to folic acid. *N. Engl. J. Med.* 260:461–468, 1959.

48. Lubby, A.L., Cooperman, J.M., and Feldman, R. Folic acid deficiency as a limiting factor in the anemias of thalassemia major. *Blood* 18:786–787, 1961.

49. Logothetis, J., Haritos-Fatouros, M., Constantoulakis, M., et al. Intelligence and behavioral patterns in patients with Cooley's anemia (homozygous beta-thalassemia): A study based on 138 consecutive cases. *Pediatrics* 48:740–744, 1971.

50. Chatterjea, J.B. Thalassemia: Clinical and hematological aspects. *Sandoz J. Med. Sci.* 7:101, 1965.

51. Hazell, J.W., and Modell, C.B. E.N.T. complications in thalassemia major. *J. Laryngol. Otol.* 90:877–881, 1976.

52. Dines, D.M., Canale, V.C., and Arnold, W.D. Fractures in thalassemia. *J. Bone Joint Surg.* 58A:662–666, 1976.

53. Johnston, F.E., and Roseman, J.M. The effects of more frequent transfusions upon bone loss in thalassemia major. *Pediatr. Res.* 1:479–483, 1967.

54. Jurkiewicz, M.J., Pearson, H.A., and Furlow, L.T., Jr. Reconstruction of the maxilla in thalassemia. *Ann. NY Acad. Sci.* 165:437–442, 1969.

55. Luyendijk, W., Went, L., and Schaad, H. Spinal cord compression due to extramedullary hematopoiesis in homozygous thalassemia. *J. Neurosurg.* 42:212–216, 1975.

56. Sorsdahl, O.E., Taylor, P.E., and Noyes, W.D. Extramedullary hematopoiesis, mediastinal masses, and spinal cord compression. *JAMA* 189:343–347, 1964.

57. Gatto, I., Terrana, V., and Biondi, L. Compressione sul midollo spinale du proliferazione di midollo osseo nella spazio epidurale in sagetto affeto da malattia di Cooley splenectomizzato. *Haematologica* 38:61, 1954.

58. Estes, J., Farber, E., and Stickney, J. Ulcers of the leg in Mediterranean disease. *Blood* 3:302–306, 1948.

59. Ganor, S., and Cohen, T. Leg ulcers in a family with beta-thalassemia and G-6-PD deficiency. *Br. J. Dermatol.* 95:203–206, 1976.

60. Pascher, F., and Keen, R. Ulcers of the leg in Cooley's anemia. *N. Engl. J. Med.* 256:1220–1222, 1957.

61. Craig, R.P., Bate, C.M., and Humphries, G. Surgical aspects of beta-thalassemia. *Br. J. Surg.* 64:277–280, 1977.

62. Afifi, A.M., Ellis, L., Huntsman, R.G., et al. High dose ascorbic acid in the management of thalassemic leg ulcers—a pilot study. *Br. J. Dermatol.* 92:339–341, 1975.

63. Witzleben, C. The pathogenesis of iron toxicity. *Ann. NY Acad. Sci.* 165:105–110, 1969.

64. Brown, E.B., Dubach, R., and Smith, D. Studies in iron transportation and metabolism. Long term iron overload in dogs. *J. Lab. Clin. Med.* 50:862–893, 1959.

65. Lisboa, P.E. Experimental hepatic cirrhosis in dogs caused by chronic massive iron overload. *Gut* 12:363–368, 1971.

66. Wasi, P. Streptococcal infection leading to cardiac and renal involvement in thalassemia. *Lancet* 1:949–950, 1971.

67. Economidou, J., and Constantoulakis, M. Streptococcal infection in thalassemia. *Lancet* 2:1160–1161, 1971.

68. Necheles, T.F., Beard, M.E.J., and Allen, D.M. Myocardial hemosiderosis in hypoxic mice. *Ann. NY Acad. Sci.* 165:167–170, 1969.

69. Beard, M.E.J., Necheles, T.F., and Allen, D.M. Clinical experience with intensive transfusion therapy in Cooley's anemia. *Ann. NY Acad. Sci.* 165:415–422, 1969.

70. Risdon, R., Barry, M., and Flynn, D. Transfusional iron overload. Relationship between tissue iron concentration and hepatic fibrosis in thalassemia. *J. Pathol.* 116:83–95, 1975.

71. Hilgartner, M.W., and Smith, C.H. Coagulation studies as a measure of liver function in Cooley's anemia. *Ann. NY Acad. Sci.* 119:631–640, 1964.

72. Sinniah, O., White, J.C., Omar, A., et al. Digital clubbing, a clinical sign in thalassemia. *J. Pediatr.* 92:597–599, 1978.

73. Okon, E., Levy, I., and Rachmilewitz, E.A. Splenectomy, iron overload, and liver cirrhosis in β-thalassemia major. *Acta Haematol.* 56:142–150, 1976.

74. Masera, G., Jean, G., Gazzola, G., et al. Role of chronic hepatitis in development of thalassemic liver disease. *Arch. Dis. Child.* 51:680–685, 1976.

334

75. McIntosh, N. Endocrinopathy in thalassemia major. *Arch. Dis. Child.* 51:195–201, 1976.

76. Saudek, C., Hemm, R., and Peterson, C. Abnormal glucose tolerance test in thalassemia major. *Metabolism* 26:43–52, 1977.

77. Costin, G., Kogut, M., Hyman, C., et al. Carbohydrate metabolism and pancreatic islet cell function in thalassemia major. *Diabetes* 26:230–240, 1977.

78. Lassman, M.N., O'Brien, R.T., Pearson, H.A., et al. Endocrine evaluation in thalassemia major. *Ann. NY Acad. Sci.* 232:226–237, 1974.

79. Zaino, E.C., Kuo, B., and Rozinski, M.S. Growth retardation in thalassemia major. *Ann. NY Acad. Sci.* 165:394–399, 1969.

80. Constantoulakis, M., Panagopolous, G., and Augoustaki, O. Stature and longitudinal growth in thalassemia major. *Clin. Pediatr.* 14:355–357, 1975.

81. Wolff, J.A., and Luke, K.H. Management of thalassemia, a comparative program. *Ann. NY Acad. Sci.* 165:423–427, 1969.

82. Piomelli, S., Danoff, M.H., Becker, M.J., et al. Prevention of bone malformations and cardiomegaly in Cooley's anemia by early hypertransfusion regimen. *Ann. NY Acad. Sci.* 165:427–436, 1969.

83. Canale, V.C., Steinherz, P., New, M., et al. Endocrine function in thalassemia major. *Ann. NY Acad. Sci.* 232:333–345, 1974.

84. Anoussakis, C., Alexiou, D., Abatyos, D., et al. Endocrinological investigation of pituitary gonadal axis in thalassemia major. *Acta Paediatr. Scand.* 66:49–51, 1977.

# 15 Iron Overload in Children with Hemoglobinopathies*

Alan Cohen, M.D.
Elias Schwartz, M.D.

Repeated red cell transfusions and excessive gastrointestinal iron absorption may lead to the accumulation of massive iron stores in children with disorders of hemoglobin. Iron deposition in critical organs, particularly the heart, liver, and endocrine glands, causes severe clinical problems, often culminating in death. Since body iron losses are minimal under normal conditions and fail to increase in the face of iron overload, the major therapeutic thrust has been directed toward reducing iron intake when possible and removing stored iron by the use of chelating agents. If such measures are successful, there will be vast improvements in the quality of life for many children with hemoglobinopathies.

In this chapter we will consider the contribution of transfusional and dietary iron to iron overload and will examine in depth the use of

*The authors wish to thank Carol Way for preparation of the manuscript. This work was supported by NIH grants AM 16691 and HL07150, a contract from the Commonwealth of Pennsylvania, and gifts from The Cooley's Anemia Fund and Ciba-Geigy Pharmaceutical Company. The studies were conducted in the Clinical Research Center of The Children's Hospital of Philadelphia, supported by the Division of Research Resources grant FR-240.

335

deferoxamine and other iron chelating agents for the removal of excessive iron stores.

## TRANSFUSIONAL IRON

Among the childhood hematologic disorders, secondary hemochromatosis most commonly occurs in patients with homozygous $\beta$ thalassemia who require regular transfusions. Since each 250 ml unit of packed red cells contains approximately 250 mg of iron, most of these patients will have accumulated more than 50 g of iron by the age of 10 years. Although it was once believed that hemoglobin iron would be stored exclusively in the reticuloendothelial cells with little organ dysfunction, it is now clear that in iron overload of this magnitude, storage occurs in both parenchymal and reticuloendothelial cells and organ damage is usually severe.[1]

The use of transfusion regimens to maintain hemoglobin levels above 8 to 9 g/dl has increased the rate of iron accumulation in comparison with previous methods of transfusing only for clinical need. However, death does not occur at an earlier age. Rather, patients have improved growth rates and less malformation of bones. Furthermore, there is some evidence that gastrointestinal iron absorption is reduced in most patients when hemoglobin concentrations are kept at this level.[2] Recently it has been demonstrated that hemoglobin levels can be maintained above 12 g/dl with no increase in transfusion requirements once this level is attained.[3] Since the transfusional iron would not be appreciably increased, potential benefits of this higher hemoglobin concentration should not be outweighed by an increased rate of iron loading. Children with thalassemia major should not be denied the benefits of transfusion above levels of at least 8 to 9 g/dl in order to conserve iron. No improvement in life expectancy will be gained and the recognized advantages of such a program will be lost.

Although regular red cell transfusions are not used routinely in the management of sickling disorders, specific complications such as strokes, leg ulcers, and recurrent severe infections may require multiple transfusions.[4,5,6] Iron stores, as measured by serum iron concentration, ferritin levels, and deferoxamine-induced urinary iron excretion, are directly related to the number of transfusions.[7] Several of our patients have been regularly transfused following strokes in a study to assess the effect of suppression of Hb S below 30% on cerebral arterial changes and the recurrence of neurologic findings.[4] Iron stores in these children are comparable to those found in 6- to 10-year-old children with transfusion-dependent thalassemia major.[7] One can thus anticipate the development of secondary hemochromatosis after several years of transfusion therapy in the absence of effective iron removal.

Urinary iron excretion without chelating agents is slightly increased in some patients with sickle cell anemia, but it is unrelated to the degree of iron overload and would account for an insignificant amount of the transfused iron.[8] Hepatic hemosiderosis has been attributed to transfusion iron loading in several patients.[9,10] Congestive heart failure, the most common fatal complication of iron overload in patients with thalassemia major, has occurred in at least one multiply transfused patient with sickle cell anemia in whom extensive iron deposition was found throughout the myocardium at autopsy.[11]

## IRON ABSORPTION

The absorption of inorganic iron is increased in patients with homozygous thalassemia when the hemoglobin level is below 8.5 g/dl.[2] When the hemoglobin level is raised above 9.5 g/dl the absorption of iron salts is reduced, frequently into a normal range. Iron in the form of hemoglobin, on the other hand, is normally absorbed in most patients with homozygous thalassemia, even at low hemoglobin levels.[12]

The role of absorbed iron in the clinical syndrome of iron overload in homozygous thalassemia is difficult to assess. Body iron stores at autopsy may be higher than one would predict on the basis of transfusional iron.[13] At the present time, however, most transfusion-dependent patients receive red cells to maintain minimum hemoglobin levels above 9 g/dl, a level at which the contribution of iron from food stores may be of little consequence. Furthermore, the administration of subcutaneous deferoxamine suppresses the retention of iron salts.[14] Of four regularly transfused patients studied when their hemoglobin levels were between 9.7 and 10.9 g/dl, three absorbed less than 1% and one absorbed 8% of a 5 mg ferrous sulfate test dose. For these patients, the maintenance of higher hemoglobin levels or the careful avoidance of iron-containing foods would have little impact on their total iron balance.

Iron absorption may be markedly increased in patients with homozygous thalassemia who are not regularly transfused.[14] Serum iron and ferritin concentrations are frequently elevated and hepatic iron stores may be increased. Although the use of a 12-hour subcutaneous deferoxamine infusion had little effect on the absorption of a test dose of ferrous sulfate in three such patients, 4% to 23% of the absorbed iron was excreted within 24 hours so that the actual amount of retained iron was, in fact, reduced.[14]

Increased iron stores in anemic patients with heterozygous thalassemia have been reported, although the treatment of some patients with sporadic red cell transfusions and iron preparations may be primarily responsible for these findings.[15,16] The absorption of inorganic iron was normal in two groups of patients with heterozygous thalassemia and hemoglobin levels greater than 10 g/dl.[2,17] Similarly, in a third study, the absorption of both hemoglobin iron and inorganic iron was normal in patients, although hemoglobin levels were not reported.[12] Those patients with a more severe form of heterozygous thalassemia characterized by low hemoglobin levels and reticulocytosis[18] are probably at greater risk of accumulating excessive iron, and their iron stores should be regularly evaluated. Medicinal iron should be scrupulously avoided unless there is definite evidence of iron deficiency. Although a therapeutic trial of iron may be useful in the management of patients with mild anemia and microcytosis, a lack of response should be followed by cessation of oral iron and further laboratory studies to distinguish iron deficiency from other causes of microcytosis, particularly heterozygous $\beta$ thalassemia. Widespread organ failure and death from secondary hemochromatosis has occurred following many years of ferrous sulfate administration.[19]

The gastrointestinal absorption of inorganic iron is increased several-fold in patients with sickle cell anemia in comparison with normal individuals.[2] Two patients with Hb SC and hemoglobin levels of 12.8 g/dl and 13.6 g/dl had normal iron absorption, suggesting that both anemia and increased erythropoiesis are required for increased iron absorption.[2] Elevated ferritin levels and serum iron concentrations in untransfused patients with Hb SS indicate that total iron stores may be increased, even in the absence of stainable iron in the bone marrow.[20]

Clinical manifestations of increased iron absorption in sickle cell anemia are rare. Severe hepatic hemosiderosis involving both parenchymal and reticuloendothelial cells was found at autopsy in a 5-year-old girl who had never been transfused.[10] However, most patients with similar pathologic findings have received multiple red cell transfusions and the contribution of absorbed iron to the tissue damage cannot be assessed.[9]

## DEFEROXAMINE

A clinically useful iron chelating drug must have a strong affinity for iron, must be specific for this particular metal, and must be nontoxic. In addition, the drug should be easily administered and not prohibitively expensive. Many agents have been tested in animal models and a few have reached the stage of clinical trials. Although no drug has met all of the above criteria for an ideal chelating agent, deferoxamine has been successful enough to gain widespread usage while undergoing extended clinical trials.

## Source and Biochemistry

Certain bacteria have developed elaborate systems for the recovery of relatively unavailable iron in order to meet their metabolic needs. Deferoxamine, a trihydroxamic acid compound, is derived from one such microbe, *Streptomyces pilosis*.[21] Ferric iron is tightly bound within the center of its ring-like structure. One molecule of deferoxamine (molecular weight 597) binds one iron atom; 100 mg. of deferoxamine can theoretically bind 9.35 mg. of iron. the iron-containing complex is water soluble and readily excreted by the kidney. In human studies, approximately two-thirds of the iron excreted in response to deferoxamine is in the urine and the remaining one-third is in the stool.[22]

The source of iron available for binding to deferoxamine in the human is still not completely understood. Originally, the high affinity constant led workers to believe that deferoxamine could remove iron from all binding proteins, including transferrin. Recent studies, however, have demonstrated no movement of iron from transferrin to deferoxamine, despite the lower affinity constant for iron of transferrin.[23] The authors speculate that the affinity constants for both compounds are sufficiently high to prevent the accumulation of free iron which is necessary for iron transfer.

Two other body iron sources contribute little or no iron to deferoxamine. Hemoglobin iron in either washed red cells or hemolysate is not bound by the chelating agent and only a small fraction of gastrointestinal iron is bound by deferoxamine.[24,25]

The major source of chelatable iron appears to be storage iron, although there is much controversy as to whether deferoxamine binds iron directly from the storage forms of ferritin and hemosiderin or rather acts on an intermediate iron pool. In one study, reticuloendothelial and parenchymal cells in the rat were labeled with $^{59}$Fe-containing heat-denatured red cells and $^{59}$Fe-bound transferrin, respectively. Diminished radioactivity was found in both cell types within four hours of deferoxamine administration in comparison with nonchelated controls.[26] In further studies by the same investigators, hypertransfused rats which were simultaneously iron loaded with iron sorbitol citrate showed less deferoxamine-induced iron excretion in the presence of suppressed erythropoiesis than a control group of iron-loaded but untransfused rats. Since ferritin and hemosiderin concentrations remain unchanged or increase when hypertransfusion is used to suppress red cell production, the decrease in iron excretion suggests that this form of iron is not the immediate site of action of the chelating agent.

More recent studies, using heat-damaged red cells and precipitated ferritin to label reticuloendothelial cells with [59]Fe and hemoglobin-haptoglobin complexes and soluble ferritin to label parenchymal cells with [59]Fe, have found the iron excreted in response to deferoxamine to be exclusively parenchymal in origin in rats.[27] In a further study by one of the investigators, two pathways of iron chelation were found in the hypertransfused rat.[28] Parenchymal iron was chelated intracellularly by deferoxamine and excreted in the bile. Iron derived from reticuloendothelial cells was chelated extracellularly and excreted in the urine, but only if transferrin iron binding sites were fully saturated. Further clinical studies of iron distribution in the human before and after prolonged chelation therapy and of response to bolus injections or continuous infusions of the chelating agent may help resolve these issues concerning the site of action of deferoxamine.

## Routes of Administration and Dosages

Deferoxamine must be administered parenterally to achieve clinically useful iron chelation. The difficulties involved in repeated intramuscular injection in children and low urinary iron excretion in response to intramuscular deferoxamine in younger patients resulted in only sporadic use of the drug in the United States until recently. However, the successful use of intramuscular deferoxamine in long-term clinical studies in England[29,30] and the demonstration of increased iron excretion during continuous intravenous or subcutaneous deferoxamine infusion have renewed interest in this chelating agent, and improvement of means of delivery of the drug has received considerable attention.[31,32]

**Intramuscular Injection**   Negative iron balance, defined operationally as urinary iron excretion in excess of transfusional iron loading, can be achieved using daily intramuscular deferoxamine in many patients with greatly increased iron stores.[29,33] Although urinary iron excretion may be low in very young patients using this method of drug administration, negative iron balance has been achieved in 5- to 7-year-old children with thalassemia major.[29] The dose is limited by the poor solubility of deferoxamine in water. It is difficult to dissolve one gram of the drug in less than 2 ml of water, making this the maximum dose that can be administered without undue pain. Excretion of the drug following intramuscular administration occurs in 4 to 6 hours, limiting the time of exposure of iron stores to the chelating agent.[34] Although other methods of deferoxamine administration allow the use of higher doses and increase the duration of drug effect, intramuscular deferoxamine administration is simple and well-tolerated. If the injection site is alternated between the two thighs, there is little discomfort. Compliance has been excellent even in the younger children, in large part because of the minimum disruption of normal daily events.

**Intravenous Administration**    The continuous intravenous administration of deferoxamine has two major advantages. First, urinary iron excretion is increased by as much as 300% in response to a 24-hour intravenous infusion of 750 mg of deferoxamine in comparison with an intramuscular injection of the same dose.[31] Although this improved iron excretion has been attributed to the prolonged exposure of the chelating agent to a labile iron pool, the existence or form of this pool remains controversial. Second, larger doses of deferoxamine can be administered by intravenous infusion since volume limitations are not important. Iron excretion increases as the dose of deferoxamine is raised from 0.5 to 16 g per 24 hours, although the efficiency of chelation (measured iron excretion/theoretical maximum iron excretion) decreases at higher doses.[31,33] Decisions regarding appropriate intravenous doses should not be made solely on the basis of the efficiency of chelation. For some patients the increased iron excretion at higher doses may be crucial for the establishment of negative iron balance or for the rapid removal of large iron stores.

The major disadvantage of intravenous deferoxamine is the need for hospitalization. This method of therapy can be used at the time of outpatient blood transfusions, but in most centers only a few hours are needed for a transfusion, limiting the time available for deferoxamine infusion. The portable infusion pumps now being used for subcutaneous infusions are capable of delivering the drug intravenously; in outpatient trials we have administered 8 g of deferoxamine intravenously in 12 hours without difficulty or complication using the infusion pump.

**Subcutaneous Administration**    The subcutaneous administration of deferoxamine permits the use of a continuous infusion system for outpatients. The drug is delivered by a small, lightweight infusion pump which is worn on a belt or a shoulder strap. A butterfly needle is easily placed subcutaneously in the abdominal wall or the extremities. The infusion time and volume may be varied, allowing flexibility in designing chelation programs.

The 24-hour subcutaneous infusion of 750 mg of deferoxamine increases iron excretion by slightly over 100% in comparison with the same dose administered intramuscularly.[35] Using doses of 750, 1500, and 2250 mg, 24-hour subcutaneous infusions are 84% as effective as intravenous infusions.[32] A linear increase in urinary iron excretion occurs as the subcutaneous dose is raised within this range. However, some investigators have found a plateau or decrease in iron excretion when the dose is raised to 4000 mg while others have found a continuing linear increase.[36,37]

A 24-hour infusion may be difficult for many patients, particularly adolescents who are reluctant to wear the pump during school hours. As a result, 12-hour infusion times have been evaluated and have been found to be equally as effective as 24-hour infusions at doses of 750 mg of deferoxamine.[36] Equal iron excretions have been found using 12-hour and 24-hour subcutaneous infusions of higher doses (1500 to 4000 mg) in some patients but not in others.[36,37] It is thus essential to evaluate carefully different doses of deferoxamine and different infusion times for each patient so that an optimal program of chelation can be devised and unnecessary inconvenience or cost to the patient avoided.

Erythema, induration, and tenderness are commonly found at the infusion site during subcutaneous deferoxamine administration and for up to 24 hours after completion of the infusion. Attempts to reduce the hypertonicity by adding more water to the solution have had little effect on these complications. At the present time we dissolve each 500 mg of deferoxamine in 1 ml of sterile water. When 2 g of deferoxamine are infused, the final volume is slightly more than 5 ml and the osmolarity is 1428 mOsm.[32] The addition of hydrocortisone to the infusion has been recommended to alleviate the side effects, but this makes the already tedious process of drug preparation a bit more cumbersome and has been of little value in many cases.

**Programs of Chelation Therapy**

**Thalassemia Major**    Urinary iron excretion exceeds transfusional iron intake in most children with thalassemia major using daily subcutaneous deferoxamine and in some of the older children using daily intramuscular deferoxamine. Only in children less than 5 years of age is it sometimes difficult to achieve negative iron balance using a single route of chelation therapy. This fact has prompted discussions regarding the appropriate age to institute chelation therapy. Several observations suggest that deferoxamine may be useful even in the absence of negative iron balance. First, iron stores are markedly increased in very young children with thalassemia major. Cardiac studies of patients in whom hemoglobin concentrations were consistently maintained above 9.0 g/dl from the time of diagnosis have shown increased left ventricular wall thickness, probably due to iron storage, even before the age of 3 years.[38] Excessive hepatic iron deposition was found in three children less than a year of age and early cirrhotic changes were seen by light and electron microscopy.[39] Similarly, bone marrow iron may be increased even prior to transfusion therapy.[39]

Second, daily subcutaneous deferoxamine therapy in the first 5 years of life will retard iron accumulation. At least 50% of the transfused iron may be excreted in the urine in young patients receiving 20 mg/kg of deferoxamine as a 10-hour subcutaneous infusion.[41] The inclusion of fecal iron may increase the measured iron losses by an additional 50%.

Third, the early introduction of chelation therapy as an integral part of the management of thalassemia will increase patient acceptance. Patients who have received intramuscular deferoxamine at 2 to 3 years of age have little difficulty continuing the injections in later years.[42]

These observations suggest that the use of deferoxamine in children with thalassemia major as young as 1 to 2 years of age may be beneficial. The subcutaneous infusion of the drug is the most effective method of administration in these children. The intravenous infusion of higher doses of deferoxamine for several days each month will further retard iron accumulation.

In older patients several factors must be carefully considered before iron chelation is undertaken. The magnitude of previous iron accumulation, the rate of ongoing iron loading from transfusions, and the severity of organ dysfunction all will influence the intensity of a program of iron removal. Attention must also be paid to patient compliance. The physician may feel quite comfortable knowing that negative iron balance can theoretically be achieved for a particular patient using daily subcutaneous deferoxamine, but the patient may in fact infrequently use the drug because of doubts about its effectiveness or concerns about possible social stigmata. Finally, urinary iron excretion must be carefully measured in response to various dosages and routes of administration so that maximum effectiveness of the drug is achieved within the bounds of acceptable costs and patient compliance.

We have previously emphasized that older patients with very large iron stores and imminent or actual cardiac disease are unlikely to benefit from the prevention of further iron accumulation alone.[43] If chelation therapy is to have a major therapeutic impact on their lives, its use must be designed to deplete body iron stores rapidly. This can be accomplished by combining different routes of administration. Assuming constant rates of iron excretion as iron stores diminish, a chelation regimen in which an intramuscular injection is given in the morning, subcutaneous deferoxamine is infused overnight, and high doses of intravenous deferoxamine are administered two days each month will theoretically remove more than 70 g of iron in less than three years.[43] There is no evidence that even this intensive an approach will rescue these severely iron-overloaded patients from death; the achievement of negative iron balance without diminution of the massive iron stores may be a costly undertaking with little reward.

**Sickle Cell Anemia**   Chelation therapy may retard the accumulation of iron in repeatedly transfused children with sickle cell anemia. Iron stores may be markedly increased in these children. We have studied eight children, 8 to 16 years old, who have been transfused for two to five years following cerebral vascular accidents. Ferritin levels are greater than 2000 ng/ml in all eight patients. All but the least frequently transfused patient would be in negative iron balance using 2.0 g of deferoxamine as a 12-hour subcutaneous infusion. Urinary iron excretion in response to this method of therapy is 13.0 to 39.0 mg/24 hours.

## Vitamin C

Urinary iron excretion in response to deferoxamine increases by 20% to 250% after repletion of vitamin C in most patients with thalassemia major who have excessive iron stores and low white cell vitamin C concentrations.[36,44,45] The precise dose of vitamin C needed to achieve and maintain this higher level of iron excretion is uncertain and may vary between patients. We have studied two patients before vitamin C supplementation and following the use of 100 mg and 250 mg of vitamin C daily. Iron excretion in response to intravenous, intramuscular, and subcutaneous deferoxamine did not change after three weeks of the 100 mg dose but rose sharply after the dose was increased to 250 mg for three weeks. Other investigators have found increased iron excretion in response to deferoxamine after supplementation with 200 mg of vitamin C daily.[29] It seems clear that it is difficult to predict the dose of vitamin C that will produce normal leukocyte vitamin C concentrations. It seems probable that additional vitamin C beyond that required to maintain normal leukocyte vitamin C concentrations is unnecessary.

When daily vitamin C supplementation was stopped in a group of patients with thalassemia major, leukocyte vitamin C concentrations decreased to subnormal levels in two weeks.[29] However, changes in deferoxamine-induced iron excretion were inconsistent when vitamin C was stopped after two months of supplementation; iron excretion decreased in two patients but rose in one patient. In another study, there was a parallel decrease in leukocyte vitamin C concentration and deferoxamine-induced iron excretion after withdrawal of vitamin C.[46]

We have found low leukocyte vitamin C levels in three of eight repeatedly transfused patients with sickle cell anemia. In one of these patients, urinary iron excretion in response to intravenous and subcutaneous deferoxamine rose by 35% and 140%, respectively, after 250 mg of vitamin C daily for three weeks. Urinary iron excretion in response to deferoxamine was elevated prior to vitamin C supplementation in another patient but did not increase further after vitamin C levels had returned to normal. The third patient still had low leukocyte vitamin C levels after three weeks of vitamin C therapy, and deferoxamine-induced urinary iron excretion did not change.

The association of iron overload and low leukocyte vitamin C levels was first noted in the South African Bantus. The high incidence of scurvy among the males was related to the large consumption of beer which was fermented in iron pots and had an iron concentration of 4 mg/100 ml.[47] Low leukocyte vitamin C levels have since been found in patients with transfusional iron overload.[44] Plasma clearance times for vitamin C are increased in siderotic patients even once the tissue stores are replete. Experimental evidence has established that vitamin C is oxidized in the presence of large iron stores with the formation of oxalic acid as well as several other products.[47]

The mechanism by which vitamin C supplementation increases deferoxamine-induced iron excretion is uncertain. A greater proportion of iron is stored as insoluble hemosiderin in comparison with soluble ferritin in vitamin C-deficient guinea pigs.[48] If ferritin iron is more readily available for chelation, the redistribution of storage iron after vitamin C therapy would increase iron excretion in response to deferoxamine. Vitamin C deficiency also inhibits the release of iron from reticuloendothelial cells.[49] The replenishment of vitamin C may increase the deferoxamine-induced iron excretion by releasing this iron directly to the chelating agent or by shifting more iron into parenchymal tissue where chelation may occur more readily. Finally, it has been suggested that vitamin C is necessary for the reduction of ferric iron to ferrous iron in order to facilitate transport between storage sites and a site readily available to the chelating agent.[45]

Questions regarding the safety of vitamin C therapy have been raised. Cardiac ejection fractions decreased in 8 of 11 patients receiving intramuscular deferoxamine and 500 mg of vitamin C daily.[50] When the vitamin C was discontinued and the deferoxamine administered subcutaneously rather than intramuscularly, cardiac function returned to normal in five patients. However, the use of digoxin and other supportive measures for the management of heart failure makes it difficult to assess the role of the discontinuation of vitamin C in the eventual improvement of these patients.

The theoretical basis of the concern about vitamin C toxicity lies in its potentiation of the ability of iron to generate free radicals.[51] These free radicals may damage cell membranes by lipid oxidation, eventually causing cell death and organ dysfunction. Because intramuscular deferoxamine is excreted rapidly, unbound iron may be present between injections and this iron may combine with vitamin C to increase the generation of free radicals. Presumably the use of a continuous deferoxamine infusion would prevent the circulation of free iron and the toxic interaction of iron and vitamin C. However, there is no evidence in vivo to confirm this theory of vitamin C intramuscular deferoxamine toxicity. Furthermore, no clinical evidence of toxicity has been reported after several years of such a chelation program In many patients in Great Britain. A reasonable approach at present would be to use the smallest dose of vitamin C necessary to achieve the level of iron excretion required for the ultimate goals of the chelation program. It makes little sense to subject a child to the rigors of chelation therapy if the amount of iron removed is of little or no consequence.

## Effects of Deferoxamine Therapy
## on Organ Structure and Function

The usefulness of iron chelating agents in the treatment of iron overload will ultimately be based on their ability to prevent or reverse organ damage and prevent early death from hemochromatosis. Several patients with thalassemia major have died despite being in negative iron balance for as long as two years, indicating that the rate of iron removal from critical organs was insufficient to prevent progressive deterioration. Careful long-term studies are necessary to assess the effect of iron chelation therapy on the severe morbidity and early mortality of patients with iron overload. However, preliminary results suggest that improved hepatic histology, cardiac function, and survival are associated with chronic use of deferoxamine.

**Liver** In 1974 investigators from Great Britain published the results of a study in which hepatic iron content and histology were compared in nine chelated and nine control patients with thalassemia major.[30] The chelation regimen, begun in 1966, consisted of intramuscular injections of 500 mg of deferoxamine six out of every seven days and, in some patients, intravenous infusion of 2 g of diethylenetriamine penta-acetate with each unit of blood. Liver biopsies performed after five to six years of chelation therapy showed a significant difference in iron content and fibrosis in comparison with non-chelated controls. Interestingly, liver iron concentrations continued to increase in most chelated patients with initial concentrations less than 2.4% dry weight but did not rise above 3.2%, a level at which hepatic fibrosis begins to accelerate. The serum ferritin levels were closely related to the liver iron concentrations and the authors proposed the use of serum ferritin levels as an alternative to liver biopsy for assessing hepatic iron content. No major clinical differences between the two groups were detected.

In another study of long-term chelation therapy, liver size decreased and function improved after ten months to eight years of intramuscular deferoxamine injections administered six days per week.[52] We and others have not found similar evidence of improvement. Problems of methodology, such as variation in liver size according to hemoglobin concentration and the influence of hemolysis on serum glutamic oxaloacetic transaminase (SGOT) levels, make this type of assessment of liver function difficult.

**Heart**   Few data concerning the effect of chelation therapy on the multiple cardiac abnormalities of iron-overloaded children are available. Twenty-four hour electrocardiographic monitoring has been used to compare the incidence of cardiac arrhythmias in regularly chelated (0.5 to 1.0 g deferoxamine daily for at least two years) and irregularly chelated or nonchelated patients.[53] The mean transfusion load since infancy for both groups was 283 units of blood per patient, although the mean age was 16.1 years for the regularly chelated patients and 17.6 years for the inadequately treated patients. Major arrhythmias (frequent supraventricular ectopic beats or any number of ventricular ectopic beats) were found in none of seven adequately chelated patients and in five of six inadequately chelated patients.

Significant improvement of congestive heart failure and electro-cardiographic abnormalities has been reported in five patients with thalassemia major who were receiving 1.0 g of deferoxamine intra-muscularly six days each week. However, the authors give few details of concomitant drug therapy or alterations in transfusion regimens which may have influenced the cardiac disease.[52]

**Endocrine**   Changes in endocrine function have been reported in only a few patients. Slightly increased prepubertal height velocity was found in patients receiving 500 mg of deferoxamine intramuscularly six days out of seven, in comparison with nonchelated controls.[30] Delayed puberty was less common in the former group. Extensive endocrine evaluations are presently being done in several centers in order to more fully assess the effects of long-term chelation on endocrine function.

**Mortality**   Survival has been compared in two groups of patients with thalassemia major who are 17 years of age or older.[53] Patients in the first group had a mean age of 18.9 years and were not treated regularly with chelating agents. Patients in the second group had a mean age of 18.5 years and received 500 mg of deferoxamine in-tramuscularly at least six of seven days each week for two years. Eight of 20 unchelated patients have died in comparison with none of the 10 chelated patients. The authors found these results to be significant at the 5% level.

Further studies of the effects of chelation therapy on organ func-tion in iron-overloaded patients are now underway in several medical centers. The inclusion of a larger number of patients and the use of more sensitive techniques to evaluate cardiac and endocrine function in particular will greatly assist the study of this problem and the effort to improve longevity in patients with iron-overload by the optimal use of chelating agents.

**Drug Toxicity**

Few side effects of deferoxamine have been reported despite its increasingly widespread use for acute and chronic iron poisoning. Pain at the site of intramuscular injection may occur frequently but is short-lived and has caused only rare compliance problems in our patients. The injection of volumes as high as 2 ml seems to be well tolerated. Some patients have experienced flushing, dizziness, anxiety, and throbbing headache immediately upon intramuscular injection of deferoxamine. The appearance of blood in the syringe tip or flowing from the injection site in many cases has suggested direct access of the concentrated drug to the intravascular space. Patients should be warned about this kind of reaction and taught to aspirate to test for accidental puncture of a vein before injecting the drug. The occurrence of urticaria during deferoxamine therapy has been reported in several patients. One patient developed an anaphylactic reaction characterized by itching, laryngospasm, wheezing, and cyanosis during desensitization injections with deferoxamine.[54] Only 1.6 mg of the drug was administered, suggesting that the drug itself or a contaminating substance might be a very potent allergen in some people. The occurrence of pruritis, painful induration, and erythema at the site of subcutaneous infusions has been discussed previously.

The formation of cataracts has been associated with prolonged (three weeks to six months) intravenous deferoxamine administration in dogs at doses of 100 mg/kg/day.[55] Cataracts have also occurred in humans receiving deferoxamine; however, several of these patients were simultaneously receiving corticosteroids. No reports of cataract formation due to deferoxamine have been published despite the recent intensive use of the drug in many patients. Routine slitlamp examinations during deferoxamine therapy are nonetheless recommended by the manufacturer of the drug.

A particularly disturbing feature of deferoxamine toxicity studies is our present inability to separate clearly drug effects from abnormalities related to the underlying disease of iron overload. Four of our patients with thalassemia major and exposure to deferoxamine have died during a two year period. Two of these patients had received one or two initial 18-hour intravenous infusions of 1.5 g of deferoxamine to evaluate the extent of iron stores. The remaining two patients had received daily intramuscular or subcutaneous deferoxamine for five months in one case and two years in the other. All four patients were 16 years of age or older and severely iron-overloaded. Death was from cardiac failure or arrhythmia and could not be directly related to deferoxamine administration. Similar cases have occurred elsewhere.[56] In most instances, cardiac disease was evident at the time of institution of chelation.

Two possible roles of chelation therapy in the development of cardiac toxicity have been proposed. First, if transferrin binding sites are fully saturated, iron mobilized from the usual storage sites during deferoxamine therapy might theoretically remain unbound once the drug has been excreted. This free iron might be directly toxic or, alternatively, might be moved from less toxic sites such as reticuloendothelial cells to potentially dangerous locations such as the myocardium. Second, experimental evidence has shown that ascorbic acid enhances the cytotoxicity of iron. It is encouraging to note that no reported deaths have occurred in younger patients with less iron accumulation. However, until these issues are resolved it will be difficult to determine whether similar deaths in patients receiving deferoxamine are due to drug effects or represent the natural course of iron overload.

## Cost

It is not realistic to design a program of iron chelation without consideration of the very high costs. The price of deferoxamine is approximately $3.50 per 500 mg vial. The yearly cost of deferoxamine for a patient receiving daily subcutaneous infusions of 2.0 gm is more than $5000. In addition, the infusion pump costs $850 to $1150, and the needles and syringes an additional $135 each year. Few families can afford such expenses. Many patients have been included in studies of iron chelation so that drugs and supplies have been provided at no charge. In Pennsylvania, a bill has been passed by the legislature allocating funds for the treatment of iron overload in children with thalassemia major, but this bill must be voted on each year for refunding. Health insurance companies have been generally unwilling to pay for outpatient treatment. The present sources of funds for chelation therapy are clearly tenuous. It is important to re-emphasize the need for long-range cost planning and the development of less expensive chelating agents and methods of drug administration.

## OTHER CHELATING AGENTS AND DELIVERY SYSTEMS

### Rhodotorulic Acid

Rhodotorulic acid, like deferoxamine, is a hydroxamic acid compound of microbial derivation. Although this iron chelating compound must also be administered parenterally, it possesses three properties which may ultimately make it clinically useful.[58] First, iron excretion in response to rhodotorulic acid is more than twice as high as that obtained in response to deferoxamine in the Iron-overloaded rat, suggesting greater efficacy at equivalent doses. Second, rhodotorulic acid is relatively insoluble in water. If it were administered intramuscularly as a suspension, release of the drug would be slower, allowing increased duration of exposure of iron to the chelating agent. Under these conditions, a single intramuscular injection might be as effective as a continuous subcutaneous infusion. Finally, rhodotorulic acid can be obtained from cultures more efficiently than deferoxamine, and would presumably be less expensive.

## 2,3-Dihydroxybenzoic Acid

2,3-Dihydroxybenzoic acid is the parent compound of a second class of chelators in which iron is bound to the hydroxyl groups of the benzene ring. The major advantage of this drug is its oral absorption. In addition, it is highly specific for iron and well tolerated. Unfortunately, mean 24-hour iron excretion was only 6.5 mg per day in response to 2,3-dihydroxybenzoic acid administered four times daily.[59] When deferoxamine and 2,3-dihydroxybenzoic acid were given simultaneously to iron-overloaded rats, iron excretion was increased in comparison with the use of either agent alone, suggesting the presence of two distinct sites or mechanisms of iron chelation.[60] This observation, in addition to the unexplained wide variation in iron excretion in humans following 2,3-dihydroxybenzoic acid (1.4 to 19.0 mg), may warrant clinical trials using deferoxamine and 2,3-dihydroxybenzoic acid in combination in some patients.

## METHODS OF DRUG DELIVERY

An intriguing approach to the problem of iron chelation is the development of delivery systems which will carry the drug directly to the most severely iron-loaded organs. Deferoxamine has been successfully incorporated into human and rat red cell ghosts which are normally taken up by reticuloendothelial cells.[61] Experiments in vitro have shown that unbound deferoxamine is released as the red cell undergoes autohemolysis, suggesting that the drug would be available for binding iron within the reticuloendothelial system. When iron-overloaded rats were given red cell ghosts containing deferoxamine, the urine and fecal excretion of $^{59}$Fe-labeled reticuloendothelial iron increased four-fold in comparison with a similar intravenous dose.

Liposomes carrying therapeutic agents have been used to enhance drug delivery to specific organs, particularly the liver and spleen. By blocking liver and spleen uptake or by coating the liposome with organ-specific antibody, it may be possible to deliver drugs directly to such critical areas as the myocardium. Furthermore, deferoxamine entrapped in a liposome may be absorbed in the gastrointestinal tract, permitting effective oral administration.

## OTHER METHODS OF PREVENTING IRON ACCUMULATION

### Transfusional Iron

Since the major portion of excessive iron stores in patients with thalassemia major comes from red cell administration, any program designed to prevent iron overload must focus on transfusion requirements as well as chelation therapy. The proper identification and management of patients with abnormally high transfusion requirements may significantly reduce the rate of iron accumulation and may increase the effectiveness of iron chelation by raising the net iron excretion.

In the absence of isoimmune or autoimmune hemolysis, rapidly increasing transfusion requirements are most commonly due to hypersplenism. Investigators in Great Britain, by plotting the amount of administered whole blood per kilogram per year against mean hemoglobin concentration, have found that transfusion requirements in splenectomized patients with thalassemia major fall within a narrow range.[57] We have performed similar calculations using the amount of packed red cells and the pretransfusion hemoglobin concentration and have found the range of transfusion requirements to be 80 to 155 cc/kg/yr in 18 splenectomized patients.[62] It is thus possible to predict accurately the potential reduction in transfusion requirements and resulting iron loading after splenectomy in patients with thalassemia major on the basis of the current red cell requirements and the predicted requirements postsplenectomy.

Because splenectomy removes a relatively safe reservoir of excessive iron, there has been concern that more critical organs such as the heart and liver will accumulate iron more rapidly in splenectomized patients, possibly leading to earlier death. However, the maintenance of negative iron balance by chelation therapy obviates the problem of iron redistribution since there is no net iron accumulation. Even in the absence of chelation therapy the reduction in transfusional iron following splenectomy may result in less hepatic and cardiac iron accumulation despite the absence of the spleen. For example, a 7-year-old boy weighing 25 kg may receive 500 cc of red cells every three weeks (or 340 cc/kg/yr), thus accumulating 8.5 g of transfusional iron each year. If one-third of this iron is stored in the spleen, 5.7 g is distributed in other organs. Following removal of the spleen, predicted transfusion requirements would be no greater than 150 cc/kg/yr, so that maximum transfusional iron delivery is 3.75 g and iron accumulation by organs other than the spleen is reduced by 34%.

Despite the acknowledged benefits of transfusion programs in which the hemoglobin concentration is kept above 8 to 9 g/dl, hemoglobin levels are allowed to drop much lower in some patients. Massive splenic enlargement under these conditions may actually increase transfusion requirements. Once the hemoglobin concentration is raised above 8 to 9 g/dl, spleen size decreases, less blood is required to maintain the higher hemoglobin level, and the rate of iron accumulation decreases. Although there may be long-term benefits of maintaining hemoglobin concentrations above 12 to 13 g/dl,[3] there is no evidence that iron accumulation is significantly retarded in such a program.

The major obstacle to the long-term survival of children with transfusion-dependent disorders of hemoglobin is the development of iron overload. If iron chelation therapy is successful in preventing secondary hemochromatosis, young patients with thalassemia major will have a vastly improved prognosis. Of equal importance, new therapeutic approaches will be available for patients with disorders such as sickle cell anemia in which regular blood transfusions can eliminate many of the most serious complications. To rescue the severely iron-overloaded adolescents from death will, however, be a formidable task. It is therefore crucial that such problems as drug cost and cumbersome delivery systems be quickly resolved so that chelation therapy can be instituted for affected children as early as clinically useful. Such a program will enable many children with hemoglobinopathies to remain as healthy and active as possible until advances in bone marrow transplantation and the molecular biology of hemoglobin synthesis lead to the cure of these disorders.

## REFERENCES

1. Risdon, R.A., Barry, M., and Flynn, D.M. Transfusional iron overload: The relationship between tissue iron concentration and hepatic fibrosis in thalassemia. *J. Pathol.* 116:83–95, 1974.

2. Erlandson, M.E., Walden, B., Stern, G., et al. Studies on congenital hemolytic syndromes. IV. Gastrointestinal absorption of iron. *Blood* 19:359–378, 1962.

3. Propper, R.D., and Nathan, D.G. Persistent maintenance of normal hematocrits (HCT) in thalassemia major (THAL). *Blood* 50(suppl):116, 1977.

4. Russell, M.O., Goldberg, H.I., Reis, L., et al. Transfusion therapy for cerebrovascular abnormalities in sickle cell disease. *J. Pediatr.* 88:382–387, 1976.

5. Chernoff, A.L., Shapleigh, J.B., and Moore, C.V. Therapy of chronic

ulceration of the legs associated with sickle cell anemia. *JAMA* 155:1487–1491, 1954.

6. Nathan, D.G., and Pearson, H.A., Sickle cell syndromes and hemoglobin C disease. Edited by D.G. Nathan and F.A. Oski. *Hematology of Infancy and Childhood.* Philadelphia: W.B. Saunders Co., 1974.

7. Cohen, A., and Schwartz, E. Excretion of iron in response to deferoxamine in sickle cell anemia. *J. Pediatr.* 92:659–662, 1978.

8. Washington, R., and Boggs, D.R. Urinary iron in patients with sickle cell anemia. *J. Lab. Clin. Med.* 86:17–23, 1975.

9. Bogoch, A., Casselman, W.G.B., Margolies, M.P., et al. Liver disease in sickle cell anemia. *Am. J. Med.* 19:583–609, 1955.

10. Song, Y.S. Hepatic lesions in sickle cell anemia. *Am. J. Pathol.* 33:331–351, 1957.

11. Buja, L.M., and Roberts, W.C. Iron in the heart. *Am. J. Med.* 51:209–221, 1971.

12. Bannerman, R.M., Callender, S.T., Hardisty, R.M., et al. Iron absorption in thalassemia. *Br. J. Haematol.* 10:490–495, 1964.

13. Ellis, J.T., Schulman, I., and Smith, C.H. Generalized siderosis with fibrosis of liver and pancreas in Cooley's (Mediterranean) anemia, with observations on the pathogenesis of the siderosis and fibrosis. *Am. J. Pathol.* 30:287–309, 1954.

14. Pippard, M.J., Warner, G.T., Callender, S.T., et al. Iron absorption in iron-loading anemias: Effect of subcutaneous desferrioxamine infusions. *Lancet* 2:737–739, 1977.

15. Lewis, M., Lee, G.R., and Haut, A. The association of hemochromatosis with thalassemia minor. *Ann. Intern. Med.* 63:122–128, 1965.

16. Williams, C.E., and Siemsen, A.W. Hemosiderosis in association with thalassemia minor. *Arch. Intern. Med.* 121:356–360, 1968.

17. Shahid, M.J., and Haydar, N.A. Absorption of inorganic iron in thalassemia. *Br. J. Haematol.* 13:713–718, 1967.

18. Friedman, Sh., Ozsoylu, S., Luddy, et al. Heterozygous beta thalassemia of unusual severity. *Br. J. Haematol.* 32:65–77, 1976.

19. Case Records of the Massachusetts General Hospital (Case 44131). *N. Engl. J. Med.* 258:652–661, 1958.

20. Peterson, C.M., Graziano, J.H., deCiutiis, A., et al. Iron metabolism, sickle cell disease, and response to cyanate. *Blood* 46:583–590, 1975.

21. Moeschlin, S., and Schnider, U. Treatment of primary and secondary hemochromatosis and acute iron poisoning with a new, potent iron-eliminating agent (desferrioxamine-B). *N. Engl. J. Med.* 269:57–66, 1963.

22. Cumming, R.L.C., Millar, J.A., Smith, J.A., et al. Clinical and laboratory studies on the action of desferrioxamine. *Br. J. Haematol.* 17:257–263, 1969.

23. Pollack, S., Aisen, P., Lasky, F.D., et al. Chelate mediated transfer of iron from transferrin to desferrioxamine. *Br. J. Haematol.* 34:231–235, 1976.

24. Keberle, H. The biochemistry of desferrioxamine and its relation to iron metabolism. *Ann. NY Acad. Sci.* 119:758–768, 1964.

25. Brown, E.B., Hwang, Y.F., and Allgood, J.W. Studies of the site of action of deferoxamine. *J. Lab. Clin. Med.* 69:382–404, 1967.

26. Lipschitz, D.A., Dugard, J., Simon, M.O., et al. The site of action of desferrioxamine. *Br. J. Haematol.* 20:395–404, 1971.

27. Hershko, C., Cook, J.D., and Finch, C.A. Storage iron kinetics. III. Study of desferrioxamine action by selective radioiron labels of RE and parenchymal cells. *J. Lab. Clin. Med.* 81:876–886, 1973.

28. Hershko, C. Determinants of fecal and urinary iron excretion in

354

desferrioxamine-treated rats. *Blood* 51:415–423, 1978.

29. Modell, C.G., and Beck, J. Long-term desferrioxamine therapy in thalassemia. *Ann. NY Acad. Sci.* 232:201–210, 1974.

30. Barry, M., Flynn, D.M., Letsky, E.A., et al. Long-term chelation therapy in thalassemia major: Effect on liver iron concentration, liver histology, and clinical progress. *Br. Med. J.* 2:16–20, 1974.

31. Propper, R.D., Shurin, S.B., and Nathan, D.G. Re-assessment of the use of desferrioxamine B in iron overload. *N. Engl. J. Med.* 294:1421–1423, 1976.

32. Propper, R.D., Cooper, B., Rufo, R.R., et al. Continuous subcutaneous administration of deferoxamine in patients with iron overload. *N. Engl. J. Med.* 297:418–423, 1977.

33. Cohen, A., and Schwartz, E. Iron chelation therapy with deferoxamine in Cooley's anemia. *J. Pediatr.* 92:643–647, 1978.

34. Waxman, H.S., and Brown, E.B. Clinical usefulness of iron chelating agents. *Prog. Hematol.* 6:338–373, 1969.

35. Hussain, M.A.M., Green, N., Flynn, D.M., et al. Subcutaneous infusion and intramuscular injection of desferrioxamine in patients with transfusional iron overload. *Lancet* 2:1278–1280, 1976.

36. Hussain, M.A.M., Green, N., Flynn, D.M., et al. Effect of dose, time, and ascorbate on iron excretion after subcutaneous desferrioxamine. *Lancet* 1:977–979, 1977.

37. Pippard, M.J., Callender, S.T., and Weatherall, D.J. Chelation regimens with desferrioxamine. *Lancet* 1:1101, 1977.

38. Piomelli, S., Desferrioxamine B chelation in the young thalassemic. Edited by E.C. Zaino and R.H. Roberts. In *Chelation Therapy in Chronic Iron Overload.* Miami: Symposia Specialists, 1977, p. 65.

39. Discussion. Edited by E.C. Zaino and R.H. Roberts. In *Chelation Therapy in Chronic Iron Overload.* Miami: Symposia Specialists, 1977, p. 138.

41. Piomelli, S., Desferrioxamine B chelation in the young thalassemic. Edited by E.C. Zaino and R.H. Roberts. In *Chelation Therapy in Chronic Iron Overload.* Miami: Symposia Specialists, 1977, p. 70.

42. Discussion. Edited by E.C. Zaino and R.H. Roberts. In *Chelation Therapy in Chronic Iron Overload.* Miami: Symposia Specialists, 1977, p. 138.

43. Cohen, A., and Schwartz, E., Comparison of different parenteral routes of deferoxamine administration. Edited by E.C. Zaino and R.H. Roberts. In *Chelation Therapy in Chronic Iron Overload.* Miami: Symposia Specialists, 1977, p. 87.

44. Wapnick, A.A., Lynch, S.R., Charlton, R.W., et al. The effect of ascorbic acid deficiency on desferrioxamine-induced urinary iron excretion. *Br. J. Haematol.* 17:563–568, 1969.

45. O'Brien, R.T. Ascorbic acid enhancement of desferrioxamine-induced urinary iron excretion in thalassemia major. *Ann. NY Acad. Sci.* 232:221–225, 1974.

46. Nienhuis, A.W., Delea, C., Aamodt, R., et al., Evaluation of desferrioxamine and ascorbic acid for the treatment of chronic iron overload. Edited by D. Bergsma, A. Cerami, C.M. Peterson, and J.H. Graziano. In *Iron Metabolism and Thalassemia.* New York: Alan R. Liss, 1976.

47. Lynch, S.R., Seftel, H.C., Torrance, J.D., et al. Accelerated oxidative catabolism of ascorbic acid in siderotic Bantu. *Am. J. Clin. Nutr.* 20:641–647, 1967.

48. Lipschitz, D.A., Bothwell, T.H., Seftel, H.C., et al. The role of ascorbic acid in the metabolism of storage iron. *Br. J. Haematol.* 20:155–163, 1971.

49. Lynch, S.R., Lipschitz, D.A., Bothwell, T.H., et al. Iron and the

reticuloendothelial system. Edited by A. Jacobs and M. Worwood. In *Iron in Biochemistry and Medicine.* London: Academic Press, 1974.

50. Henry, W., and Nienhuis, A. Evaluation of cardiac function in patients with myocardial iron overload on chelation therapy. *Blood* 50(suppl):93, 1977.

51. Graziano, J.H., Potential usefulness of free radical scavengers in iron overload. Edited by D. Bergsma, A. Cerami, C.M. Peterson, and J.H. Graziano. In *Iron Metabolism and Thalassemia.* New York: Alan R. Liss, 1976.

52. Seshadri, R., Colebatch, J.H., Gordon, P., et al. Long-term administration of desferrioxamine in thalassemia major. *Arch. Dis. Child.* 49:621–626, 1974.

53. Modell, B., Owen, M., and Kaye, S.G., Clinical experience with the use of deferoxamine in the United Kingdom. Edited by E.C. Zaino and R.H. Roberts. In *Chelation Therapy in Chronic Iron Overload.* Miami: Symposia Specialists, 1977.

54. Athanasiou, A., Shepp, M.A., and Necheles, T.F. Anaphylactic reaction to deferoxamine. *Lancet* 2:616, 1977.

55. Report of the ad hoc working group to develop a policy position on the use of desferrioxamine in chronic iron overload. Division of Blood Diseases and Resources of the National Heart and Lung Institute, National Institutes of Health, April 22, 1976.

56. Nienhuis, A.W. Safety of intensive chelation therapy. *N. Engl. J. Med.* 296:114, 1977.

57. Modell, B. Total management of thalassemia major. *Arch. Dis. Child.* 52:489–500, 1977.

58. Graziano, J.H., and Cerami, A. Chelation therapy for the treatment of thalassemia. *Semin. Hematol.* 14:127–134, 1977.

59. Peterson, C.M., Graziano, J.H., Grady, R.W., et al. Chelation studies with 2,3-dihydroxybenzoic acid in patients with β-thalassemia major. *Br. J. Haematol.* 33:477–485, 1976.

60. Graziano, J.H., Grady, R.W., and Cerami, A. The identification of 2,3-dihydroxybenzoic acid as a potentially useful iron-chelating drug. *J. Pharmacol. Exp. Ther.* 190:570–575, 1974.

61. Green, R., Miller, J., and Crosby, W.H. Delivery of desferrioxamine to reticuloendothelial cells in red cell ghosts. *Blood* 50(suppl):78, 1977.

62. Cohen, A.R., Markenson, A., and Schwartz, E. Transfusion requirements and splenectomy in Cooley's anemia. *Pediatr. Res.* 12:462, 1978.

# 16 The Alpha-Thalassemia Syndromes

George R. Honig, M.D., Ph.D.

Thalassemia resulting from a deficiency of hemoglobin α chains was first recognized with the discovery of Hb H and Hb Bart's and the finding that these abnormal hemoglobins had no α chains, but represented tetramers of normal β chains and γ chains, respectively. It has been approximately 20 years since these observations were made, and during that time α thalassemia has been shown to be the underlying abnormality of a diverse group of hematologic disorders ranging in clinical expression from a form of congenital anemia so severe as to be incompatible with extrauterine survival, to a disorder so subtle that it totally escapes detection by the usual forms of hematologic evaluation. Alpha thalassemia has been identified in a number of population groups, and there are notable differences in the clinical and hematologic expression in these various populations of what are apparently identical genetic syndromes. Other α-thalassemia syndromes that result from the concurrence of α thalassemia and structural variants of hemoglobin have also been identified. These may differ significantly in their clinical manifestations from α thalassemia alone or from the unmodified hemoglobinopathy. In addition, in recent years it has been recognized that some acquired forms of hematologic disease may share many of the features of congenital $\alpha$ thalassemia.

The purpose of this chapter is to review the clinical and hematologic features of these syndromes, particularly those of the pediatric patient, and to present some of the current approaches to their diagnosis and therapy.

## PATHOGENESIS

The common underlying abnormality shared by all forms of $\alpha$ thalassemia is an insufficiency of hemoglobin $\alpha$ chain synthesis by the erythroid cells. In all types of $\alpha$ thalassemia except the mildest under-hemoglobinization of the erythrocytes occurs, producing anemia with microcytic, hypochromic red cells. In the more severe forms of $\alpha$ thalassemia a significant hemolytic process is also present, related largely to the instability of Hb H and Hb Bart's.

A number of genetic mechanisms appear to be responsible for the reduced rate of $\alpha$ chain synthesis in these disorders, and it seems likely that still others will be identified. Hybridization studies, using DNA derived from tissues of patients from the Far East with severe $\alpha$ thalassemia, have shown a total absence of DNA sequences that could hybridize with a synthetic DNA probe having $\alpha$ chain specificity,[1,2] indicating a congenital absence of $\alpha$ chain structural genes as the cause for this form of $\alpha$ thalassemia. More recently, a patient with well-documented $\alpha$ thalassemia was shown by hybridization studies to have a nondeletion type of defect,[3] suggesting that this form of $\alpha$ thalassemia had a different pathogenic mechanism, presumably one representing a regulative defect of $\alpha$ chain synthesis. In another group of patients having typical hematologic features of $\alpha$ thalassemia, small quantities of variant hemoglobins with structurally abnormal $\alpha$ chains have been identified. These structural variants appear to produce the hematologic picture of $\alpha$ thalassemia due to a substantially reduced rate of synthesis of the abnormal $\alpha$ chain.[4] Lastly, $\alpha$ thalassemia syndromes acquired by an unknown mechanism have been observed in association with leukemia and other hematologic disorders[5] in individuals who are genetically normal with respect to $\alpha$ chain synthesis.

## GENETICS OF $\alpha$ THALASSEMIA

Detailed studies of patients with $\alpha$ thalassemia and their families among Far Eastern populations[6] suggest that there are two types of $\alpha$-thalassemia genes; one type, $\alpha$-thal-1, responsible for a marked deficiency, and another, $\alpha$-thal-2, responsible for a milder defect. The expression of these genes, alone or in combination, appears to provide an adequate explanation for the various hematologic forms of $\alpha$ thalassemia (Table 16-1). An alternative genetic model for $\alpha$ thalassemia has been proposed, however, following the recognition that more than a single pair of $\alpha$ chain genes may be present in individuals of at least some populations.[7] By basing this theory on a model that assumes the presence of four $\alpha$ chain genes, it is possible to account for the known forms of $\alpha$ thalassemia as representing the presence of one, two, three, or four $\alpha$-thalassemia genes (Table 16-1). Although there is some experimental evidence that appears to support the four-gene model,[8] at present either of these models seems to be equally valid.[9]

## CLASSIFICATION OF THE $\alpha$-THALASSEMIA SYNDROMES

The characterization of the major forms of $\alpha$ thalassemia (Table 16-1) has come mainly from studies of Asian populations (Thai, Malayan, Chinese) in which $\alpha$ thalassemia occurs with high frequency.[6,10,11] Other groups having a substantial frequency of $\alpha$ thalassemia include Afro-Americans,[12] Indians,[13] Shiite Arabs,[14] and Yemenite and Iraqi Jews.[15] In these latter groups $\alpha$ thalassemia presents as a milder syndrome than that seen in Far Eastern populations, and in none has the most severe form of $\alpha$ thalassemia, the hydrops fetalis syndrome, been observed. The milder expression of $\alpha$ thalassemia in these populations may represent the presence of primarily $\alpha$-thal-2 genes[7] from which the hydrops fetalis disease could not develop. It has been established that the $\alpha$-thal-1 gene is present in individuals of the American black population,[16] but the relative frequency of the gene is unknown.

### Clinical and Hematologic Expression

The silent carrier and trait forms of $\alpha$ thalassemia (Table 16-1) ordinarily produce no clinical manifestations. Hemoglobin H disease, due to a combination of $\alpha$-thal-1 and $\alpha$-thal-2 or a lack of function of three of four genes, is expressed as a chronic hemolytic anemia of moderate severity; the neonate with Hb H disease usually appears normal, but by the end of the first year of life hepatosplenomegaly and anemia, often accompanied by jaundice, become apparent. Hb H disease in American blacks may be sufficiently mild to escape detection even in adults unless appropriate hematologic studies are done. Although anemia is characteristically mild in these individuals, the

**Table 16-1**
**Clinical and Hematologic Features of α Thalassemia**

| Form of α thalassemia | Genotype | | Hemoglobin findings | | Hematologic changes | Clinical features |
|---|---|---|---|---|---|---|
| | 2-gene model | 4-gene model | Newborn | Adult | | |
| Silent carrier | α-thal-2/α | αα/α- | 1% to 2% Hb Bart's | No abnormality | Usually no abnormality; mild microcytosis may be present | Clinically normal |
| α-thal trait | α-thal-1/α or α-thal-2/α-thal-2 | αα/-- or α-/α- | 2% to 10% Hb Bart's | No abnormality | Red cell microcytosis and hypochromia with mildly abnormal morphology; anemia mild or absent | Usually normal |
| Hb H disease | α-thal-1/α-thal-2 | α-/-- | 20% to 30% Hb Bart's | 5% to 25% Hb H (β4); May be traces of Hb γ4 | Moderately severe anemia with marked anisopoikilocytosis and microcytosis; red cell inclusion bodies demonstrable by supravital staining | Pallor, jaundice, hepatosplenomegaly; cholelithiasis occurs commonly in adults |
| Hydrops fetalis | α-thal-1/α-thal-1 | --/-- | > 80% Hb Bart's with the remainder Hb β4 and Hb Portland (ζ2γ2) | — | Severe anemia, markedly abnormal erythrocyte morphology with anisopoikilocytosis, hypochromia, and pronounced erythroblastemia | Massive hepatosplenomegaly, generalized edema with ascites and pleural and pericardial effusion; all have been stillborn or died shortly after birth |

erythrocyte morphology is strikingly abnormal, with hypochromia, anisocytosis, poikilocytosis, and numerous target cells.

The hydrops fetalis form of $\alpha$ thalassemia undoubtedly constitutes the most severe known anemic disorder. This syndrome, which has been observed almost exclusively among Far Eastern populations, results from a total absence of $\alpha$-globin production. Because $\alpha$ chains are common to all of the normal postnatal hemoglobins, the hemoglobin forms present in this condition are all abnormal (Table 16-1) except for the variable presence of small amounts of an embryonic hemoglobin composed of $\gamma$ and $\zeta$ chains,[17] the latter probably representing a primitive $\alpha$-like globin chain. Because Hb Bart's,[4] the predominant hemoglobin in these infants, has a very high oxygen affinity, it is virtually useless as an oxygen carrier. It therefore seems remarkable that any of the affected infants have survived gestation; most have been stillborn and those alive at birth have all died within the first day of life.[18] The appearance of these infants is similar to that of infants with severe isoimmune hemolytic disease. A marked degree of pallor, generalized edema, and extreme abdominal distention due to massive liver enlargement are characteristic features. The placenta is edematous and friable (Figure 16-1).

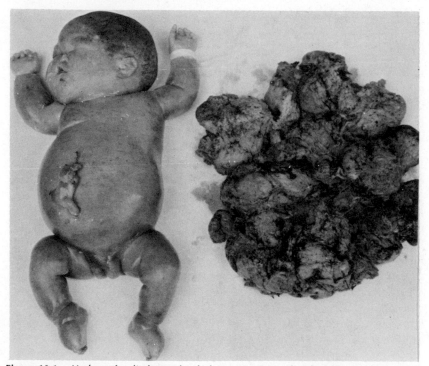

**Figure 16-1.** Hydrops fetalis form of $\alpha$ thalassemia. Generalized edema and abdominal distention due to massive liver enlargement and ascites are present. The placenta is swollen and edematous. [Photograph kindly supplied by Dr. Lie-Injo Luan Eng.]

## HEMOGLOBINS WITH ABNORMAL α CHAINS THAT PRODUCE THE HEMATOLOGIC FEATURES OF α THALASSEMIA

A group of α chain structural abnormalities have been identified which produce a disorder indistinguishable from α thalassemia. In these α chain variants (Table 16-2) there is a greatly reduced rate of synthesis and a biochemical defect comparable to that produced by an α-thal-2 gene. Most of these abnormal hemoglobins were first observed in individuals with the hematologic features of Hb H disease or in combination with another α chain variant with which it produced α-thalsssemia-like hematologic changes. Hb Constant Spring, the most widely distributed of this group of variants, has been identified in numerous population groups and is found in a significant percentage of the cases of Hb H disease, which it causes when combined with α-thal-1.

**Table 16-2**
**Structurally Abnormal α Chain Variants That Produce the Hematologic Picture of α Thalassemia**

| Hemoglobin variant | Amino acid substitution | Racial group(s) affected | Reference |
|---|---|---|---|
| Hb Constant Spring | α142 Gln | Chinese, Thai, Greek, Malayan | 4 |
| Hb Icaria | α142 Lys | Greek | 4 |
| Hb Koya Dora | α142 Ser | Indian | 4 |
| Hb Seal Rock | α142 Glu | black American | 4 |
| Hb Q | α74 His | Thai, Chinese | 19 |
| Hb Ft. Worth | α27 Gly | black American | 20 |
| Hb Petah Tikva | α110 Asp | Iraqi Jewish | 21 |

Four of the variants listed in Table 16-2 represent "terminator mutants," which result from a point mutation at amino acid position 142 of the α chain. The normal α chain contains 141 amino acids. The nucleotide triplet codon representing amino acid 141 is known to be followed normally by a codon that signals chain termination. In the terminator variants a point mutation appears to have occurred in the latter codon, causing the chain termination signal to be replaced by a codon that specifies the insertion of an amino acid. As a result of this change, additional amino acids can be added to the α-polypeptide chain until the next termination signal is reached. The α chain of Hb Constant Spring has 172 amino acids.[4] The basis for the greatly reduced rate of synthesis of the terminator mutants is unknown.

Hb Q, a variant that is relatively common in the Far East, produces a syndrome indistinguishable from Hb H disease when present in combination with an α-thal-1 gene; this syndrome is characterized by a total absence of Hb A, suggesting that an α-thalassemia gene may be closely linked to the gene for Hb Q.[19] Hb Petah Tikva,[21] which was identified in two Israeli patients with Hb H disease, appears to be synthesized actively only in nucleated red cell precursors and not in reticulocytes, and this may account for its thalassemia-like effect.

## SYNDROMES OF α THALASSEMIA IN COMBINATION WITH HEMOGLOBIN STRUCTURAL VARIANTS

A substantial group of syndromes that result from the coexistence of α thalassemia in its various forms with one or more structurally abnormal hemoglobins have been identified. In a number of these syndromes the clinical and hematologic expression of the hemoglobin abnormality appears to be significantly modified by the associated thalassemia. Studies of these doubly affected individuals and their families have aided in the understanding of the genetic pattern of α chain abnormalities.

Syndromes of α thalassemia occurring in combination with α chain structural variants are included in Tables 16-2 and 16-3. Those in Table 16-3 differ from the previously described variants in that none has been conclusively shown to produce thalassemia-like changes unless accompanied by an α-thalassemia gene. In general, the hematologic picture seen in these syndromes is one of an "interacting" thalassemia. The thalassemia is expressed in much the same manner as it is in the absence of the abnormal hemoglobin. The percentage of the hemoglobin variant in the blood, however, is characteristically increased in comparison to that seen in the simple heterozygote, presumably because of the relatively reduced production of normal α chains due to the α-thalassemia gene.

### α Thalassemia-α Structural Variant Syndromes

The hematologic expression of the α chain variant Hb G Philadelphia, alone and in combination with α thalassemia, has been the subject of considerable recent interest. This variant, which is relatively widespread in the American black population, presents in heterozygous individuals in what appears to be a trimodal distribution,[22,37] with approximately 20%, 30% or 40% of the hemoglobin in the blood being represented by Hb G. The findings in the highest percentage group, in particular, have appeared to be inconsistent with the four-gene model of α chain genetics, from which it would be predicted that only about 25% of Hb G would be present in the heterozygote. To account for this inconsistency, French and

**Table 16-3**
**Syndromes of α Thalassemia in Combination with Hemoglobin Structural Variants**

| Syndrome | % Variant Hb present | Comment | Reference |
|---|---|---|---|
| **α chain variants** | | | |
| Hb G Philadelphia + Hb H disease | > 90% | 4% to 8% Hb H present with no Hb A | 16,22 |
| Hb I + α-thal trait | 70% | Hb A present | 23 |
| Hb Grady + α-thal trait | 22% | Carriers of Hb Grady may have a greater than normal number of α loci | 24 |
| **β chain variants** | | | |
| Hb AS + α-thal silent carrier | normal range | Normal hematologic picture | 25,26 |
| Hb AS + α-thal trait | 23% to 28% | See text | 25,26 |
| Hb SS + α-thal trait | > 85% Hb S | May be clinically milder than usual SS | 26–28 |
| Hb SS + Hb H disease | Hb S 41% Hb F 44% Hb γ4 14% | Very mild sickle cell disease | 30 |
| Hb AC + α-thal silent carrier | normal range | Normal hematologic picture | 25,26 |
| Hb AC + α-thal trait | 24% to 33% | | 25,26 |
| Hb CC + α-thal trait | 77% | Hb F 23% | 31 |
| Hb SC + α-thal trait | Hb S 51% Hb C 48% | May be milder disease | 32 |
| Hb AE + α-thal trait | 15% to 22% | | 6,33 |
| Hb AE + α-thal-1/α-thal-2 | 12% to 15% E | Thalassemia of intermediate severity; γ4 present but no β4 | 6,33 |
| Hb EE + α-thal trait | > 90% E | No significant hematologic disease | 6,33 |
| Hb EE + α-thal-1/α-thal-2 | > 90% E | Cooley's anemia-like disease of moderate severity | 6,33 |
| Hb J Bangkok + α-thal trait | 64% | No significant hematologic disease | 6 |
| Hb D Punjab + α-thal trait | 41% | Moderately severe anemia ? related to this syndrome | 34 |
| Hb Camden + Hb S + α-thal trait | 22% Hb S | No significant hematologic disease | 35 |
| Hb Leslie + α-thal trait | 11.4% | | 25 |
| Hb O Arab + Hb S + α-thal trait | 54% Hb S | Appears to be milder sickle cell disease | 36 |

Lehmann[18] proposed that the $\alpha^G$ gene may be closely linked to a gene for $\alpha$ thalassemia. Subsequent efforts to examine this question experimentally[22,37] have yielded inconclusive results. Although it seems clear that individuals with relatively high percentages of Hb G have microcytic red cells, the results of globin biosynthesis studies thus far available are conflicting, one study[22] having shown an unbalanced pattern of synthesis, such as occurs in $\alpha$ thalassemia, while in another study[37] a normal, balanced pattern of synthesis was observed.

To explain the trimodal distribution of Hb G, Rucknagel and coworkers[37,39] have proposed that the $\alpha^G$ gene may occur in at least two different forms. Assuming a model in which a pair of $\alpha$ genes are closely linked on a single chromosome, in one proposed configuration a normal $\alpha$ gene is assumed to occupy one locus on the chromosome and an $\alpha^G$ gene the other. In the second proposed configuration, a type of chromosome was postulated in which only a single $\alpha$ gene locus was present, this being occupied by an $\alpha^G$ gene.[37] If a configuration of the latter type had arisen as a result of $\alpha$ gene deletion, then the final result would not, of course, differ from that originally hypothesized by French and Lehmann.[38] Further work will be required to resolve this question.

A picture of even greater complexity has been described for the Hb Grady/$\alpha$-thalassemia syndrome.[24] The structural variant, which contains three additional amino acids in its $\alpha$-polypeptide chain, may have arisen through a process of unequal crossing over.[24] A heterozygous carrier of this variant had 12% of Hb Grady, but 22% Hb Grady was present in another member of the family who also had $\alpha$ thalassemia. The findings from studies of this family are consistent with the presence of as many as five $\alpha$ chain genes in carriers of the abnormal hemoglobin. This genetic configuration could have arisen by a crossover process that involved noncorresponding $\alpha$ genes of chromosomes having a tandem pair of $\alpha$ loci. A process of this kind was postulated to have produced a chromosome that contains two normal $\alpha$ genes and a gene for the Hb Grady $\alpha$ chain as well.[24]

### $\alpha$ Thalassemia-$\beta$ Structural Variant Syndromes

The principal syndromes of $\alpha$ thalassemia with coexistent $\beta$ chain structural variants are indicated in Table 3. In most instances $\alpha$-thalassemia trait/$\beta$-hemoglobinopathy trait syndromes exhibit a significant decrease in the percentage of the abnormal hemoglobin in the blood, a feature that is often of considerable diagnostic value; $\beta$ hemoglobinopathy disease states appear in some cases to be significantly modified in their expression by the presence of $\alpha$ thalassemia.

### Sickle Cell-α-Thalassemia Syndromes

It was recognized in early studies of sickle cell trait[40] that a bimodal distribution existed in the percentages of Hb S present in heterozygous individuals, and that similar levels of Hb S tended to occur in members of a single family in which sickle cell trait was present. Detailed hematologic and genetic studies of the form of sickle cell trait with lower than usual percentages of Hb S[41,42] have shown the typical hematologic features of α thalassemia. In addition, studies of globin synthesis by peripheral blood reticulocytes (Figure 16-2) have shown the unbalanced pattern of globin synthesis characteristic of α-thalassemia trait. At least two lines of experimental evidence help to explain the lower than usual percentage of Hb S in sickle cell trait/α-thalassemia trait individuals. Shaeffer and coworkers[43] found from synthesis studies in vitro that a fraction of the newly synthesized $\beta^S$ chains undergoes rapid breakdown within the red cells of these persons. A study by Abraham et al[44] has also shown that when α chains are in limiting concentration, their combination with $\beta^A$ into tetramers occurs at a more rapid rate than with $\beta^S$, providing a possible explanation for the early destruction of the latter when α thalassemia is also present.

A reduced percentage of the variant β chain hemoglobin in the presence of α thalassemia has also been observed with hemoglobins C, E, and others (Table 16-3), most likely representing a process similar to that seen with Hb S. Hemoglobins S and C each have been observed in combination with the silent carrier form of α thalassemia. Although there is a suggestion that the percentage of the abnormal hemoglobin in these syndromes may be somewhat lower than that seen in the usual heterozygote,[25] this percentage is nevertheless entirely within the range of normal[25] and the patients studied in our laboratory do not have an abnormal hematologic picture.[26]

The combination of sickle cell anemia and α thalassemia in the form of Hb H disease was observed in a single Arab child.[30] Although sickle cell anemia appears to be a relatively mild condition in Arab populations, it was notable that this child had none of the manifestations of sickle cell disease. Her blood contained 41% Hb S, 14% Hb Bart's, and 44% Hb F; the low percentage of Hb S and considerably elevated level of fetal hemoglobin may have accounted for the benign nature of her disease. Hemoglobin H disease has also been observed in combination with the homozygous form of Hb E.[6,33] In contrast to the findings in the sickle cell anemia syndrome, the Hb H/Hb E disease appears to be at least as severe a condition as Hb H disease or Hb E disease alone, and in some cases may be significantly more severe. The reasons for these differences are not known.

Homozygous β-chain hemoglobinopathies have also been observed in combination with α-thalassemia trait. Two Ghanian patients with

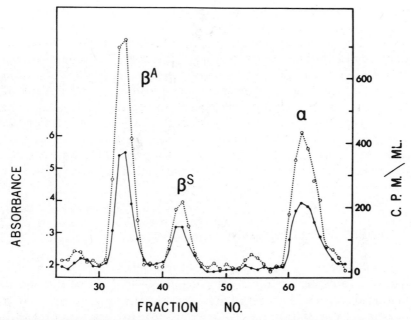

**Figure 16-2.** The pattern of globin chain synthesis in the sickle cell trait–α-thalassemia trait syndrome. Solid line: globin protein; dotted line: incorporated radioactivity after incubation of the red cells in medium containing L-leucine-$^{14}$C. The fraction representing $\beta^S$ is significantly smaller than that usually seen in sickle cell trait, and a correspondingly reduced rate of synthesis of this chain is seen. The $\alpha/\beta^A + \beta^S$ ratio of 0.68 confirms the diagnosis of α-thalassemia trait.

sickle cell anemia and α-thalassemia trait[26] were reported to have a milder clinical course than that expected for sickle cell anemia. An ameliorative effect of α thalassemia did not appear to exist, however, in a group of American children having this syndrome.[28] Studies of sickling in vitro have also suggested that α-thalassemia trait may reduce the disease potential of Hb SC disease,[32] but it remains uncertain if clinical benefit is derived from the addition of the α thalassemia. A number of other α-thalassemia syndromes representing combinations with β chain hemoglobin variants are indicated in Table 16-3. None is associated with significant clinical disease.

## OTHER α-THALASSEMIA SYNDROMES

In a number of populations both α thalassemia and β thalassemia occur with substantial frequency, and examples of doubly affected individuals representing various combinations of these syndromes have been reported. A recent review[45] summarizes the findings from many of these reports. Although the hematologic expression of these disorders may vary considerably, depending on the specific forms of thalassemia involved, in general a more nearly balanced pattern of α/non-α globin chain synthesis occurs, which in some cases appears to reduce the degree of hemolysis that may occur from either of the thalassemic disorders alone. In particular, Cooley's anemia when combined with α thalassemia[45,46] appears to be of reduced clinical severity.

Syndromes have also been described in which α thalassemia was associated with multiple congenital anomalies, including patent ductus arteriosis, cryptorchidism, hypospadias, and retardation,[47] or was present as part of a neonatal syndrome characterized by increased numbers of normoblasts in the blood.[48] It is unclear if these additional abnormalities represented part of a specific α-thalassemia syndrome or were present only by chance association.

## ACQUIRED α THALASSEMIA

A number of examples have been reported of a syndrome hematologically indistinguishable from congenital Hb H disease occurring in individuals with a variety of myeloproliferative disorders.[49,50] Those affected have shown no evidence of pre-existing features of α thalassemia, nor has there been evidence of α-thalassemia genes in family members. In some cases[51] evidence has been found that the Hb H producing cells are derived from an antigenically distinct hematopoietic clone. All of the reported cases have been adults, most of whom were elderly when the features of α thalassemia were identified.

## DETECTION AND DIAGNOSIS OF α-THALASSEMIA SYNDROMES

### Diagnosis of α Thalassemia in the Older Child and Adult

The diagnostic feature common to all forms of thalassemia, underhemoglobinization of the erythrocytes with microcytosis, represents in some forms of α thalassemia the only reliable hematologic evidence of this disorder. In general, the finding of microcytosis in an individual whose iron stores are adequate, particularly if other family members show similar findings, can be taken as presumptive evidence of thalassemia. It is quite clear, however, that significant microcytosis may be absent in individuals with well-documented α thalassemia. In the silent carrier form of α thalassemia, microcytosis of sufficient degree to be of diagnostic value is not usually found. Even in α-thalassemia trait microcytosis may not be reliably seen; whereas in a Greek population α-thalassemia trait appeared to be generally accompanied by significant microcytosis,[52] studies of black children[53] and adults[41] with α-thalassemia trait showed that their MCV values overlapped considerably with the normal range of values. The blood smear in α-thalassemia trait may show morphologic changes, such as hypochromia, anisopoikilocytosis, and target cells, that are associated with other forms of heterozygous thalassemia. Rare cells containing inclusions, presumably representing Hb H, may also be seen in supravitally stained red cells, but this type of determination for diagnostic purposes is unreliable. The levels of Hbs F and $A_2$ are characteristically normal.

From the foregoing it is apparent that the diagnosis of α-thalassemia trait in the older child and adult may be difficult or even impossible by the usual hematologic criteria. Family studies, including determination of α and β chain synthetic ratios, may be required to establish the diagnosis with certainty.

More severe α thalassemia, in the form of Hb H disease, can usually be diagnosed readily by relatively simple laboratory testing. Hb H disease produces a moderate degree of anemia in most patients and is usually accompanied by jaundice, hepatosplenomegaly, and often by cholelithiasis. The reticulocyte count is typically elevated to between 5% and 10%, the red cell indices are significantly microcytic, and the red cell morphology is strikingly abnormal. Supravital staining with brilliant cresyl blue produces coarse inclusions representing precipitated Hb H; this procedure is a useful screening test when this diagnosis is suspected. Electrophoresis of a freshly prepared hemolysate shows 5% or more of very rapidly migrating Hb H and may also show traces of Hb Bart's, which migrates slightly less rapidly. Hb H is quite unstable, and in hemolysates stored for any substantial length of time the Hb H will precipitate and no longer be detectable by electrophoresis. Hb H also may undergo total precipitation if the hemolysate is treated with toluene, carbon tetrachloride, or other organic solvents. In laboratories that routinely employ such solvents for removal of red cell stroma, an alternative procedure is required for the preparation of the hemolysate when Hb H is suspected, or its presence may escape detection.

## Diagnosis of α Thalassemia in the Neonate

In contrast to the diagnostic difficulties that accompany α thalassemia in the older child and adult, the α-thalassemia syndromes in the neonate can usually be identified relatively readily by the presence in the blood of significant quantities of Hb Bart's ($\gamma_4$) (Figure 16-3). Cord blood studies representing a number of populations[6,53-56] have shown an excellent correlation between the quantity of Hb Bart's present at birth and the presence of α thalassemia. In an extensive study from Thailand,[6] 1% to 2% of Hb Bart's was shown to correspond to $\alpha$-thal-2, 5% to 6% to $\alpha$-thal-1, and about 25% to Hb H disease. Studies of other population groups have indicated a similar correlation. Although $\alpha$ thalassemia in the newborn appears reliably to produce Hb Bart's at birth, cord blood studies from Nigeria[57] suggest that in some instances elevated levels of Hb Bart's may be present at birth as a developmental abnormality in infants not having thalassemia.

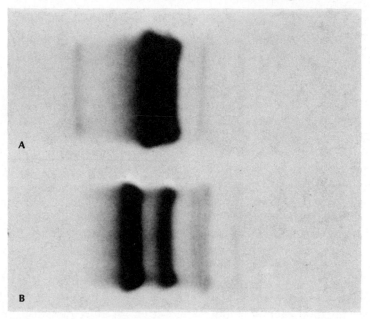

**Figure 16-3.** Hb Bart's ($\gamma$4) in cord blood of an infant with the $\alpha$-thalassemia trait–sickle cell anemia syndrome. Hemoglobin from the infant **(A)** included 3.9% Hb Bart's and 13.4% Hb S, with the remainder being Hb F. No Hb A was present. The father of the infant **(B)** had sickle cell trait with a lower than usual percentage of Hb S. The mother's hemoglobin (not shown) contained equal quantities of Hb S and C.

A recent study by Schamaier et al[58] suggested that significant microcytosis may be a reliable feature of $\alpha$-thalassemia trait at birth, and it was proposed that measurements of the MCV and MCH in the neonate might provide an adequate means of screening for $\alpha$-thalassemia trait. In a study by Friedman et al,[4] however, these indices of newborns with $\alpha$-thalassemia trait showed overlap into the normal range, casting doubt on the validity of this type of measurement as a screening test.

The diagnosis of the hydrops fetalis form of $\alpha$ thalassemia is made by identification of mainly Hb Bart's in the blood. By clinical criteria this syndrome may be difficult to distinguish from hydrops fetalis due to isoimmunization or other causes. Of value in this regard has been the finding that in infants with $\alpha$-thalassemia hydrops fetalis, massive liver enlargement is typically present, with the spleen showing little or no enlargement,[10,18] in contrast to the usual findings in isoimmune disease of the newborn. The direct antiglobulin test is characteristically negative in α-thalassemia hydrops fetalis. The hemoglobin findings that accompany this disorder are listed in Table 16-1.

## Prenatal Diagnosis of α Thalassemia

The feasibility of establishing the diagnosis of α thalassemia in the fetus in utero was demonstrated by Kan et al.[59] These investigators, in a remarkable tour de force, diagnosed α-thal-1 by hybridization of a radioactive DNA probe having α chain specificity with DNA derived from amniotic fluid fibroblasts obtained by amniocentesis. Testing of this kind will most certainly be confined to the very highly specialized research laboratories.

## MANAGEMENT OF THE CHILD WITH α THALASSEMIA

Relatively few principles need to be considered regarding the medical management of the α-thalassemia patient. In the child with α-thalassemia trait no treatment is required; the primary requirement when this diagnosis has been established is to convey to the patient and his family a thorough understanding of the nature of the condition. Especially when anemia is present, it is important that the family understand that this disorder is refractory to hematinics, particularly iron, so that needless therapeutic attempts can be avoided. A thorough explanation of the genetic implications of α thalassemia should be given to adolescent and postadolescent patients.

The patient with Hb H disease is subject to any of the complications that accompany chronic hemolytic disease. Cholelithiasis is a relatively common complication in the older child and adult and may require cholecystectomy. Hypersplenism, with worsening anemia as its principal complication, may also occur in the patient with Hb H disease and is an indication for splenectomy.[60] As in other chronic hemolytic disorders, folic acid deficiency may develop, and daily administration of an oral folic acid preparation is recommended for these patients.[60] Hemoglobin H, in common with other unstable hemoglobins, has increased susceptibility to chemical injury from oxidizing drugs and chemicals, and exposure of patients with Hb H disease to such agents may precipitate hyperhemolytic episodes; therefore, physicians should avoid giving these patients sulfonamides and other drugs having oxidizing potential.[61]

For the infant with α thalassemia hydrops fotalis, no form of therapy has thus far been successful, and none of these infants has survived more than a few hours. If such infants could in fact be salvaged, their condition would unquestionably require lifelong transfusions to sustain life and they would therefore be subject to all of the complications that are associated with transfusion-dependent β thalassemia and perhaps others. Counseling of couples who are at risk of having offspring with this condition may be the most practical available measure. Most such couples are identified as a result of having had an affected infant; if each of a pair of prospective parents could be identified by hematologic testing to carry an α-thal-1 gene, however, then appropriate counseling could be given before an infant with hydrops is born. Apart from the trauma to a family that results from having a stillborn or moribund infant with this disorder, the frequent association of this condition with toxemia[6] adds further to the desirability of preventing such pregnancies. If antenatal testing techniques[59] become a practical reality, these couples will be provided with the opportunity of having offspring without taking the risk of carrying a pregnancy with an affected fetus to term.

## REFERENCES

1. Ottolenghi, S., Laynon, W.G., Paul, J., et al. Gene deletion as the cause of α-thalassemia. *Nature* 251:389–392, 1974.

2. Taylor, J.M., Dozy, A.M., Kan, Y.W., et al. Genetic lesion in homozygous α-thalassemia (hydrops fetalis). *Nature* 251:392–393, 1974.

3. Kan, Y.W., Dozy, A.M., Trecartin, R., et al. Identification of a nondeletion defect in α-thalassemia. *N. Engl. J. Med.* 297:1081–1084, 1977.

4. Clegg, J.B., and Weatherall, D.J. Molecular basis of thalassemia. *Br. Med. Bull.* 32:262–269, 1976.

5. Hamilton, R.W., Schwartz, E., Atwater, J., et al. Acquired Hemoglobin H disease. *N. Engl. J. Med.* 285:1217–1221, 1971.

6. Wasi, P., Na-Nakorn, S., Pootrakul, S., et al. Alpha and beta-thalassemia in Thailand. *Ann. NY Acad. Sci.* 165:60–82, 1969.

7. Lehmann, H. Different types of alpha-thalassemia and significance of hemoglobin Bart's in neonates. *Lancet* 2:78–80, 1970.

8. Kan, Y.W., Dozy, A.M., Varmus, H.E., et al. Deletion of α-globin genes in hemoglobin H disease demonstrates multiple α-globin structural loci. *Nature* 255:255–256, 1975.

9. Koler, R.D., Jones, R.T., Wasi, P., et al. Genetics of hemoglobin H and α-thalassemia. *Ann. Hum. Genet.* 34:371–377, 1971.

10. Lie-Injo, L.E. Alpha-chain thalassemia and hydrops fetalis in Malaya: Report of five cases. *Blood* 20:581–590, 1962.

11. McFadzean, A.J.S., and Todd, D. Distribution of Cooley's anemia in China. *Trans. R. Soc. Trop. Med. Hyg.* 58:490, 1964.

12. Stamatoyannopoulos, G., Heywood, D., and Papayannopoulou, T. Hemoglobin H disease in the Afro-American: Phenotypic and genetic considerations. *Birth Defects* 8:29–38, 1972.

13. Walford, D.M., and Deacon, R. Alpha-thalassemia trait in various racial groups in the United Kingdom: Characterization of a variant of alpha-thalassemia in Indians. Br. J. Haematol. 34:193–200, 1976.

14. Pembrey, M.E., Weatherall, D.J., Clegg, J.B., et al. Hemoglobin Bart's in Saudi Arabia. Br. J. Haematol. 29:221–234, 1975.

15. Zaizov, R., Kirschmann, C., Matoth, Y., et al. The genetics of α-thalassemia in Yemenite and Iraqi Jews. Isr. J. Med. Sci. 9:1457–1460, 1973.

16. Rieder, R.F., Woodbury, D.H., and Rucknagel, D.L. The interaction of α-thalassemia and hemoglobin G Philadelphia. Br. J. Haematol. 32:159–160, 1976.

17. Todd, D., Lai, M.C.S., Beaven, G.H., et al. The abnormal hemoglobins in homozygous α-thalassemia. Br. J. Haematol. 19:27–31, 1970.

18. Lie-Injo, L.E., Lopez, C.G., and Dutt, A.K. Pathological findings in hydrops fetalis due to alpha-thalassemia: A review of 32 cases. Trans. R. Soc. Trop. Med. Hyg. 62:874–879, 1968.

19. Lorkin, P.A., Charlesworth, D., Lehmann, H., et al. Two hemoglobins Q, α74 (EF3) and α75 (EF4) aspartic acid→histidine. Br. J. Haematol. 19:117–125, 1970.

20. Schneider, R.G., Brimhall, B., Jones, R.T., et al. Hb Ft. Worth: α27 glu→gly (B8). A varient present in unusually low concentration. Biochim. Biophys. Acta 243:164, 1971.

21. Honig, G.R., Shamsuddin, M., Kirschmann, C., et al. Hemoglobin Petah Tikva (α 110 ala→asp), an electrophoretically silent variant associated with α-thalassemia. Proc. XVII Cong. Internat. Soc. Hematol. 321, 1978.

22. Milner, P.F., and Huisman, T.H.J., Studies on the proportion and synthesis of hemoglobin G Philadelphia in red cells of heterozygotes, a homozygote, and a heterozygote for both hemoglobin G and α-thalassemia. Br. J. Haematol. 34:207, 1976.

23. Atwater, J., Schwartz, I.R., Erslev, A.J., et al. Sickling of erythrocytes in a patient with thalassemia-hemoglobin-I disease. N. Engl. J. Med. 263:1215, 1960.

24. Huisman, T.H.J., and Miller, A. Hb Grady and α-thalassemia: A contribution to the problem of the number of Hb$_\alpha$ structural loci in man. Am. J. Hum. Genet. 28:363, 1976.

25. Huisman, T.J.H. Trimodality in the percentages of β chain variants in heterozygotes: The effect of the number of active Hb$_\alpha$ structural loci. Hemoglobin 1:349, 1977.

26. Honig, G.R., Mason, R.G., et al. α-Thalassemia silent carrier with hemoglobins S and C. Pediatr. Res. 12:465, 1978.

27. van Enk, A., Lang, A., White, J.M., et al. Benign obstetric history in women with sickle-cell anemia associated with α-thalassemia. Br. Med. J. 4:524–526, 1972.

28. Honig, G.R., Koshy, M., Mason, R.G., et al. Sickle cell syndromes. II. The sickle cell anemia-α-thalassemia syndrome. J. Pediatr. 92:556–561, 1978.

29. Kim, H.C., Weierbach, R.G., Friedman, Sh., et al. Detection of sickle α- or β⁰-thalassemia by studies of globin biosynthesis. Blood 49:785–792, 1977.

30. Weatherall, D.J., Clegg, J.B., and Blankson, J. A new sickling disorder resulting from interaction of the genes for hemoglobin S and α-thalassemia. Br. J. Haematol. 17:517–526, 1969.

31. Steinberg, M.H. Hemoglobin C/α thalassemia. Hematological and biosynthetic studies. Br. J. Haematol. 30:337–342, 1975.

32. Honig, G.R., Gunay, U., Mason, R.G., et al. Sickle cell syndromes. I. Hemoglobin SC-α-thalassemia. Pediatr. Res. 10:613–620, 1976.

33. Wasi, P., Sookanek, M., Pootrakul, S., et al. Hemoglobin E and alpha

thalassemia. *Br. Med. J.* 4:29–32, 1967.

34. Cavdar, A.O., and Arcasoy, A. Hb D Punjab-alpha thalassemia combination in a Turkish family. *Scand. J. Haematol.* 13:313–319, 1974.

35. Honig, G.R., Koduri, P.R., et al. In preparation.

36. Ballas, S.K., Atwater, J., and Burka, E.R. Hemoglobin S-O Arab-α-thalassemia: Globin biosynthesis and clinical picture. *Hemoglobin* 1:651–662, 1977.

37. Baine, R.M., Rucknagel, D.L., Dublin, P.A., Jr., et al. Trimodality in the proportion of hemoglobin G Philadelphia in heterozygotes: Evidence for heterogeneity in the number of human alpha chain loci. *Proc. Natl. Acad. Sci. USA* 73:3633–3636, 1976.

38. French, E.A., and Lehmann, H. Is hemoglobin G α-Philadelphia linked to α-thalassemia? *Acta Haematol.* 46:149–156, 1971.

39. Rucknagel, D.L., and Rising, J.A. A heterozygote for Hb$_\beta^S$, Hb$_\beta^C$ and Hb$_\alpha^G$ Philadelphia in a family presenting evidence for heterogeneity in the number of alpha chain loci. *Am. J. Med.* 59:53–60, 1975.

40. Neel, J.V., Wells, I.C., and Itano, H.A. Familial differences in the proportion of abnormal hemoglobin present in the sickle cell trait. *J. Clin. Invest.* 30:1120–1124, 1951.

41. Steinberg, M.H., Adams, J.G., III., and Dreiling, B.J. Alpha thalassemia in adults with sickle-cell trait. *Br. J. Haematol.* 30:31–37, 1975.

42. Shaeffer, J.R., De Simone, J., and Kleve, L.J. Hemoglobin synthesis studies of a family with α-thalassemia trait and sickle cell trait. *Biochem. Genet.* 13:783–788, 1975.

43. Shaeffer, J.R., Kleve, L., and De Simone, J.B. $\beta^S$ chain turnover in reticulocytes of sickle trait individuals with high or low concentrations of hemoglobin S. *Br. J. Haematol.* 32:365–372, 1976.

44. Abraham, E.C., Cope, N.D., and Huisman, T.H.J. Differences in affinity of variant $\beta$ or $\alpha$ chains for normal $\alpha$ or $\beta$ chains: A possible explanation for the variations in the relative quantities of hemoglobin variants in heterozygotes. *Blood* 50(suppl):100, 1977.

45. Altay, C., Say, B., Yetgin, S., et al. α-Thalassemia and β-thalassemia in a Turkish family. *Am. J. Hematol.* 2:1–15, 1977.

46. Bate, C.M., and Humphries, G. Alpha-beta thalassemia. *Lancet* 1:1031–1034, 1977.

47. Borochovitz, D., Levin, S.E., Krawitz, S., et al. Hemoglobin-H disease in association with multiple congenital abnormalities. *Clin. Pediatr.* 9:432–435, 1970.

48. McCormack, M.K., Geller, G.R., Zak, S., et al. Complex α-thalassemia-like syndrome: A cause of neonatal normoblastemia. *J. Pediatr.* 89:446–451, 1976.

49. Rosenzweig, A.I., Heywood, J.D., Motulsky, A.G., et al. Hemoglobin H as an acquired defect of alpha-chain synthesis. *Acta Haematol.* 39:91–101, 1968.

50. Veer, A., Rowley, P.T., Kosciolek, B.A., et al. Acquired hemoglobin H disease in idiopathic myelofibrosis: Extreme imbalance of globin synthesis and of messenger RNA activity. *Blood* 50(suppl):120, 1977.

51. André, R., Najman, A., Duhamel, G., et al. Erythro Leucémie avec hémoglobine H acquise et anomalies des antigénes érythrocytaires. *Nouv. Rev. Fr. Hematol.* 12:29–42, 1972.

52. Pearson, H.A., McPhedran, P., O'Brien, R.T., et al. Comprehensive testing for thalassemia trait. *Ann. NY Acad. Sci.* 232:135, 1974.

53. Charache, S., Conley, C.L., Doeblin, T.D., et al. Thalassemia in black Americans. *Ann. NY Acad. Sci.* 232:125, 1974.

54. Friedman, Sh., Atwater, J., Gill, F., et al. α-Thalassemia in Negro infants. *Pediatr. Res.* 8:955–959, 1974.

55. Lopez, C.G., and Lie-Injo, L.E. Alpha thalassemia in newborns in West Malaysia. *Hum. Hered.* 21:185–191, 1971.

56. Zaizov, R., and Matoth, Y. α-Thalassemia in Yemenite and Iraqi Jews. *Isr. J. Med. Sci.* 8:11–17, 1972.

57. Esan, G.J.F. Hemoglobin Bart's in newborn Nigerians. *Br. J. Haematol.* 22:73–86, 1972.

58. Schmaier, A.H., Maurer, H.M., Johnston, C.L., et al. Alpha thalassemia screening in neonates by mean corpuscular volume and mean corpuscular hemoglobin determination. *J. Pediatr.* 83:794–797, 1973.

59. Kan, Y.W., Golbus, M.S., and Dozy, A.M. Prenatal diagnosis of α-thalassemia. Clinical application of molecular hybridization. *N. Engl. J. Med.* 295:1165–1167, 1976.

60. Wasi, P., Na-Nakorn, S., and Pootrakul, S. The α-thalassemias. *Clin. Haematol.* 3:383–410, 1974.

61. Zinkham, W.H. The selective hemolytic action of drugs: Clinical and mechanistic considerations. *J. Pediatr.* 70:200–210, 1967.

# INDEX